CHAPTER 1
ANATOMY AND PHYSIOLOGY OF THE RESPIRATORY SYSTEM

Anatomy

UPPER RESPIRATORY TRACT

- Nasal cavities—cartilage and bone lined with m̲ ̲ ̲ ̲ ̲ ̲ ̲ ̲ ̲ ̲ ̲ ̲ .s (vibrissae). The cavities include the paranasal sinuses (two sphenoid and two maxillary), and the pharynx (nasopharynx and oropharynx).

LOWER RESPIRATORY TRACT

- Trachea—a flexible tube constructed with cartilage rings, lined with mucus-secreting ciliated cells, and protected by the epiglottis.

- Mainstem bronchus—forks into the left and right mainstem bronchi at the carina and branches into the lobar, segmental, and subsegmental bronchi.

- Alveoli—includes 150 to 160 million sacs; gas exchange occurs at the alveolar-capillary membrane.

- Thorax—a cavity encased by 12 pairs of ribs and the sternum.

- Diaphragm—principle muscle of ventilation.

- Pleura—membranes that encase the lungs and line the thoracic cavity.

CHAPTER 2
ASSESSMENT OF THE RESPIRATORY SYSTEM

History (prior medical and surgical history)

- Current symptoms—cough, nasal secretions, dyspnea, and pain.

- Lifestyle and behavior patterns—cigarette smoking (# packs per day x 3 years smoking = 3 pack years).

- Occupation—exposure to chemicals, molds, dust, asbestos, and other tobacco products.

- Genetic history—asthma, emphysema, cystic fibrosis.

Physical Assessment (respiratory rate, rhythm, depth)

- Normal rate—12 to 20 breaths per minute (<12 = bradypnea; >20 = tachypnea).

- Presence of central (lips, inside eyelids) or peripheral (nail beds) cyanosis.

- Examination of mouth, nose, sinuses, posterior oropharynx, neck, thorax (shape and expansion during normal breathing).

- Palpation for tactile fremitus.

- Percussion for air-filled (resonant) or solid-filled (dullness) areas.

- Auscultation with stethoscope for breath sounds (tracheal—windy sounds over trachea; bronchial—harsh sounds over bronchi; vesicular—soft sounds over lung tissue).

CHAPTER 1
ANATOMY AND PHYSIOLOGY OF THE RESPIRATORY SYSTEM

Physiologic Concepts

- Ventilation—inhalation occurs when air is drawn into the thorax as the diaphragm contracts; exhalation is normally passive.

- Compliance—the ease with which the lungs are inflated.

- Surface tension—surfactant lowers the tension, allowing even inflation.

- Pressures—normal atmospheric pressure is 760 mmHg; intrathoracic pressure varies 3 to 5 mmHg during ventilation; air is composed of 20.8% O_2 and 79.6% N_2.

- Ventilatory rate—controlled by central and peripheral chemoreceptors.

- Diffusion—ability of gas molecules to cross a membrane from areas of high concentration to areas of lower concentration.

This card refers to the following book:
Sheldon LK. *Oxygenation*. Thorofare, NJ: SLACK Incorporated; 2001.

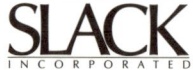 SLACK INCORPORATED

6900 Grove Road • Thorofare, NJ 08086 • 856-848-1000
An innovative information, education and management company

CHAPTER 2
ASSESSMENT OF THE RESPIRATORY SYSTEM

- Adventitious (abnormal) breath sounds (crackles [rales]: popping sounds of air in fluid; wheezes: whistling sounds over partially obstructed airways; sonorous wheezes [rhonchi]: rough, gurgling sounds).

Diagnostic Tests

SPIROMETRY

- Airflow rates or pulmonary mechanics.

- Lung volumes—tidal volume (TD) 550 mL; inspiratory reserve volume (IRV) 3300 mL; expiratory reserve volume (ERV) 1100 mL; residual volume (RV) 100 mL.

- Lung capacities—vital capacity (VC) 5000 mL; inspiratory capacity (IS) 3000 mL; functional residual capacity (FRC) 1200 mL; total lung capacity (TLC) 6000 mL.

- TLC = TV + IRV + ERV + RV.

- Arterial blood gases—PO_2 (80 to 100 mmHg); PCO_2 (35 to 45 mmHg); pH 7.35 to 7.45; SaO_2 85% to 100%.

This card refers to the following book:
Sheldon LK. *Oxygenation*. Thorofare, NJ: SLACK Incorporated; 2001.

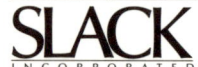 SLACK INCORPORATED

6900 Grove Road • Thorofare, NJ 08086 • 856-848-1000
An innovative information, education and management company

Chapter 3
Management of Adults with Respiratory Disorders

Many disorders can compromise oxygenation including asthma, pneumonia, chronic obstructive pulmonary disease (COPD), respiratory failure, and pulmonary embolism. Nursing diagnoses can be used to direct treatment and evaluate outcomes.

Impaired gas exchange is an imbalance between oxygen uptake and carbon dioxide elimination at the alveolar-capillary membrane.

Interventions

- Monitor for signs of hypoxemia.
- Check mental status for irritability, somnolence.
- Provide assistance in clearing secretions.
- Administer supplemental oxygen as ordered.
- Monitor respiratory rate, pattern, and oxygen saturation.
- Position patient to optimize ventilation and perfusion.
- Monitor pulmonary artery pressures for increasing resistance.

Outcomes

- Patient will maintain a clear airway, PaO_2 >60 mmHg.
- SaO_2 >90%, pH between 7.35 and 7.45, $PaCO_2$ 35 to 45 mmHg.

Chapter 4
Common Interventions to Improve Oxygenation

- Maintaining respiratory health—healthy lifestyle, adequate nutrition and hydration, regular exercise, no smoking, avoid secondhand smoke, reduce exposure to noxious fumes.
- Care of patients with chronic obstructive pulmonary diseases—decrease oxygen consumption (pace activities, eat light meals, avoid breath-holding and Valsalva's maneuvers, decrease temperature); teach diaphragmatic and pursed lip breathing, cascade "huff" or quad coughing.
- Chest physical therapy (CPT)—percussion, vibration, postural drainage.
- Closed chest drainage—tubes to drain fluid and air from pleural space and allow re-expansion of the lung.
- Maintaining a patent airway—oral, nasal, and nasopharyngeal airways.
  - Endotracheal tube—past trachea into bronchus.
  - Tracheostomy tube—placed in surgically created opening in trachea.
- Oxygen therapy—delivers more oxygen to prevent hypoxemia, decreases work of breathing, and maximizes tissue oxygen supply.
  - Low-flow devices—nasal cannula, oropharyngeal catheter, face mask, face mask with oxygen reservoir, transtracheal catheter.
  - Continuous positive airway pressure (CPAP)—greater than atmospheric pressure.

Activity Intolerance is defined as a patient not having enough physiological or psychological energy to perform the required or desired activities.

Interventions

- Monitor oxygen levels for signs of desaturation with activity.
- Monitor blood pressure, respiratory rate, and pulse during activity.
- Schedule activities to avoid fatigue and dyspnea.
- Teach patient pursed lip breathing and energy conservation measures.
- Teach patient proper administration of medications.

Outcome

- Patient will be able to perform required or desired activities.

This card refers to the following book:
Sheldon LK. *Oxygenation*. Thorofare, NJ: SLACK Incorporated; 2001.

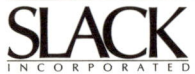 6900 Grove Road • Thorofare, NJ 08086 • 856-848-1000
An innovative information, education and management company

- Hazards of oxygen therapy—pulmonary oxygen toxicity, hypoventilation, ciliary dysfunction, and alveolar fibrosis.
- Mechanical ventilation—provides oxygen to lungs, maintain alveolar ventilation, and reduce work of breathing.
  - Types—negative pressure (uncommon), positive pressure (most common; inspiration cycled by volume, pressure, or time).
  - Positive end expiratory pressure (PEEP)—enhances gas exchange.

This card refers to the following book:
Sheldon LK. *Oxygenation*. Thorofare, NJ: SLACK Incorporated; 2001.

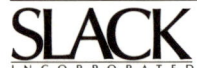 6900 Grove Road • Thorofare, NJ 08086 • 856-848-1000
An innovative information, education and management company

CHAPTER 5
ANATOMY AND PHYSIOLOGY OF THE CARDIOVASCULAR SYSTEM

Heart

- Muscular organ within the pericardial sac in the thorax.

- Three layers: epicardium, myocardium, endocardium; four chambers: two atria and two ventricles.

- Right side pumps blood to the pulmonary circulation; left side pumps blood to the systemic circulation.

- Four valves control flow of blood: tricuspid, mitral, aortic, and pulmonic.

- Conduction system allows contraction of myocardium through electrical impulses originating at the sino-atrial (SA) node.

Vascular System

- Arterial system—high pressure with thick vessels.

- Capillaries—tiniest vessels; thin walls allow diffusion of gases and exchange of nutrients and waste products.

- Venous system—low pressure system, thinner walled vessels, valves to maintain one-way flow.

CHAPTER 6
ASSESSMENT OF THE CARDIOVASCULAR SYSTEM

History—heart disease, diabetes, hypertension, hyperlipidemia, rheumatic fever.
Common signs and symptoms of disorders—chest pain, pain in extremities on exertion, dypsnea on exertion, orthopnea, palpitations, edema of extremities, dizziness or fainting.

Assessment

- Skin for cyanosis, ulcers, swelling, or redness.

- Peripheral pulses.

- Pulse rate regularity (normal 60 to 100 beats per minute).

- Blood pressure (normal 120/80 mmHg).

- Examination of chest—inspection, palpation, auscultation, jugular vein distention (>3 to 4 cm above sternal notch may indicate increased CVP).

Cardiac Assessment

- Palpate cardiac landmarks (aortic, pulmonic, Erb's point, tricuspid, and mitral areas).

- Locate apical pulse and note location, amplitude, and regularity.

- Auscultate using bell and diaphragm of stethoscope.

Pulmonary circulation—pulmonary artery takes deoxygenated blood from right side of heart to lungs for gas exchange and returns reoxygenated blood via the pulmonary vein to the left side of the heart.

Factors Affecting Blood Flow

- Pressure—blood flows from areas of higher pressure to areas of lower pressure.

- Resistance—force that opposes movement (ie, viscosity, turbulence).

Blood pressure—systolic/diastolic (normal: 120/80 mmHg.

Pulse pressure—(SBP - DBP = PP).

Cardiac output (CO)—volume of blood pumped every minute (CO = stroke volume x heart rate).

Stroke volume—amount of blood ejected during systole 50 to 100 cc.

Heart rate—normal (60 to 100 beats per minute); tachycardia >100; bradycardia <60.

This card refers to the following book:
Sheldon LK. *Oxygenation*. Thorofare, NJ: SLACK Incorporated; 2001.

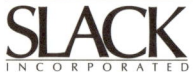 **SLACK** INCORPORATED   6900 Grove Road • Thorofare, NJ 08086 • 856-848-1000
An innovative information, education and management company

- Listen to first (S1) and second (S2) heart sounds as heart valves close, assessing rate, rhythm, and quality.

- Extra heart sounds—S3, S4, heart murmurs, clicks, rubs, opening snaps. Murmurs are described by timing in cardiac cycle, pitch, intensity, and radiation.

Diagnostic Tests

- Blood tests (electrolytes, cholesterol, cardiac enzymes, CBC, troponin, arterial blood gases, clotting studies).

- Electrocardiograms (measure electrical activity in the heart).

- Cardiac catheterization (study coronary arteries).

- Radionuclide scans (detect perfusion defects in heart muscle).

- Hemodynamic monitoring (measure pressures in the great vessels and heart; arterial lines measure BP, pulmonary artery lines measure pulmonary artery pressure (PA), central venous pressure (CVP), pulmonary artery wedge pressure (PAWP), and cardiac output (CO).

This card refers to the following book:
Sheldon LK. *Oxygenation*. Thorofare, NJ: SLACK Incorporated; 2001.

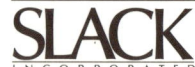 **SLACK** INCORPORATED   6900 Grove Road • Thorofare, NJ 08086 • 856-848-1000
An innovative information, education and management company

CHAPTER 7
DISORDERS OF THE CARDIOVASCULAR SYSTEM

Atherosclerosis—causes arterial walls to thicken, lose elasticity; accumulates lipids, overgrowth of smooth muscle, formation of connective tissue within vessel; and leads to hypertension, arterial insufficiency, and coronary artery disease.

Coronary artery disease—narrowed coronary arteries with tissue hypoxia, angina, myocardial infarction; treatment includes thrombolytics, angioplasty, and bypass surgery.

Heart failure—left-sided: pulmonary edema, decreased cardiac output with fatigue, weakness, and dyspnea on mild exertion; right-sided: peripheral edema, engorged venous system.

Decreased Cardiac Output (related to heart failure)

- Expected outcomes—cardiac function will improve, vital signs will stabilize, and fluid volume balance will improve with decreasing edema and increasing output if on diuretics.

- Supplemental oxygen, avoid breath-holding and Valsalva's maneuver.

- Promote rest, increase activity as tolerated.

- Semi-Fowler's position.

- Small meals, avoid excessive fluid intake, avoid salt, no smoking.

- Daily weights, intake and output.

- Assess for crackles, increased dyspnea, tachycardia.

- Medications to increase cardiac output, and to decrease excess fluid, preload, vascular resistance, and cardiac workload.

CHAPTER 8
ROLE OF THE HEMATOLOGIC SYSTEM IN OXYGEN TRANSPORT

Red Blood Cells or Erythrocytes (carry hemoglobin which binds to oxygen)

- 40% to 50% of blood is RBCs, 4.2 to 5.4 million RBC/μl.

- Produced in bone marrow by stimulation from erythropoetin (hormone produced by the kidneys), 120-day life span.

Hemoglobin (heme unit composed of iron)

- Binds with O_2 to become oxyhemoglobin.

- Carries 98% to 99% of oxygen in the blood.

- Affinity for O_2 varies with blood pH and certain enzymes.

- Normal Hgb = 13.5 to 17.5 g/100 mL.

- Mean Corpuscular Volume (MCV) 87 to 103 fl/red cell.

- Mean Corpuscular Hemoglobin Concentration (MCHC) 31 to 37 Hgb/dl.

- Anemia—decreased circulating RBCs due to nutritional deficiencies (iron, folic acid, B12, malabsorption), bone marrow failure, hemolysis, excessive bleeding, drugs. Symptoms include fatigue, weakness, pallor, tachypnea, dizziness, and syncope.

CHAPTER 7
DISORDERS OF THE CARDIOVASCULAR SYSTEM

Peripheral arterial disease—decrease in blood flow to the extremities due to atherosclerotic plaque.

- Symptoms—intermittent claudication, leg pain relieved with rest.

- Assessment—symptoms, pulses, color of extremities, ulcers.

- Altered tissue perfusion related to peripheral arterial disease.

- Expected outcome—circulation will be maintained.

- Fastidious foot care.

- Walk 60 minutes per day, stop if pain develops, then resume.

- No tobacco products or caffeine.

- Control diabetes.

- Use medications to improve circulation.

- Head of bed up 4 to 6 inches.

This card refers to the following book:
Sheldon LK. *Oxygenation*. Thorofare, NJ: SLACK Incorporated; 2001.

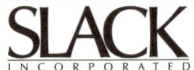 SLACK INCORPORATED 6900 Grove Road • Thorofare, NJ 08086 • 856-848-1000
An innovative information, education and management company

CHAPTER 8
ROLE OF THE HEMATOLOGIC SYSTEM IN OXYGEN TRANSPORT

Altered Nutritional Intake (related to iron deficiency anemia)

- Expected outcome—hematocrit and hemoglobin will rise in 4 weeks and return to normal levels in 3 months.

- Increase intake of iron-rich foods, such as lean red meat, dark green leafy vegetables, liver, egg yolks, raisins.

- Take supplemental ferrous sulfate as ordered with stool softener (stools will be black).

- Pace activities and allow for rest periods.

- Hemoglobinopathies—defect in hemoglobin structure that can cause RBC destruction and blood vessel occlusion.
- Sickle-cell anemia—congenital defect in hemoglobin molecule that results in "sickle-shaped" RBC that can block vessels.
- Thalassemia—inherited anemia in those of Mediterranean descent; reduced hemoglobin synthesis.

This card refers to the following book:
Sheldon LK. *Oxygenation*. Thorofare, NJ: SLACK Incorporated; 2001.

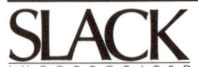 SLACK INCORPORATED 6900 Grove Road • Thorofare, NJ 08086 • 856-848-1000
An innovative information, education and management company

Oxygenation

Oxygenation

Lisa Kennedy Sheldon, RN, MS, ARNP

St. Joseph's Hospital
Nashua, New Hampshire

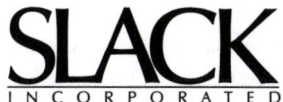

SLACK
INCORPORATED

an innovative information, education, and management company
6900 Grove Road • Thorofare, NJ 08086

Cover illustration by Thom Sevalrud

Freelance Illustrators: Robert Hochgertel, Joe Kulka, Barbie Minnick-Maglio

Sheldon, Lisa Kennedy.

    Nursing concepts : oxygenation / Lisa Kennedy Sheldon.

       p. ; cm. -- (Nursing concepts series)

    Includes bibliographical references and index.

    ISBN 1-55642-523-6 (alk. paper)

    1. Inhalation therapy. 2. Oxygen--Therapeutic use. 3. Respiratory organs--Diseases--Nursing. I. Title. II. Series.

    [DNLM: 1. Oxygen Inhalation Therapy--methods--Case Report. 2. Oxygen Inhalation Therapy--methods--Nurses' Instruction. 3. Biological Transport--Case Report. 4. Biological Transport--Nurses' Instruction. 5. Cardiovascular Diseases--therapy--Case Report. 6. Cardiovascular Diseases--therapy--Nurses' Instruction. 7. Oxygen Consumption--Case Report. 8. Oxygen Consumption--Nurses' Instruction. 9. Respiration Disorders--therapy--Case Report. 10. Respiration Disorders--therapy--Nurses' Instruction. WF 145 S544n 2001]

    RC735.I5 S525 2001

    615.8'36--dc21

                                       2001042890

Printed in the United States of America

Published by: SLACK Incorporated

                    6900 Grove Road

                    Thorofare, NJ 08086 USA

                    Telephone: 856-848-1000

                    Fax: 856-853-5991

                    www.slackbooks.com

Contact SLACK Incorporated for more information about other books in this field or about the availability of our books from distributors outside the United States.

Last digit is print number: 10 9 8 7 6 5 4 3 2 1

DEDICATION

To my husband, Tom, for his patience and love.

CONTENTS

ACKNOWLEDGMENTS

It would have been impossible to write this book without the help of many people. First of all, I want to thank Joanne Farley for giving me the opportunity to write this book. I am truly grateful for your insight and confidence. A special thank you to my students for their inspiration and enthusiasm. From you, I learned what I needed to teach. For all the ongoing support, I want to thank Jill Tweedie at SLACK Incorporated for teaching me the way. To my friend, Dr. Paul DelGiudice, I am very grateful for your suggestions, reviews, and ideas. To my children, Brad, Greg, Andrea, and Luke: you are the lights in my life. Thanks for letting me clog up the computer. And to my husband, Tom, thank you for more reasons than I can write here.

Lisa Kennedy Sheldon, RN, MS, ARNP

About the Author

Lisa Kennedy Sheldon, RN, MS, ARNP graduated from Saint Anselm College in Manchester, NH with a bachelor of science degree in nursing. She attended Boston College and graduated as a clinical nurse specialist and later did a postgraduate program to complete an adult nurse practitioner certification. Ms. Sheldon worked in a variety of clinical settings, including gastrointestinal surgery, postoperative intensive care, and radiation oncology, as well as in research regarding health care reimbursement. She taught at Saint Anselm College as a clinical professor on a cardiovascular progressive care unit. Ms. Sheldon currently practices as a nurse practitioner in oncology at St. Joseph's Hospital in Nashua, NH. She lives with her husband and four children in New Hampshire.

CONTRIBUTING AUTHOR

Mary M. Sanford, RN, MSN, ANP-C, ACNP-C, CCRN
Catholic Medical Center
Manchester, NH

INTRODUCTION

Does my patient need oxygen just because he is anemic? How does O_2 saturation differ from the PO_2 on an arterial blood gas? What are some interventions for a nursing diagnosis of Impaired Gas Exchange?

As I sat with my nursing students at our postclinical conference, I began to realize how difficult it was for my students to synthesize their coursework with the clinical experience. With previous classes in anatomy, physiology, physics, and chemistry, I knew the foundations were in place, but the students were confused about how to apply the concepts to their patient's nursing care. The blending of the basic sciences with the art of nursing is not a new problem. Perhaps an integrated curriculum, combining the scientific facts with the nursing process, is one solution.

The concept of oxygenation is fundamental to the nursing care of many types of patients—from those with the common cold to patients recovering from coronary artery bypass grafting. Certain basic aspects of oxygenation apply to the care of all patients. Oxygenation refers to the processes of ventilation, diffusion, perfusion, and transportation. The respiratory system is only part of oxygenation. The circulatory and hematologic systems also play essential roles.

Integrating the care of patients with disorders of oxygenation requires a collaborative view of health care. Nursing plays a large role in teaching our patients and the general public about healthy behaviors, such as avoiding the use of tobacco products. There are many different health problems that require nursing interventions so that the patient can recover and become fully functional. This book takes a holistic approach to the care of patients with disorders of oxygenation. This allows the reader to become familiar with the nursing interventions for a specific problem, as well as specific medical interventions and alternative therapies. Patients benefit from a nurse who approaches the treatment plan with a comprehensive background and who can explain about all the interventions including testing, medications, and self-help techniques. In this book, nursing diagnoses and interventions are used to help plan the nursing care and organize documentation.

While no book could fully cover all aspects of oxygenation, I have tried to present this concept by systems—first, by reviewing the anatomy and physiology, then defining scientific concepts and describing common disorders of oxygenation, and finally, outlining nursing and medical interventions. I hope it is helpful to students and nurses to have this concept covered in a single text. I especially hope it helps our patients' recovery.

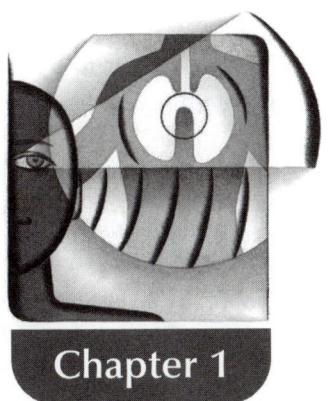

Chapter 1

Anatomy and Physiology of the Respiratory System

Code Blue! Room 622! Code Blue! Room 622!

Hearing those words over the intercom always perks up a nurse's ears and attention. Everyone moves quickly to assure the best outcome for the patient. But much of what goes on during a code involves understanding the anatomy and physiology of the respiratory system. Let's return to the code and watch the interventions of the staff.

Mrs. T. is a 68-year-old woman who had a colectomy 2 days ago. The surgery was uncomplicated, but her oxygen saturation levels were low, so she was receiving oxygen via nasal cannula at 4 liters (L) per minute. Her vital signs 1 hour ago were: blood pressure (BP)—168/88 mmHg, pulse—92 beats per minute, respiration—24 breaths per minute, and her temperature was 100.8°F orally. Her prior medical history includes hypertension, obesity, and smoking one pack of cigarettes per day for 50 years. Mrs. T. had just ambulated in the hall with the nursing assistant and felt short of breath, so she was returned to bed. The nursing assistant came to find the nurse to report Mrs. T's symptoms. The nurse entered the room and found the patient unresponsive and not breathing. She yelled for help and began cardiopulmonary resuscitation (CPR). As she hyperextended the patient's neck and listened for breathing, she watched the chest and did not observe any movement. Pinching the patient's nose, she tried to deliver a breath but could not get air into the patient. She repositioned the head, pulling the jaw forward and was then able to deliver a breath and see the chest rise and fall. As she was checking for the carotid pulse, the anesthesiologist arrived and determined that Mrs. T. needed to be intubated. The nurse felt for a carotid pulse and felt a faint pulse. Using the laryngoscope, the anesthesiologist visualized the vocal cords and inserted the endotracheal tube. After inflating the cuff on the tube, lungs were ventilated by manual inflation. Listening with the stethoscope, the anesthesiologist noted that there were no breath sounds on the left side of the chest.

- Why did changing the position of the head allow the nurse to ventilate the patient?
- If rescue breathing involves exhalation, why does it help oxygenate the patient?

- Why are the vocal cords visualized prior to intubation?
- After intubation, why were breath sounds not heard on the left side of the chest?

The primary function of the respiratory system is gas exchange. In aerobic organisms, oxygen is required for the production of energy. This efficient system provides the body with oxygen for metabolism and removes carbon dioxide, the waste product of metabolism. The lungs provide an extensive area for the exchange of gases between air and circulating blood. The respiratory system also performs several secondary functions, including regulation of acid-base balance, humidification and filtration of air, speech production, as well as taste and smell perception.

THE ANATOMY OF THE RESPIRATORY SYSTEM

The respiratory tract is divided into the upper and lower respiratory tracts (Figure 1-1). The upper respiratory system includes the nasal cavities, the pharynx, and the larynx. The lower respiratory tract includes the trachea, bronchi, bronchioles, lungs, and alveoli. The lower respiratory tract is encased in the thoracic cage and utilizes multiple muscles, including the diaphragm, to facilitate ventilation.

The Upper Respiratory Tract

The Nasal Cavities

The nasal cavities are composed of bone and cartilage (Figure 1-2). The upper third of the nose, the bridge, is bony. The lower third is cartilaginous and divided into two passages by the nasal septum. The nostrils or nares are lined with skin and hair follicles (vibrissae). The vibrissae are the first line of defense for filtering out foreign objects and preventing them from being inhaled. The interior portion of the nasal passages and nasopharynx is lined with a mucus membrane which is well supplied with blood. The mucus membrane serves to warm, filter, and humidify air. It is composed of columnar epithelial cells and goblet cells and produces mucus, which forms

> The mucus membranes of the nasal cavities serve to warm, filter, and humidify air. They are composed of columnar epithelial cells and goblet cells that produce mucus, forming the mucociliary blanket. The cilia move the mucociliary blanket and its entrapped particles toward the oropharynx to be expelled or swallowed.

the mucociliary blanket. This blanket protects the respiratory system by entrapping foreign particles and pathogens. The cilia, tiny hair-like projections which are constantly in motion, move the mucociliary blanket and its entrapped particles toward the oropharynx where it can either be expelled or swallowed. Anatomically, the nasal passages make a 90-degree angle down into the oropharynx, allowing additional filtering of particles from inspired air.

The mucus membrane, located at the top of the nasal cavity just beneath the cribriform plate of the ethmoid bone, is called the *olfactory epithelium*. It provides the sense of smell. The region is supplied by the first cranial nerve—the olfactory nerve—which passes through holes in the cribriform plate. Along the sides of the nasal vestibule are bony projections covered with mucus membrane called *turbinates*. They are highly vascular and serve to cleanse, warm, and humidify inspired air. They also increase the turbulence of inspired air, enhancing capture of particles in the mucociliary blanket.

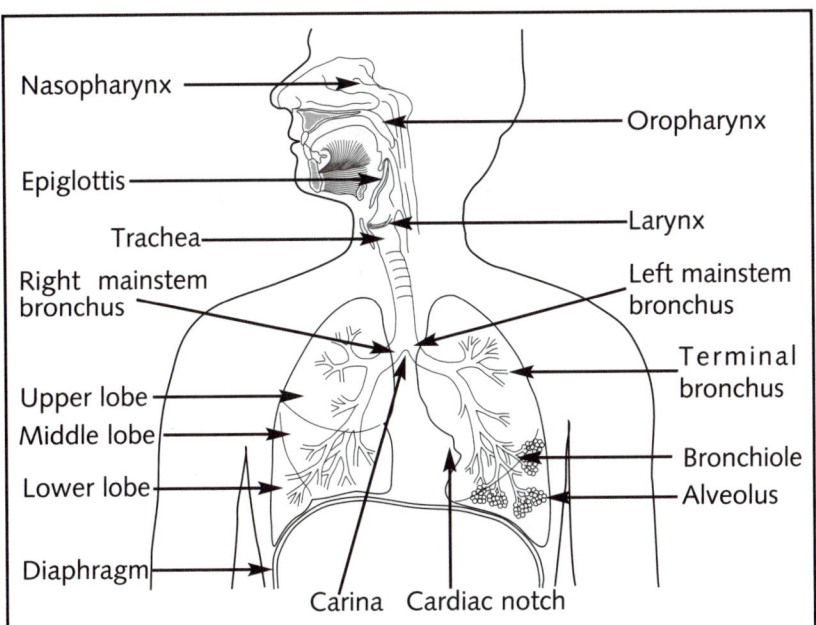

Figure 1-1. Structures of the respiratory tract.

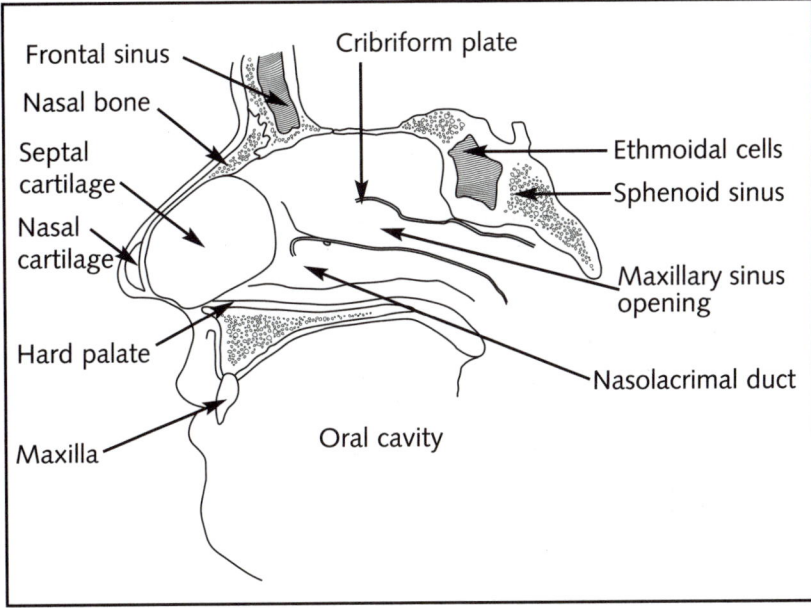

Figure 1-2. Anatomy of the nose.

The paranasal sinuses are hollow spaces in the bones surrounding the nasal passages. The sinuses are named for the bones in which they are located: sphenoid, ethmoid, and maxillary. The paranasal sinuses drain into the nasal cavities, as do the nasolacrimal ducts which drain tears from the surface of the eyes.

The Pharynx

The pharynx is located behind the oral and nasal cavities and extends down to the larynx (Figure 1-3). This tunnel shaped passageway is shared by the respiratory and digestive systems. It is divided into three parts:

Figure 1-3. Upper respiratory tract.

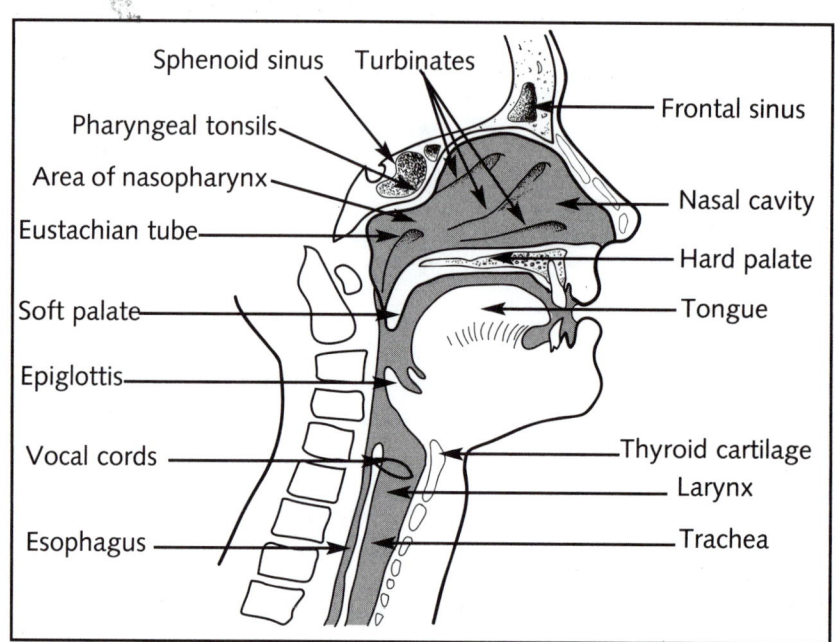

1.   The nasopharynx, located above the margin of the soft palate
2.   The oropharynx, located behind the tongue
3.   The laryngopharynx, located from the base of the tongue to the larynx

The openings for the eustachian tubes are located on either side of the oropharynx. There are lingual, palatine, and pharyngeal tonsils in the pharynx, which are nubs of lymphatic tissue. The mouth serves as an alternative airway when either the nasal passages are obstructed or when high volumes are needed, such as during exercise. It is less efficient than the nose at humidifying, filtering, and warming air. The pharynx is the only opening from the nasal passages, the mouth, and the lungs, so that any obstruction of the pharynx immediately causes ventilation to cease.

The epiglottis is a thin, leaf-shaped structure of elastic cartilage which helps to protect the larynx during swallowing (Figure 1-4). The epiglottis covers the larynx during swallowing to prevent food and fluids from entering the lungs. The closed vocal cords are the final lines of defense for the lungs. At the point where the epiglottis covers the larynx, the pharynx divides into the larynx and the esophagus.

The Larynx

The larynx—voice box—connects the pharynx with the trachea (Figure 1-5). It has two purposes:

1.   Creation of speech
2.   Protection of lungs from entrance by substances other than air

It lies in the midline of the neck and contains two folds of mucus membrane known as the *vocal cords*. Vibration of the tightened vocal cords allows phonation to occur. The arytenoid cartilage is used in vocal cord movement. The epiglottis is attached at the top of the larynx. The esophagus is just posterior to the larynx. Should anything other than air enter the larynx, the cough reflex and laryngeal spasms would reflexively try to expel it. The epiglottis is essential in creating the cough reflex. Nine cartilage rings form the larynx; the largest of which, the *thyroid cartilage,* is sometimes called the Adam's apple. The

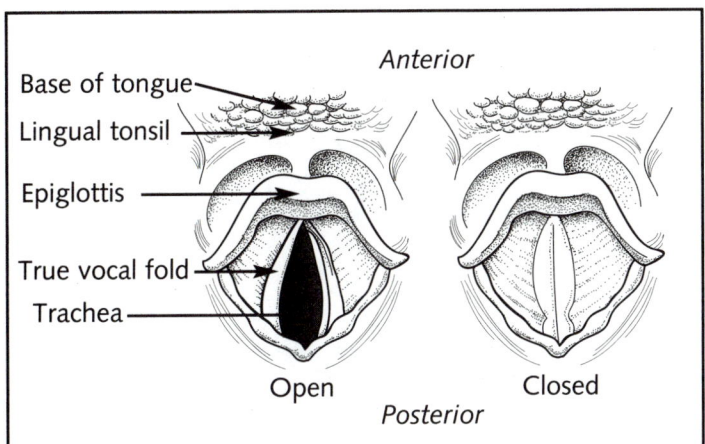

Figure 1-4. A view down the larynx, visualizing the vocal cords.

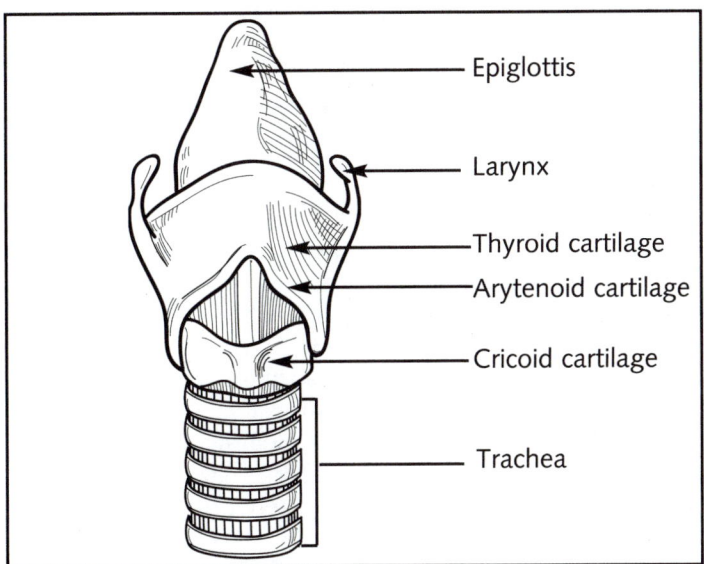

Figure 1-5. Larynx and trachea.

cricoid cartilage, which lies below the thyroid cartilage, contains the vocal cords. The cricothyroid membrane connects the cricoid and thyroid cartilage and is used for emergency access to the airway.

The Lower Respiratory Tract

The lower respiratory tract consists of the trachea, the two mainstem bronchi, lobar, segmental and subsegmental bronchi, bronchioles, alveolar ducts, and alveoli. The tracheobronchial tree can be viewed as a system of branching tubes, each smaller, carrying air to the site of gas exchange: the *alveolar membrane*. There are about 23 levels of branching from the trachea down to the alveolar sac. Smooth muscle is found wound about all the structures of the lower respiratory tract and constricts airways in disorders such as asthma.

The Trachea

The trachea or windpipe is a flexible tube which connects the larynx with the major bronchi of the lungs. It begins at the lower border of the cricoid cartilage and extends

Figure 1-6. The alveoli with the network of capillaries.

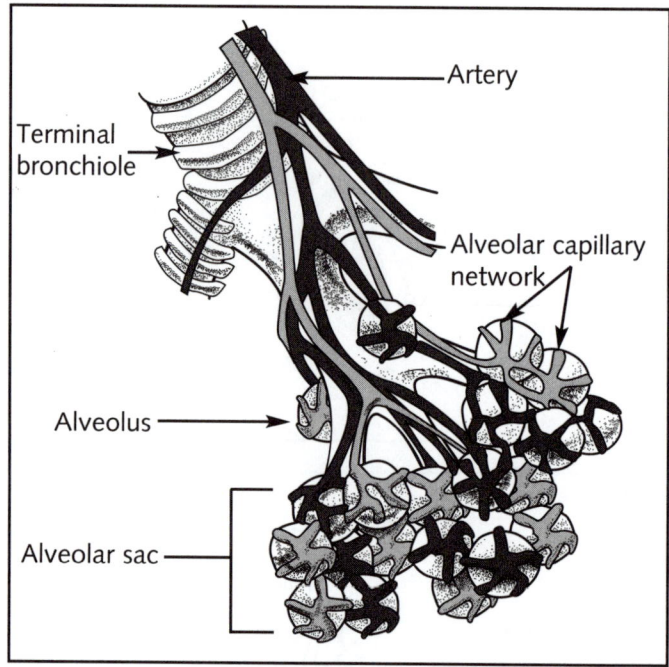

down to the level of the posterior fifth or sixth thoracic vertebrae or the anterior sternal angle, where it branches into the left and right mainstem bronchi. The site of this bifurcation is referred to as the *carina*. The strongest cough reflex is at the carina. The walls of the trachea contain about 20 horseshoe-shaped cartilage that stiffen the trachea, preventing collapse or expansion of the trachea when intrathoracic pressures change. The cartilage are open posteriorly to allow bolus of food to pass down the esophagus. The walls of the trachea are comprised of mucus-secreting, ciliated cells which carry particles away from the lungs and up to the pharynx. These cells are destroyed in those who smoke, resulting in the loss of this valuable function.

The Bronchi and Bronchioles

The right and left mainstem bronchi begin at the carina. These bronchi are similar in structure to the trachea, with cartilage surrounding the airway and maintaining the shape. Smooth muscle, which is controlled by the parasympathetic nervous system, wraps around the bronchi. The right mainstem bronchus is more like a linear extension of the trachea, and is shorter and more vertically downward than the left. Therefore, aspirated foreign bodies and even accidental intubations are more likely to occur in the right mainstem bronchus. The bronchioles spread in an inverted tree-like formation throughout each lung. The segmental and subsegmental bronchi further branch into smaller and smaller bronchioles until they reach the terminal bronchioles. These bronchioles are only about 1 mm in diameter. They do not have cartilage rings and therefore depend on the elastic recoil of the lungs to maintain patency. They do not have cilia or participate in gas exchange.

The Alveoli

The alveoli are cup-shaped structures which are grouped like clusters of grapes at the end of the terminal bronchioles (Figure 1-6). There are 150 to 300 million alveolar sacs in an adult's lungs. Thin walls separate the alveoli from each other, and within the walls is

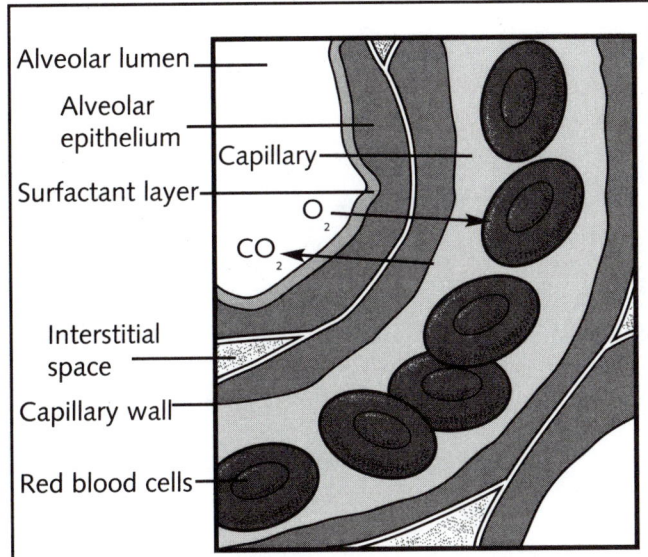

Figure 1-7. Diffusion of gases across the alveolar membrane.

Labels in figure: Alveolar lumen, Alveolar epithelium, Surfactant layer, Capillary, O_2, CO_2, Interstitial space, Capillary wall, Red blood cells

an extensive network of capillaries that is so dense that it has been referred to as a sheet of blood. It is within these walls that the actual gas exchange takes place. Oxygen in the alveoli diffuses across the alveolar capillary membrane into the blood, and carbon dioxide in the blood diffuses back into the alveoli (Figure 1-7). *Surfactant*, a phospholipid protein, is secreted by cells called type II pneumocytes within the alveoli. Surfactant reduces the surface tension in the alveoli, allowing more surface area for gas exchange and preventing collapse of the sac. Lack of surfactant can cause respiratory failure in premature infants and has been implicated in adult respiratory distress syndrome (ARDS). Since there are no mucus-secreting glands in the alveoli, the majority of particle removal is done by alveolar macrophages and the lymphatic channels of the lungs.

The Lungs

The lungs are the functional units of the respiratory system. They are spongy, cone-shaped organs located within the chest cavity on either side of the heart. Between the two lungs is a space called the *mediastinum*, which contains the heart and great vessels, the esophagus, part of the trachea and bronchi, and the thymus gland (Figure 1-8). The lungs are divided into lobes, two in the left lung and three in the right. They are further divided into 10 bronchopulmonary segments. The upper part of the lung is called the *apex*, and the lower part, which rests upon the diaphragm, is called the *base*. The lungs are elastic-like structures which are capable of inflation from within, as well as external pulling sources. Elastic and collagen fibers are contained within the alveolar walls and allow the lungs to stretch in all directions and recoil to return to their normal resting state.

The Thorax, Diaphragm, and Pleura

The thorax contains the lungs, heart, and great vessels. The outer shell of the thorax is comprised of 12 pairs of ribs, which are connected to the thoracic vertebrae of the posterior spine. The first seven pairs are connected to the sternum by cartilage, the next three pairs are connected to each other by costochondral cartilage, and the last two are unattached, the so-called floating ribs, which allow complete expansion of the lungs during inspiration (Figure 1-9).

Figure 1-8. The mediastinum, lungs, and pleural cavity.

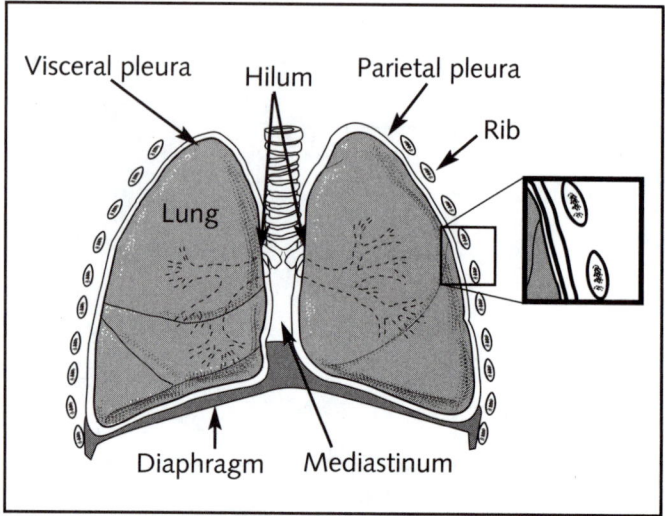

Many muscles are used during inspiration. The scalene and sternocleidomastoid muscles elevate the upper thorax. The intercostal muscles between the ribs pull the ribs upward and forward, increasing the anteroposterior and transverse diameters.

The diaphragm is the principle muscle of respiration. It serves as the lower boundary of the thorax and is attached to the xiphoid process and the lower ribs. When it is relaxed, the diaphragm is dome-shaped. Contraction of the diaphragm allows the chest to expand from top to bottom. The diaphragm is innervated by the phrenic nerve, which originates from the spinal column at the third cervical vertebrae. This is why cervical injuries may result in paralysis of the diaphragm and an inability to ventilate.

The pleura are thin, serous membranes which encase the lungs and the thoracic cavity. The visceral pleura cover the lungs and the fissures between the lobes. The parietal pleura lines the thoracic cavity (see Figure 1-8). The visceral and parietal pleurae allow the lungs to remain against the thoracic wall, creating a pulling force to hold the lungs in the expanded position. A thin film of serous fluid separates the visceral and parietal pleura, acting as a lubricant and allowing the two to glide over each other without any separation. The space between the two pleura, the pleural cavity, is considered a potential space because air, blood, and fluid can accumulate in this area.

RESPIRATORY PHYSIOLOGY

The exchange of gases in the respiratory system requires the integration of multiple processes. During respiration, the conducting airways of the upper and lower respiratory tracts deliver air to the alveolar membrane, the site of actual gas exchange. The mechanics of breathing or ventilation, the effect of respiratory pressures and airflow, the control of ventilation, the relationship of ventilation to perfusion in the exchange of gases, and the system of gas transport will be discussed.

Ventilation

The term *ventilation* refers to the entire process of gas exchange between the human body and the atmosphere. *Pulmonary ventilation* or breathing is the actual flow of gases into and out of the respiratory tract. *Alveolar ventilation* is the exchange of gases across the alveolar membrane into the circulatory system.

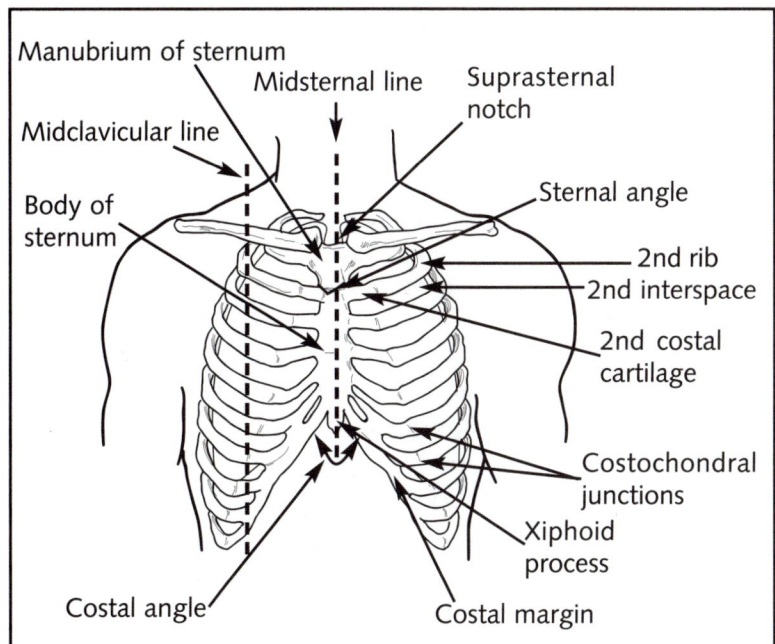

Figure 1-9. Anterior thorax, ribs, and sternum.

Manubrium of sternum
Midsternal line   Suprasternal notch
Midclavicular line
Body of sternum
Sternal angle
2nd rib
2nd interspace
2nd costal cartilage
Costochondral junctions
Xiphoid process
Costal angle   Costal margin

Pulmonary Ventilation

Breathing or pulmonary ventilation is controlled by the movement of the chest cavity, the compliance of the lungs, and the surface tension within the alveoli. A single cycle of ventilation consists of inhalation (or inspiration) followed by exhalation (or expiration). During ventilation, the accessory diaphragm muscles enlarge the thoracic cavity, creating negative pressure within the chest. Air is drawn into the lungs because the intrathoracic pressure is less than the atmospheric pressure. The diaphragm is the principal muscle of inspiration. Normal, quiet breathing is almost entirely performed by the diaphragm. When the diaphragm contracts during inspiration, the abdominal contents are pushed downward and the chest expands. The diaphragm moves down about 1 to 3 cm on normal inspiration and as much as 10 cm on forced inspiration. The lungs are pulled outward as they are adhered to the pleural lining of the thorax. The scalene muscles and the sternocleidomastoid are the accessory muscles of inspiration. The scalene raises the first two ribs and the sternocleidomastoid pulls the sternum slightly forward, increasing the anteroposterior diameter. The trapezius and pectoralis muscles also play a minor role by fixing the shoulders. The accessory muscles contribute little to normal ventilation but are used more intensively during physical exertion or when air exchange is hampered in disease states, such as chronic obstructive pulmonary disease (COPD).

Whereas inhalation requires the active involvement of muscles, exhalation is normally a passive activity. The elastic components of the lungs and chest wall recoil, increasing the pressure in the chest to more than atmospheric pressure, thereby forcing air out of the lungs. The abdominal and intercostal muscles can be used to increase the force of expiration. The use of these muscles may be seen in disorders, such as asthma, which narrow the airways. In asthmatic lungs, the narrowed air passages necessitate greater pressure during exhalation so the accessory muscles are used to force air out of the lungs.

Alveolar Ventilation

The rate at which new air reaches the gas exchange areas of the lungs is referred to as *alveolar ventilation*. During quiet inhalation, very little new air reaches as far as the alveoli.

The air which remains in the nose, pharynx, trachea, bronchi, and bronchioles is not involved in gas exchange and is called dead air space. An inspiration with a tidal volume of 500 mL results in approximately 150 mL of dead space in a 70 kg person. The remaining 350 mL are involved in gas exchange in the alveoli.

Lung Compliance

Lung compliance refers to the ease with which the lungs are inflated. The elastic nature of the lungs causes them to stretch when the lungs are inflated and recoil when the lungs are deflated. The force required to expand the lungs to a particular volume is referred to as compliance. The normal lung compliance for an adult is 200 mL per cm of water pressure. Diseases, such as emphysema, increase compliance, perhaps because the elastic tissues have been overdistended or destroyed. Other disorders, such as pulmonary fibrosis, result in a "stiffer" lung with decreased compliance.

> The diaphragm is the principle muscle of inspiration. When this muscle contracts during inspiration, the abdominal contents are pushed downward and the chest expands. The diaphragm moves down about 1 to 3 cm on normal inspiration and as much as 10 cm on forced inspiration.

Surface Tension

Lung compliance is affected by the surface tension of the alveoli. As mentioned previously, the alveoli are lined with surfactant, which is produced by the type II cells in the alveoli. Surfactant lowers the surface tension of the alveoli, providing stability and even inflation of the alveoli. Without surfactant, lung inflation would be very difficult.

Respiratory Pressures

The pressure difference between the atmosphere and the pulmonary system affects the flow and diffusion of gases. The pressure within the respiratory tract is referred to as the *intrapulmonary pressure* (Figure 1-10). Normal atmospheric pressure is 760 millimeters of mercury (mmHg). When air is not moving into or out of the lungs and the glottis is open, the difference between the intrapulmonary pressure and the atmospheric pressure is 0 mmHg. During quiet breathing, the difference between the atmospheric and intrapulmonary pressures is about 3 mmHg, dropping 3 mmHg below atmospheric pressure during inspiration and increasing 3 mmHg above atmospheric pressure during expiration. Variations in pressure increase from 3 to 5 mmHg during normal activity. During extreme exertion, these pressure differentials may increase dramatically to -80 mmHg during inspiration and +100 mmHg during expiration.

The pressure in the slim space between the visceral and parietal pleura is known as the *intrapleural pressure*. A thin layer of fluid separates the visceral and parietal membranes, providing a powerful force that holds the lung against the chest wall. This force is similar to what happens when a piece of glass is placed on a wet surface. It slides easily back and forth but is very difficult to lift off the surface. Intrapleural pressure falls about 6 mmHg during inspiration and rises as air fills the lungs. It always remains negative relative to the alveolar pressure. This negative pressure holds the lungs against the chest wall.

Although the intrapleural space is considered a potential space, air can enter the space due to a perforation in the lung or chest wall. When air accumulates in this potential space, causing the lung to collapse, this is called a *pneumothorax*. Blood can also accumulate in this space, which is known as a *hemothorax*. If serous fluid accumulates in the

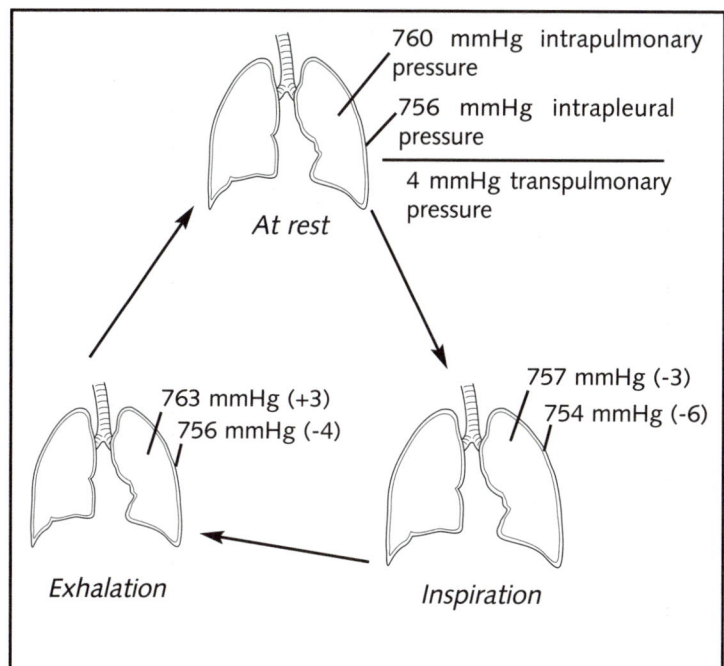

760 mmHg intrapulmonary pressure

756 mmHg intrapleural pressure

4 mmHg transpulmonary pressure

At rest

763 mmHg (+3)
756 mmHg (-4)

757 mmHg (-3)
754 mmHg (-6)

Exhalation

Inspiration

Figure 1-10. Respiratory pressures within the lungs and pleural space during breathing.

intrapleural space, it is referred to as a *pleural effusion*. When any of these accumulate in the pleural space, the intrapleural pressure exceeds the atmospheric pressure, causing a collapse of the alveoli, also called *atelectasis*. Removal of the air or liquid and the reestablishment of negative pressure in the intrapleural space are required to prevent complete collapse of the lung and shifting of the thoracic contents toward the opposite side of the chest. This is called a *mediastinal shift*.

Gas Pressures

The air in the atmosphere is composed of different gases, which move because of changes in pressure. It is composed of roughly 20.8% oxygen and 78.6% nitrogen. Each gas comprises a portion of the total atmospheric pressure, which is 760 mmHg. So if nitrogen comprises 78.6% of atmospheric air, then nitrogen makes up 600 mmHg of that total pressure of 760 mmHg. Likewise for the other components, each contributing their partial pressure to the total pressure. This can be stated in a formula with P representing the partial pressure of each component:

$$PO_2 + PCO_2 + PN_2 + PH_2O = 760 \text{ mmHg}$$

Alveolar air differs in composition from atmospheric air because of humidification, which occurs in the upper airways and by the partial replacement of air with each inspiration (Table 1-1). Not all alveolar air is replaced during each inspiration. Rather, a portion of the remaining air in the alveoli mixes with the fresh air. Even at the end of expiration, air remains within the pulmonary structures and is referred to as the residual volume. Carbon dioxide and oxygen are rapidly and constantly diffusing across the alveolar membrane, making exact measurements of these concentrations difficult.

Table 1-1			
Composition of Atmospheric and Alveolar Air			
	Atmospheric Air	*Alveolar Air*	*Expired Air*
N_2	78.6%	74.5%	75%
O_2	20.8%	15.7%	14%
CO_2	0.04%	3.6%	5%
H_2O	0.5%	6.2%	6%

Air Flow

The movement of air into and out of the lungs is directly related to the difference between the pressure in the lung, the *intrapulmonary pressure*, and the atmospheric pressure. It is inversely related to resistance in the airways. Airway resistance is normally small, and only 1 mmHg of pressure change is required to move 500 mL of air into and out of the lungs. But in conditions such as asthma, where the airways are narrowed by swelling and bronchospasm, the resistance is markedly increased. Airway resistance is influenced by lung volumes and is less during inspiration and more during expiration. For the patient with asthma, the combination of narrowed airways and increased resistance during expiration requires far greater pressure changes to effectively move air into and out of the lungs.

Control of Ventilation

As automatic as it is to breathe, there are higher functions that maintain adequate oxygenation in the body. Breathing is controlled by the brain and the peripheral chemoreceptors. The respiratory center of the brain is located in the medulla oblongata and the pons. It adjusts the respiratory rate and volumes to maintain appropriate oxygen and carbon dioxide levels. Excess carbon dioxide levels cause a lowering of the blood's pH and stimulate the respiratory center to increase inspiratory and expiratory effort. Carbon dioxide is easily diffused across the blood-brain barrier and the neurons can sense small changes in carbon dioxide levels and quickly adjust respiratory effort. The central respiratory center is a very effective and rapid control center because of the ease with which carbon dioxide molecules diffuse across the blood-brain barrier. Oxygen levels do not directly affect the central respiratory center. Rather, they affect the peripheral chemoreceptors near the carotid sinus and the aortic arch (Figure 1-11). The aortic and carotid bodies are sensitive to levels of dissolved oxygen in the plasma. They do not respond to conditions like anemia or carbon monoxide poisoning where the hemoglobin is less saturated with oxygen.

Stimulation of the carotid and aortic bodies by decreased oxygen levels results in increased inspiratory effort. In certain disease states, such as COPD, the central respiratory center becomes desensitized to high carbon dioxide levels and the peripheral chemoreceptors, using arterial oxygen levels, regulate respiration. Therefore, oxygen should be administered cautiously in patients with COPD and the effect should be assessed fre-

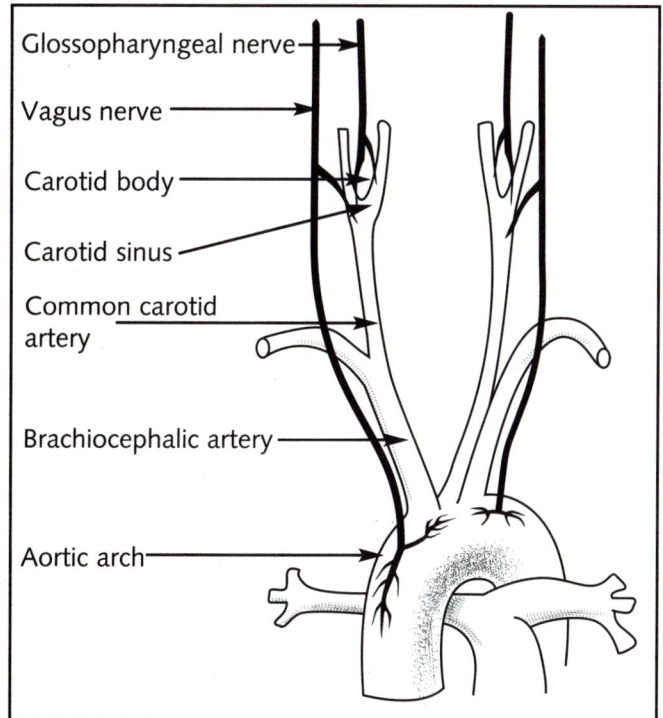

Glossopharyngeal nerve

Vagus nerve

Carotid body

Carotid sinus

Common carotid artery

Brachiocephalic artery

Aortic arch

Figure 1-11. Location of peripheral chemoreceptors.

quently. In these patients, the administration of high-flow oxygen may decrease the respiratory rate and increase the carbon dioxide levels in the blood.

Ventilation and Perfusion

As described previously, alveolar ventilation is crucial for gas exchange to take place. Diffusion is the process by which oxygen and carbon dioxide molecules are exchanged across the alveolar membrane. But diffusion requires not only that the alveoli are ventilated with fresh air but that the ventilated alveoli are perfused by pulmonary capillaries. When there is a discrepancy between ventilation and perfusion, then optimum gas exchange does not occur. A review of the concepts of diffusion and the pressures of gases will clarify this concept.

Diffusion is the random movement of molecules from areas of high concentration to areas of lower concentration. The source of energy for diffusion is the random movement and collisions of the gas molecules (see Table 1-1). Gases move from areas of high concentration to areas of lower concentration. When air enters the alveoli, it has a higher concentration of oxygen than the blood in the pulmonary capillaries. The oxygen molecules move across the alveolar membrane to the red blood cells in the capillary. Likewise, when venous blood reaches the alveolar membrane, the carbon dioxide levels in the blood are higher than the alveolar air, and the carbon dioxide molecules move into the alveoli. Carbon dioxide diffuses 20 times more rapidly than oxygen. The exchange of gases across the alveolar membrane depends on the perfusion of the pulmonary capillaries, as well as the ventilation of the alveoli. The effect of perfusion of these capillaries (Q) on alveolar ventilation (V) is quantifiable as a ratio—the ventilation/perfusion ratio (V/Q). If the alveoli are well ventilated and the capillaries are well perfused, then the ratio is approximately 1. Usually, there is relatively more perfusion than ventilation, yielding a V/Q ratio of 0.8. But when there is a mismatch between the perfusion and the ventilation, there are serious respiratory consequences.

In the case of adequate alveolar ventilation but poor capillary perfusion, there would be no blood flow to carry away the fresh oxygen or dispose of the carbon dioxide, and the

> Diffusion is the random movement of molecules from areas of high concentration to areas of lower concentration. The diffusion of gases across the alveolar membrane depends on the perfusion of the capillary membranes (Q) and the ventilation of the alveoli (V). The effect of perfusion on ventilation is quantifiable as the ventilation/perfusion ratio (V/Q).

V/Q ratio would be equal to infinity. For example, when a pulmonary embolus blocks a pulmonary artery, circulation to lung tissue distal to the blockage is impaired. The ventilation of the alveoli is useless because no gas exchange can take place without perfusion of the affected lung tissue. When the reverse situation occurs, adequate perfusion without ventilation, then the V/Q ratio is said to be 0. An example of this would be the obstruction of a bronchiole by a mucus plug. Circulation of the alveoli would be normal, but ventilation of the lung tissue distal to the blockage would be impaired. Therefore, a certain portion of blood returning via the pulmonary veins to the left side of the heart would not be oxygenated. This is known as shunting, and the quantity of unoxygenated blood is described as the physiologic shunt. Normally, the physiologic shunt is about 5 mL/dL.

Even in normally perfused and ventilated lungs, the V/Q ratio differs between the upper and lower portions of the lungs. When the body is upright, gravity affects the amount of blood flow to the upper and lower portions of the lungs. The upper lobes receive less perfusion, resulting in physiologic dead space that is adequately ventilated but has underperfused areas of the lung. During exercise, circulation to the upper lobes is increased, increasing the effectiveness of gas exchange. Conversely, the lower lobes are well perfused but somewhat underventilated. For these reasons, when the lungs are mechanically ventilated, frequent changes of position help to increase ventilation and perfusion to all parts of the lungs.

Let's return to Mrs. T. as she is being resuscitated by the nurse and the anesthesiologist. When the anesthesiologist could not hear breath sounds on the left side of the chest, she deflated the cuff of the endotracheal tube and withdrew the tube 1 to 2 cm. Then the cuff was reinflated and breath sounds could be auscultated on both sides of the chest. This maneuver solved the problem because the tube had traveled past the carina and into the right mainstem bronchus. This is a common scenario, as the right mainstem bronchus is straighter and more vertical than the left one.

During manual ventilation of Mrs. T., the nurse noticed that the lungs were difficult to inflate. Due to many years of smoking, the lung compliance was decreased, making it more difficult to ventilate. Breath sounds were distant in both lower lobes, and the nurse also heard a lot of gurgling, coarse sounds (rhonchi) that she assessed as phlegm in the airways, and decided to suction the patient. Suctioning through the endotracheal tube produced large amounts of thick sputum. Smokers frequently have large amounts of sputum because the lung's reaction to foreign particles is to produce sputum and move it out of the system. But the decrease in ciliated cells (also due to smoking) available to move mucus out of the respiratory tract resulted in accumulation of mucus in the lungs. The surgery and anesthesia further complicated the problem, as the patient had some atelectasis of the alveoli resulting in decreased oxygenation. Nursing interventions, such as assisted coughing and deep breathing, as well as instruction on the use of the incentive spirometer may have prevented this event. Pain from her abdominal incision was probably preventing Mrs. T. from deep breathing, so adequate pain medication would have made these interventions more effective.

After suctioning, breath sounds were heard in both bases. After 5 minutes of ventilation with oxygen, Mrs. T. started to respond and opened her eyes. She was transferred to the intensive care unit for further ventilatory support.

The answers to the questions listed in the introduction are as follows:

- *Why did changing the position of the head allow the nurse to ventilate the patient?*

Pulling the jaw forward brought the tongue away from the posterior oropharynx and allowed ventilation.

- *If rescue breathing involves exhalation, why does it help oxygenate the patient?*

Exhaled air contains 15.7% oxygen (atmospheric air has 20.8% oxygen), so rescue breathing still delivers oxygen to the victim.

- *Why are the vocal cords visualized prior to intubation?*

The vocal cords are visualized prior to intubation so that the endotracheal tube passes through the vocal cords into the trachea.

- *After intubation, why were breath sounds not heard on the left side of the chest?*

Breath sounds were not heard on the left side after intubation because the endotracheal tube was located in the right mainstem bronchus, and ventilation was only passing into the right lung.

BIBLIOGRAPHY

Bates B. *A Guide to Physical Examination and History Taking*. Philadelphia, Pa: J.B. Lippincott Co; 1995.

Black J, Matassarin-Jacobs E. *Medical-Surgical Nursing: Clinical Management for Continuity of Care*. Philadelphia, Pa: W.B. Saunders Co; 1997.

Guyton AC, Hall JE. *Textbook of Medical Physiology*. Philadelphia, Pa: W.B. Saunders Co; 1996.

Martini F. *Fundamentals of Anatomy and Physiology*. Englewood Cliffs, NJ: Prentice Hall; 1992.

Porth CM. *Concepts in Metered Health States*. Philadelphia, Pa: J.B. Lippincott Co; 1994.

MULTIPLE-CHOICE QUESTIONS

1. What structures prevent foreign bodies from being aspirated into the lungs?
    A. Tongue
    B. Epiglottis, vocal cords, mucociliary blanket
    C. Carina, bronchioles
    D. Teeth, tonsils, adenoids

2. In the patient with chronic obstructive pulmonary disease (COPD), why can it be dangerous to give supplemental oxygen?
    A. Supplemental O_2 may decrease respiratory drive from peripheral chemoreceptors
    B. Oxygen levels in the blood increase respiratory rate in patients with COPD
    C. Hyperventilation may occur if supplemental oxygen is given
    D. Supplemental oxygen may increase mucus production

3. If a child accidentally inhales a peanut, what lung does it usually lodge in?
    A. Either lung because the force of inspiration is equal in both lungs
    B. Inhaled objects follow the straightest path, usually the right mainstem bronchus into the right lung
    C. The left lung and the left mainstem bronchus is wider than the right
    D. Neither lung because the carina stops the object

4. Is quiet expiration active or passive (no muscle work required)?
    A. Expiration requires the use of accessory muscles, so it is active
    B. The diaphragm contracts during expiration so it is active
    C. Expiration during quiet breathing is usually passive
    D. The abdominal muscles actively contract during quiet expiration

5. When upright, what force of nature makes blood flow greater in the lower portions of the lungs?
    A. Pressure from the left ventricle increases blood flow to the lower lungs
    B. Diffusion of gases is greater in the lower lungs in the upright position
    C. Ventilation is better in the lower lungs in the upright position
    D. Gravity increases blood flow to the lower lungs when in the upright position

6. What functions of the nasal cavity are lost during mouth breathing?
    A. The nasal turbinates provide amplification of vocal sounds
    B. The nasal cavity has no function in breathing
    C. The mucus membrane of the mouth functions as well as those in the nasal cavity
    D. The nasal cavity provides humidification and warming of inspired air

7. When speaking, are the vocal cords open or shut?
   A. The vocal cords are open, allowing breathing and talking at the same time
   B. The vocal cords are completely open, allowing air to pass through and make sounds
   C. The vocal cords are closed during speaking, allowing tiny amounts of air through
   D. The vocal cords open to allow the mucociliary blanket to function

CHAPTER 1 ANSWERS

1. B
2. A
3. B
4. C
5. D
6. D
7. C

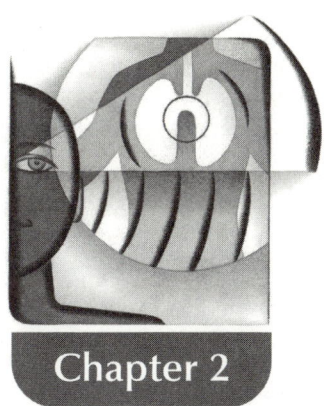

Chapter 2

Assessment of the Respiratory System

Mr. Z. is a 58-year-old man who comes to the emergency department because his wife says he "can't catch his breath." Mr. Z. is sitting in the chair beside the stretcher with his elbows propped on the arms of the chair. His wife is standing beside him, rubbing his arm. At first glance, he is working hard at breathing, with his shoulders stiff and high and his lips pursed on exhalation. His color is somewhat dusky, especially around the mouth. The nurse takes his vital signs and finds that his temperature is 100.8°F, his heart rate is 94 beats per minute, his respiratory rate is 32 breaths per minute, and his blood pressure is 168/92 mmHg. Using the pulse oximeter, the nurse measures the oxygen saturation (SaO_2) at 87%. A round chest circumference and rib retraction is noted on chest examination. Listening with the stethoscope, the nurse notes distant breath sounds with expiratory wheezes throughout his lung fields and rhonchi scattered throughout his right lung. It is difficult to hear breath sounds at the bases of the lungs.

Taking a quick history from his wife, the nurse finds that Mr. Z. has smoked 1.5 packs of cigarettes a day for 35 years. He has had "trouble catching his breath for several years," but last week he had a cold, and now he can "hardly sleep because he cannot breathe." He has no known allergies and takes atenolol, a beta-blocker, for his high blood pressure. A co-worker suggests that Mr. Z. be put on the stretcher and given oxygen via nasal prongs.

- Why is Mr. Z. sitting in the chair, and should he be on the stretcher?
- What should be considered before starting oxygen therapy?
- What changes might be seen on an arterial blood gas, given Mr. Z.'s smoking history and oxygen saturation?
- What anatomic changes cause wheezes?
- What side effect of beta-blockers is making Mr. Z.'s breathing more difficult?

To gain an accurate picture of a patient's respiratory functioning, the nurse must combine knowledge of the anatomy and physiology of the respiratory tract with data from the patient's assessment. Every patient has a unique combination of previous history, current symptoms, lifestyle and behavior patterns, and genetic history. The goal is to gather data from the history, physical assessment, and diagnostic tests, and compile a complete picture of the patient's respiratory status.

THE PATIENT HISTORY

Many aspects of an individual's life impact the functioning of the respiratory system. To gather the necessary information about the factors that affect respiratory health, the nurse must begin by taking a thorough history. Gathering an accurate database provides the nurse with the information that will direct the physical assessment and guide the planning of appropriate interventions. Possible sources of information include the patient, his family or significant others, the patient's appearance and posture, and the medical record(s).

General questions would begin the process of taking a health history. The nurse might begin by asking the following questions:

- What brings the patient to seek health care at this visit?
- What is the predominant symptom?
- How long has the patient had it?
- Has the patient tried to alleviate the problem?
- What makes it better or worse?
- How does it affect the patient's functioning in daily life?

The assessment should include demographic data, such as age, sex, and race. Aging not only affects the functioning of the respiratory tract, but disorders such as emphysema also are more age specific. Gender can influence the incidence of certain diseases of the respiratory tract; oral cancers are more common in men than in women. Race may affect such parameters as normal respiratory volumes; Caucasians have larger lung volumes than Native Americans or Asian Americans.

Symptoms

Many respiratory problems begin with similar symptoms. Clarifying the nature of these symptoms narrows the possible problems and directs the remainder of the assessment and examination. Some common presentations of respiratory problems include cough, nasal secretions, dyspnea (difficult breathing), and pain. Each presentation requires further questioning to ascertain the nature of the symptom and how it affects the patient's functioning.

Cough

Coughing is a protective mechanism for clearing the airways. It also can be a reflexive response to irritating stimuli in the tracheobronchial tree or the larynx. The cough may be described as coming in spurts (paroxysmal) or chronic, tickling, hacking, dry, or productive. Some further questions might include:

- How long has the patient had the cough?
- Is the cough productive and, if so, what does the sputum look like: clear, white, yellow, green, or blood-tinged?
- Is the cough worse at certain times of the day or night?

Nasal Secretions

Allergies, rhinitis, infection, and irritants can cause excessive secretions. Allergies may cause thin, watery secretions and pale nasal mucosa. Infection can cause yellow to greenish secretions with reddened mucosa. Some further questions might include:

- Does the patient have problems with excessive nasal secretions?
- What do the secretions look like?
- Do they increase at certain times of the year?
- Do plants or animals affect the amount of secretions?
- Do certain "triggers," such as pollen, dust, or food additives make the secretions begin or increase?

Dyspnea

Patients do not usually come in complaining of "dyspnea," but they may describe difficulty breathing in a variety of ways. Dyspnea is a common presentation of respiratory problems, but it is a subjective symptom and varies from person to person. It can be graded as to its impact on the patient's functioning using a dyspnea scale (Table 2-1). The nurse should ask about fatigue and level of activity to gather information about activity tolerance. Some more specific questions might include:

- Was the onset abrupt or gradual?
- What relieves the dyspnea—medication, cessation of activity, or change of position?
- Is the breathing rapid, labored, or noisy?
- Is the patient assuming certain positions to make the breathing easier, such as sitting upright (orthopnea)?
- In observing the patient, is he using accessory muscles in the shoulders, neck, or abdomen to make the breathing easier?
- Is breathing more difficult at certain times of the day or night?
- Does shortness of breath awaken the patient at night (paroxysmal nocturnal dyspnea)?
- Does the patient appear anxious?
- Is he gasping for breath?
- Are there any signs of cyanosis (bluish-gray tinge) or pallor of the lips, mucosal lining of the mouth, inner eyelid, skin, or nail beds?
- How does the dyspnea affect the patient's performance of normal activities?

Pain

Any pain associated with breathing needs to be assessed as to when and where it occurs. Lung tissue is insensitive to pain. But the parietal pleura, the intercostal muscles, the connections between cartilage and bone in the thoracic cage, and the tracheobronchial tree can illicit pain. Pleuritic pain usually is catching in nature and is produced by movement of the thoracic cage, which irritates the pleural lining. It is commonly unilateral and brought on by deep inspiration. Intercostal pain is worse during coughing and is transient in nature. Costochondral pain occurs at the connection of the ribs and cartilage and can be illicited with pressure on the area. When assessing pain, nurses should try to differentiate between respiratory pain and pain that may be cardiac or gastrointestinal in origin. Further questions might include:

- How would the patient grade the pain on a scale of 1 to 10?
- Where is the pain located—beneath the sternum, in the gastric area, or in the shoulder?

Table 2-1

Dyspnea Scale

Grade	Degree	Description
0	None	Not troubled with breathlessness except with strenuous exercise.
1	Slight	Troubled with shortness of breath when hurrying on level ground or walking up slight hill.
2	Moderate	Walks slower than people of same age because of breathlessness or has to stop for breath when walking at pace on level ground.
3	Severe	Stops for breath after walking approximately 100 yards after a few minutes on level ground.
4	Very severe	Too breathless to leave the house or breathless when dressing.

- What is the nature of the pain—stabbing, burning, or aching?
- When does the pain occur during the respiratory cycle?
- Does coughing make the pain worse?
- Can the patient point to the area where he feels the pain?
- Is the pain constant, transient, or catching in nature?
- Do certain activities bring on the pain, and does their cessation relieve the pain?

Prior Medical History

The patient's prior medical history contains important clues for the respiratory assessment. A thorough listing of previous illnesses, surgeries, and their respective dates should be recorded. Questions should include the presence of general conditions, such as hypertension, heart disease, and diabetes. Systemic symptoms such as weight loss, night sweats, and fatigue provide valuable information. List all medications that the patient is taking, both prescription and nonprescription medicines, as well as herbal remedies and nutritional supplements. Medications for breathing problems, how they are administered, and when they are used should be detailed in the history. Nonprescription medications taken for breathing difficulties include antihistamines, decongestants, nasal sprays, cough and allergy medications, inhalants, herbs, vitamins, and home remedies.

Specific questions about respiratory disorders provide details that will direct further questioning and examination. The patient should be asked about any history of asthma, bronchitis, pneumonia, sinusitis, tuberculosis (TB), allergies, or frequent colds during the assessment. Further clarification should be obtained about allergic conditions, such as asthma, eczema, and hay fever, as well as specific allergies to dust, mold, pollen, animal dander, foods, trees, or grass. If the patient has a history of asthma, the nurse should inquire about gastroesophageal reflux disease. Allergies also may be associated with asthma. Treatment for allergies, such as desensitization, should be listed with associated dates of treatment.

Any prior surgery to the upper or lower respiratory tract and the dates of surgery should be listed in the assessment. Family history of respiratory and other problems (eg, emphysema, cystic fibrosis, lung cancer, and asthma) is important because there may be a genetic link in these conditions. The patient should be asked about recent travel and which countries were visited; TB is very common in Asian and Latin American countries. TB is also common among household members of an infected person, so it is important to ask about family illnesses. List the dates of the last chest radiograph, TB (Mantoux or PPD) test, vaccinations for influenza and pneumococcus, and pulmonary function tests, if appropriate.

One of the most important areas to cover in a respiratory assessment is the smoking history of the patient and his or her significant others. Questioning should include the use of any tobacco products, such as cigarettes, cigars, pipe tobacco, chewing tobacco, snuff, and marijuana products. Although a patient may state that he or she does not smoke, always ask about smoking in the past. A nonjudgmental attitude about smoking should be maintained to minimize the patient's guilt and encourage honesty. For cigarette smokers, the number of years the patient has been smoking should be ascertained and multiplied by the number of packs per day to obtain the number of "pack-years."

years smoking x # packs per day = pack-years

If the patient has already quit using tobacco products, the date(s) should be noted. Also, ask the patient whether anyone in the home exposes the patient to secondhand or passive smoke. There is increasing evidence that passive smoke exposure increases the risk of asthma in children and lung cancer in nonsmoking adults. Other sources of smoke exposure include wood stoves, kerosene heaters, and fireplaces.

Reviewing the patient's dietary history provides valuable information about their appetite, nutritional status, eating patterns, and food allergies. Measure and weigh the patient to obtain an accurate height and weight. Review his or her daily dietary and fluid intake. Patients with dyspnea tend to eat smaller meals because of difficulty catching their breath when eating. Chronic dyspnea may lead to inadequate food intake and weight loss.

Food additives have been linked to allergies and asthma. Beer, wine, restaurant salads, and many processed fruits and vegetables contain sulfites as preservatives. Sulfites may produce allergic responses in sensitive individuals, such as sneezing, urticaria (hives), shortness of breath and wheezing, chest pain or tightness, and rhinitis. Another food additive that has been linked to allergic responses is tartrazine, which is a component of the Food, Drug, and Cosmetic Act (FD&C) yellow #5. This is a coloring agent used in many processed foods.

Adequate fluid intake (6 to 8 oz glasses per day) is necessary for liquefying and mobilizing secretions. The daily fluid requirements of a patient can be calculated by taking their weight in pounds and dividing it in half. That number will approximate the number of fluid ounces a patient needs daily. Caffeinated beverages have a mild diuretic effect and extra fluids will be needed to compensate for this effect. The type, amount, and frequency of alcohol intake should be determined. Excessive alcohol intake has been associated with the increased incidence of head and neck cancers. It is also nonnutritive and dehydrating.

Occupational history requires careful questioning during the assessment. The patient's job(s) and date(s) of employment should be listed. Exposure to industrial fumes, chemicals, and dust may damage the respiratory tract. Dust from coal, stone, silicone, and asbestos may cause toxic lung injury. The classic case of dust exposure and disease is coal dust and black lung disease. Other occupations that involve exposure to toxic substances are jobs in dry cleaning, beauty salons, insect control, farming, and painting. Hobbies such as furniture refinishing, model airplane building, and woodworking also may expose the patient to noxious fumes or particles.

Finally, other sources of respiratory problems include pets (eg, birds, cats), time spent in the armed forces (eg, Agent Orange exposure, Gulf War syndrome), and exposure to certain farm products (eg, moldy wheat and hay).

PHYSICAL ASSESSMENT OF THE RESPIRATORY TRACT

After gathering data about the patient's current symptoms and his or her health history, it is time to perform a physical assessment. A general assessment of the respiratory system is reviewed here, but a more specific assessment of problem areas identified while taking the history further directs the examination.

Providing the patient with appropriate draping in a warm, well-lit room makes the patient more comfortable during the examination. The room should be private and quiet to facilitate hearing breath sounds. The physical examination proceeds in an orderly manner with the following steps: inspection, palpation, percussion, and auscultation.

The examination begins with a general inspection of the patient. The respiratory rate, rhythm, and depth should be noted. The breathing pattern should be assessed without the patient's awareness so as not to make the patient self-conscious, which alters the normal pattern. A normal respiratory rate ranges from 12 to 20 breaths per minute. A rate greater than 20 (*tachypnea*) may indicate hypoxemia (low serum oxygen levels), hypercapnia (high serum carbon dioxide levels), or anxiety. A low respiratory rate (less than 12 breaths per minute) is called *bradypnea* and may indicate central nervous system (CNS) depression, as seen with head injuries and drug overdoses. Other patterns of respiration are reviewed in Figure 2-1. As the patient breathes, the nurse should watch for the use of accessory muscles in the shoulders, neck, and abdomen or changes in posture that assist the patient in breathing. Normally, these muscles are not needed for respiration, and their use indicates difficulty moving air through the respiratory passages.

> The physical examination of the respiratory system proceeds in an orderly manner: inspection, palpation, percussion, and auscultation. Inspection includes noting the respiratory rate, rhythm, and depth. Normally, accessory muscles in the shoulders, neck, and abdomen are not needed for respiration.

Check the lips, skin, and nail beds for signs of peripheral cyanosis, such as blue-gray tinge or clubbing of the nails. Clubbing of the nails is a sign of long-term, impaired oxygenation. An increase in the angle between the nail bed and the digit is seen in clubbing (Figure 2-2). Central cyanosis is better assessed by examining the mucous membranes inside the mouth and the inner eyelid for pallor. Observe the face for nasal flaring and open-mouthed or pursed-lip breathing, which may indicate respiratory distress.

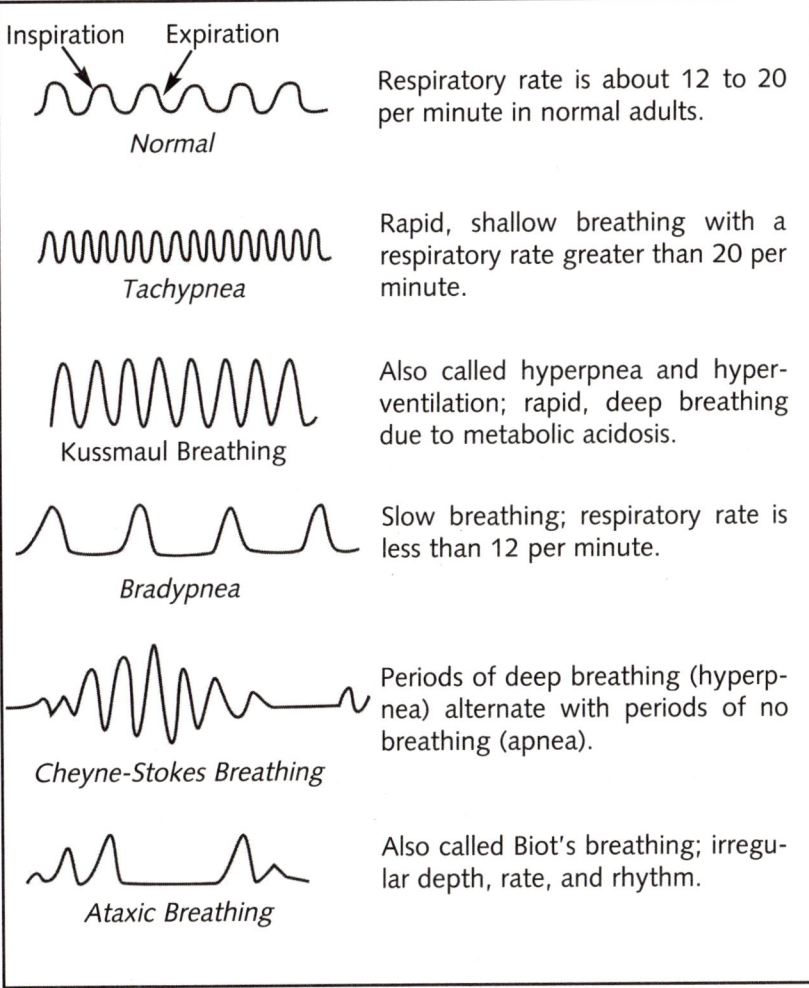

Inspiration Expiration	
Normal	Respiratory rate is about 12 to 20 per minute in normal adults.
Tachypnea	Rapid, shallow breathing with a respiratory rate greater than 20 per minute.
Kussmaul Breathing	Also called hyperpnea and hyperventilation; rapid, deep breathing due to metabolic acidosis.
Bradypnea	Slow breathing; respiratory rate is less than 12 per minute.
Cheyne-Stokes Breathing	Periods of deep breathing (hyperpnea) alternate with periods of no breathing (apnea).
Ataxic Breathing	Also called Biot's breathing; irregular depth, rate, and rhythm.

Figure 2-1. Patterns of respiration.

Nose and Sinuses

The nose and nostrils should be inspected, keeping in mind the underlying structures. The symmetry of the bony part of the nose (upper third) and the cartilaginous part (lower two-thirds) should be noted. The patient's head should be tilted back 15 to 30 degrees, and the position should be stabilized by putting a hand on the patient's forehead to prevent sudden changes of position. Using a penlight and a nasal speculum, the interior of the nose, the *nasal vestibule*, should be inspected while not touching the septum, as it is very sensitive. The outermost portion should be skin with fine hairs followed by mucous membranes, which are normally pink and moist. The mucosa may be reddened during infection or pale during allergic reactions. The nasal septum should be inspected for deviation or perforation. The middle and lower turbinates should be visible as well. The third turbinate will not be visible because of its anatomic location. The patency of each side of the nose should be assessed by pressing on one nares to block airflow, asking the patient to inhale through the other nares, and repeating on the other side. An alcohol wipe or essence of peppermint is used to assess whether the sense of smell is intact while the patient closes his eyes and is asked to identify the smell. This determines whether the first cranial nerve, the olfactory nerve, is intact.

Figure 2-2. Clubbing of the nails.

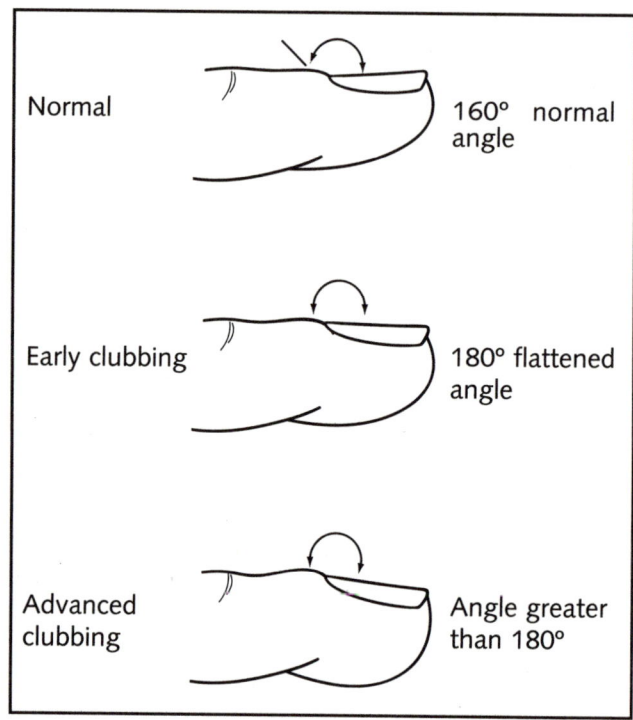

Figure 2-3. Frontal and maxillary sinuses.

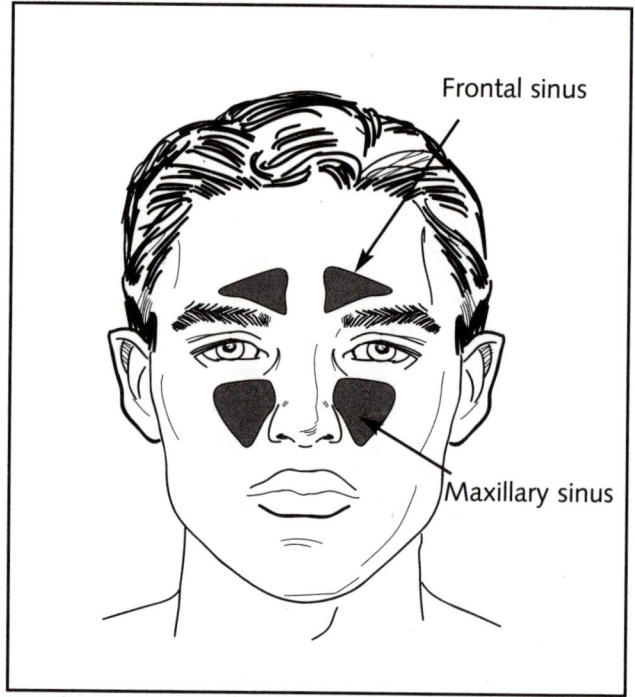

Two of the four pairs of sinuses in the head, the frontal and the maxillary, are accessible for examination (Figure 2-3). Swelling and tenderness over these sinuses is checked by palpating the area. Using the thumbs, the nurse should press up on the cheekbones to assess the maxillary sinuses and up on the brow bone to assess the frontal sinuses. Pain or tenderness in these areas may indicate infection (sinusitis).

Transillumination is another technique that may be used to assess the sinuses. In a darkened room, a penlight is placed under the brow bone to assess the frontal sinus. A dim, red glow on the forehead indicates a normally air-filled frontal sinus. Lack of this glow may indicate a fluid or mucous-filled sinus. The same technique can be used to assess the maxillary sinuses. With the patient's mouth opened and head tilted back, the light should be placed downward just under the inner aspect of the eye. A dim glow should be visible in the mouth on the hard palate. Although transillumination is not a definitive test, it may be helpful in conjunction with other findings in the physical examination and history for deciding whether radiographs or computed tomography (CT scan) are needed.

Mouth, Pharynx, Trachea, and Larynx

The examination begins by assessing the lips for cyanosis or pallor, sores, ulcers, cracks, or nodules. Look for signs of peripheral cyanosis on the lips that may indicate poor oxygenation. Sores or ulcers may be present with a herpes infection. Cracks in the corners of the mouth (cheilitis) may indicate nutritional deficiencies. The teeth, the quality of the dental hygiene, and the presence of dentures and other dental appliances should be noted. The patient should remove the dentures, if they are present. A penlight and tongue blade should be used to check the gums for soreness or redness, which may indicate poorly fitting dentures, gingivitis, or aphthous ulcers (canker sores). Check the mucous membranes of the mouth for pallor. Because the tongue may interfere with a thorough examination, a dry 4x4 gauze should be used to hold the tongue and gently move it side to side to examine the mouth. The mucous membranes should be moist, and their color may vary from coral pink in light skinned people to a brownish-pink tone in darker skinned people. Any redness, especially along the gum line, white patches (candida or leukoplakia), ulcers, sores, or growths should be noted.

The tongue should have pinkish papillae and be without redness or white patches. A shiny surface also is an abnormal finding on the tongue and may indicate nutritional deficiencies. With the tongue wrapped in gauze, the tongue should be moved side to side in order to examine the base of the tongue and the floor of the mouth. This is especially important for people at high risk for oral cancers, such as smokers, alcohol abusers, and those who chew tobacco. Any redness, white patches, or ulcerations should be noted.

The posterior oropharynx is visualized with a tongue blade and a penlight. While gently pressing on the middle of the tongue (not too far back, as this may cause gagging), the palate, uvula, tonsils, and posterior oropharynx should be inspected. The color and symmetry from one side to the other should be noted. Abnormal findings include swelling, exudate, and ulceration. Enlargement of the tonsils is an abnormal finding in the adult, because tonsils should be small to nonexistent in adults. Pushing gently down on the tongue and having the patient say "ahhhh" or yawn elevates the soft palate, allowing visualization of the posterior oropharynx. Asymmetric elevation of the soft palate and the uvula indicates a problem with the 10th cranial nerve.

The neck should be inspected for alignment, symmetry, nodules, or masses. The lymph nodes in the neck should be palpated, assessing their size and mobility and whether they are tender (Figure 2-4). Tender lymph nodes usually indicate inflammation, whereas hard, fixed nodes may indicate malignancy. The trachea should be palpated gently so coughing is not stimulated. The thyroid cartilage (Adam's apple) and the cricoid cartilage beneath it should be identified. The trachea should be uniform and midline, and it should elevate smoothly during swallowing. Palpation should be gentle to prevent coughing or gagging.

Figure 2-4. Cervical lymph node chains.

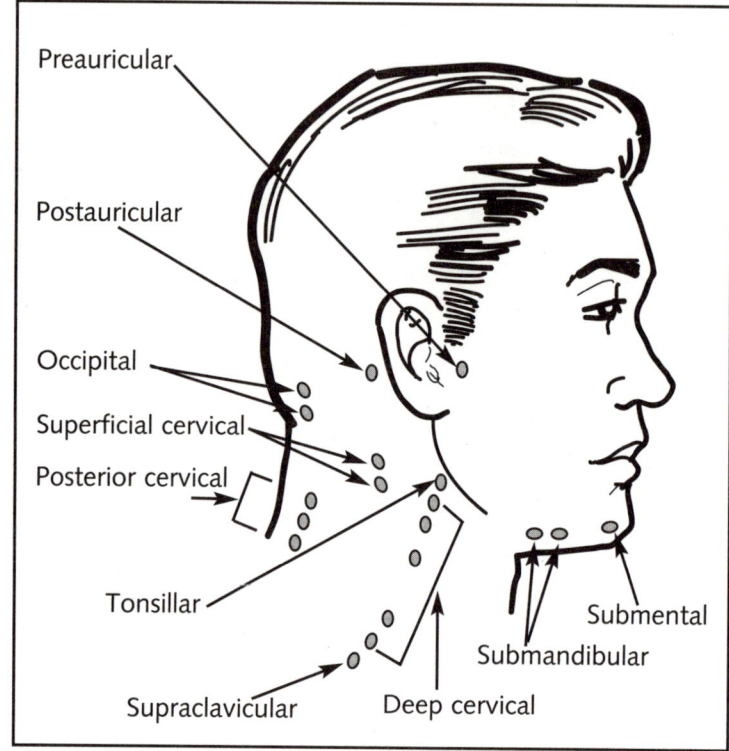

Thorax and Lungs

Before examining the lungs, the anatomy of the underlying structures in the thorax should be reviewed. Anatomic landmarks are useful for identifying organs within the thoracic cavity and for labeling abnormal findings (Figures 2-5 through 2-8). The midsternal line is an imaginary line that runs vertically through the sternum. The midclavicular line runs vertically down the anterior chest wall beginning at the center of each clavicle. The anterior axillary line is another landmark that runs vertically along the anterior aspect of the chest at the anterior fold of the axilla. The posterior axillary line, which also starts at the axilla, extends vertically down the posterior chest. Also remember that each intercostal space is numbered by the rib just above it. Finally, the bases of the lungs are the lowest portions of the lungs. Anteriorly, the bases of the lungs begin at the sixth intercostal space at the midclavicular line, the eighth space laterally, and the 10th to 12th intercostal spaces posteriorly. The apex of the lung refers to the uppermost portion of the lung located above the clavicle anteriorly.

The examination begins at the posterior chest with the patient sitting with his arms folded across his chest. The posterior chest should be uncovered, taking care to cover the anterior chest, particularly on female patients. If the patient has difficulty sitting up, ask for assistance or roll the patient side to side. The chest is examined by following the same step-wise examination: inspection, palpation, percussion, and auscultation. One side of the patient should be compared with the other side to assess physical symmetry and similarity of breath sounds.

Inspection of the chest begins with observing the patient's breathing, watching for chest expansion, and the use of accessory muscles. The rate, rhythm, and regularity of the ventilations, and the length of inspiration and expiration should be noted. Expiration is

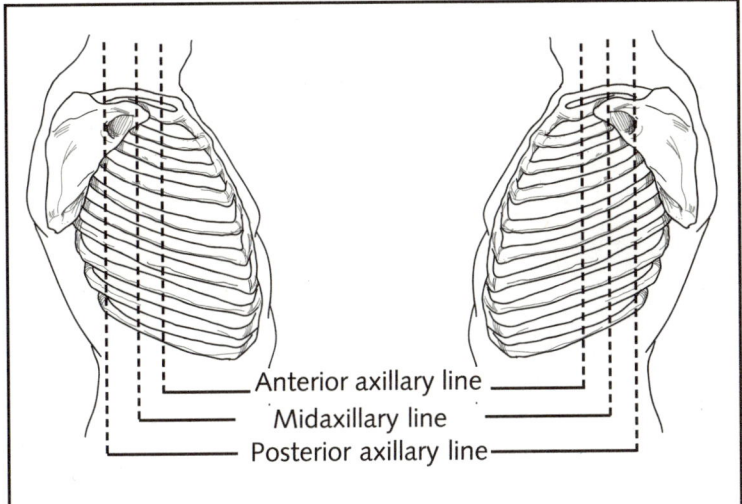

Figure 2-5. Lateral landmarks of the thorax.

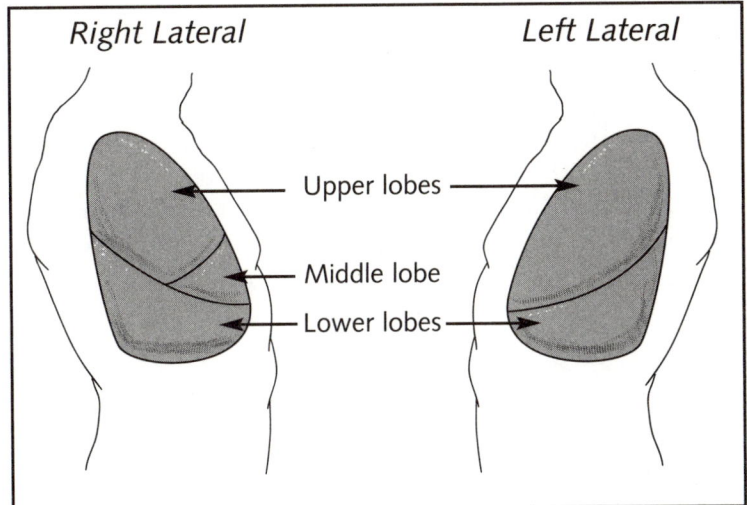

Figure 2-6. Lateral lung structures.

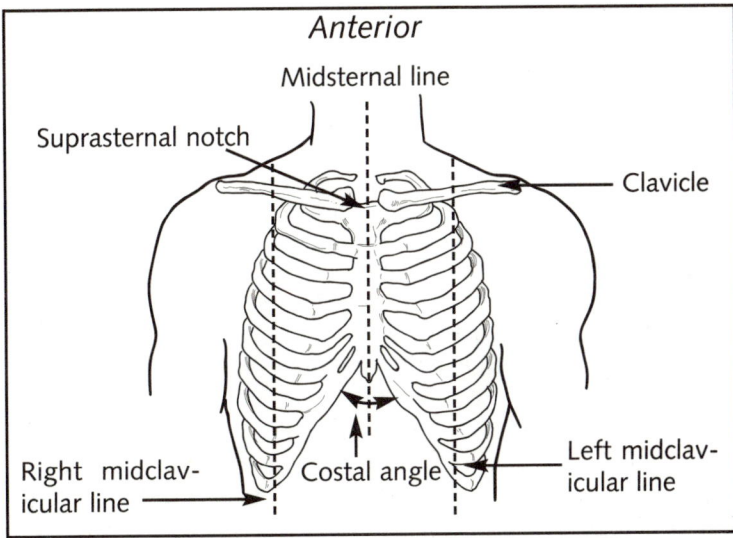

Figure 2-7. Anterior landmarks of the thorax.

Figure 2-8. Anterior lung structures.

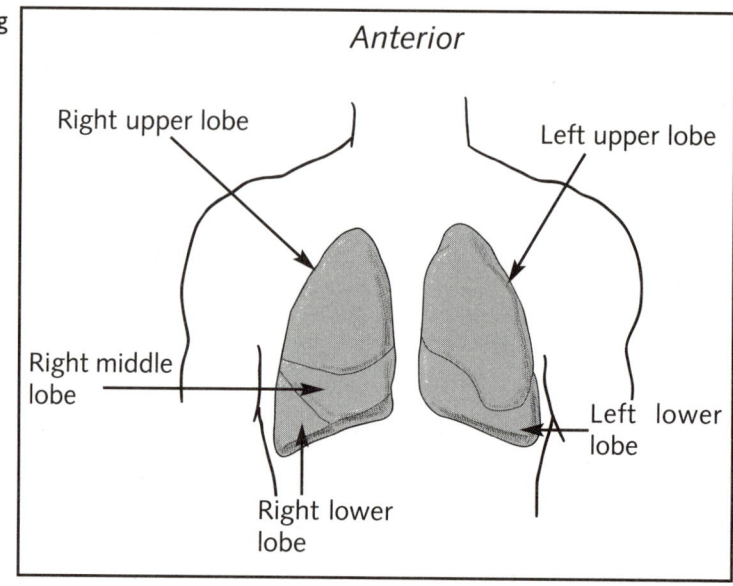

Anterior

Right upper lobe

Left upper lobe

Right middle lobe

Left lower lobe

Right lower lobe

normally 1.5 times longer than inspiration. Prolonged expiration indicates narrowed airways or difficulty moving air out of the lungs (air trapping), as seen in emphysema. Slight retraction of the intercostal spaces is normal in thin people during quiet breathing, but any more than slight retraction indicates difficulty moving air, which may occur with chronic obstructive pulmonary disease (COPD) or an obstructed airway. Accessory muscles in the neck and shoulders normally are not used during breathing; their use indicates respiratory distress.

A normal chest has a lateral (side-to-side) diameter, which is twice as large as the anteroposterior (front-to-back) diameter. In patients with emphysema or in infants, the ratio of the lateral to anteroposterior (A-P) diameter may be increased and equal the transverse diameter. Some common abnormalities of the chest as seen in Figure 2-9, are:

- **Barrel chest.** The chest appears round, and the sternum appears pulled out. The A-P diameter is normally increased with aging or in diseases such as emphysema.
- **Funnel chest (pectus excavatum).** This is a congenital depression of the sternum that decreases the A-P diameter.
- **Kyphosis and scoliosis.** This is abnormal curvature of the spine with vertebral rotation that distorts the thorax.

Palpation of the thorax provides information about respiratory excursion, tender areas or masses on the chest, and the presence of tactile fremitus. Keeping the patient warm and draped, the posterior chest is examined beginning with any areas that the patient reports as problematic. The chest wall is gently palpated with the palm of the hand, and any painful areas and their anatomic location are noted. Respiratory excursion is assessed by placing the thumbs at the level of the 10th rib at the vertebra (Figure 2-10) and stretching the hands around the rib cage. The patient is asked to inhale deeply while the nurse watches the thumbs separate and feels the symmetry of the chest expansion. The thumbs should separate 5 to 8 cm during inspiration. Any asymmetry or diminished excursion should be noted in the assessment and direct further examination.

Tactile fremitus, the palpable vibrations of the voice that are transmitted down the tracheobronchial tree and through the chest wall, are assessed by placing the palm of the hand on the chest wall and having the patient repeat a phrase or word like "ninety-nine."

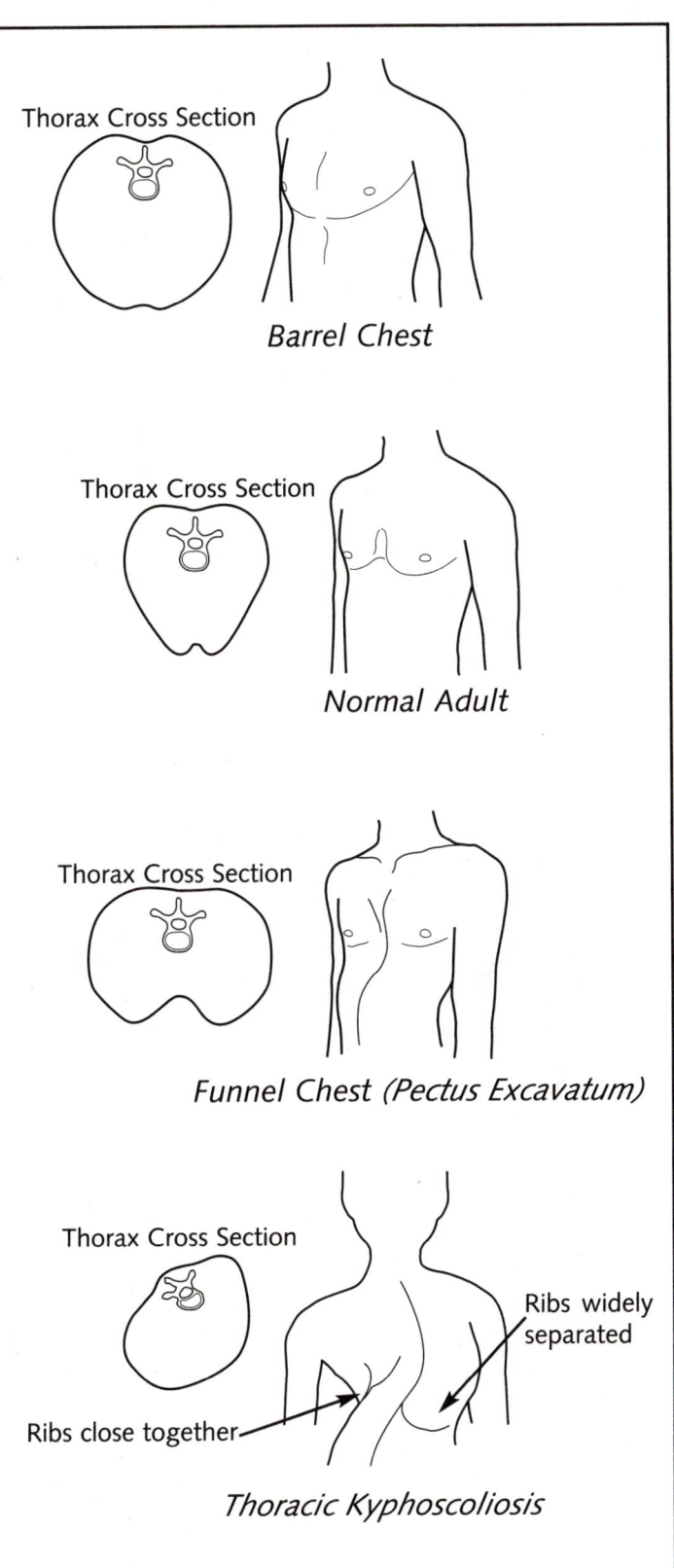

Figure 2-9. Abnormalities of the chest.

Thorax Cross Section

Barrel Chest

Thorax Cross Section

Normal Adult

Thorax Cross Section

Funnel Chest (Pectus Excavatum)

Thorax Cross Section

Ribs widely separated

Ribs close together

Thoracic Kyphoscoliosis

Figure 2-10. Assessing respiratory excursion.

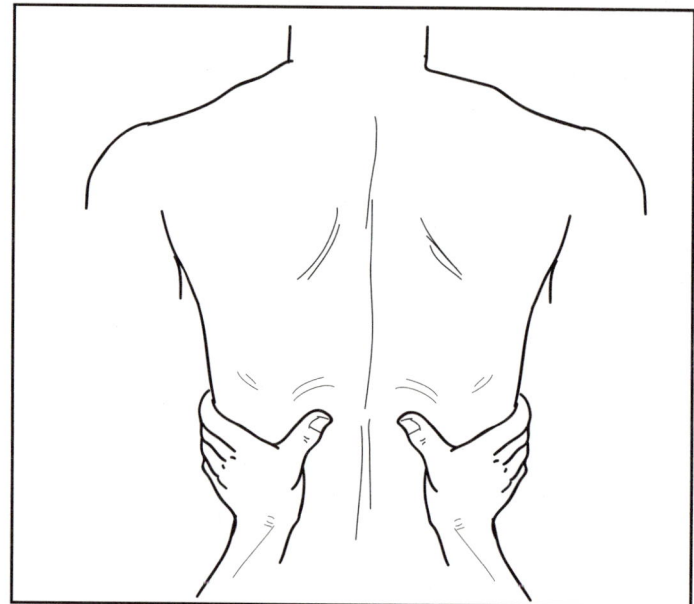

Figure 2-11. Assessing for tactile fremitus.

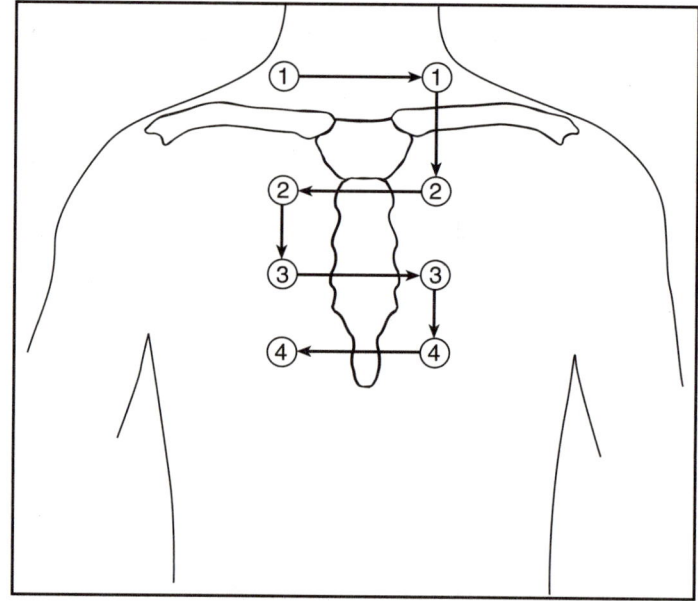

One side of the chest is compared with the other at several locations (Figure 2-11) to assess the symmetry of the vibrations. The transmission of voice sounds is decreased when the tracheobronchial tree is obstructed by pleural effusion, tumors, or even a thick chest wall.

Fremitus may be increased when part of the lung is consolidated, as seen in pneumonia. Percussion of the chest wall produces vibrations that may help in determining whether the underlying tissue is filled with air or fluid or is solid. Percussion also assesses lung size and position and diaphragmatic excursion. It involves a technique that requires some practice to become proficient and to differentiate the different vibration. Using the distal joint of the middle finger of the left hand, the joint is placed on the inter-

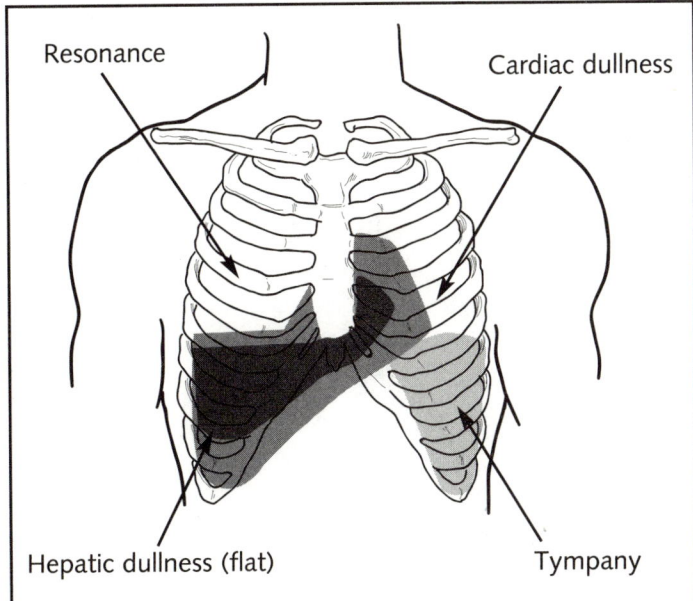

Figure 2-12. Different vibrations with percussion of the thorax.

Resonance

Cardiac dullness

Hepatic dullness (flat)

Tympany

costal space to be percussed and the middle finger of the right hand is used to strike the left with a quick, short stroke. The chest is percussed from the apices down to the bases moving from side to side. With time, the different vibrations of air, liquid, and solid can be detected by noting the intensity, pitch, duration, and quality of the sound. Using one side of the chest as a comparison to the other, the symmetry of the sounds is noted (Figure 2-12). Normal lung tissue sounds hollow and low-pitched when percussed. The sound is dull and flat over solid tissue such as muscle and bone. The anatomic location of areas that do not have the expected percussion sound should be noted.

Percussion may be used to assess diaphragmatic excursion, which is the downward movement of the diaphragm as it contracts during inspiration. The distance between the relaxed diaphragm (after expiration) and the contracted diaphragm (after inspiration) is a measure of diaphragmatic excursion. The patient is asked to take a deep breath, and the nurse percusses downward until resonance (lung tissue) is replaced by dullness (diaphragm). This spot is marked. Then, the patient is asked to exhale forcefully and hold it. The nurse then percusses upward until resonance is detected again. This spot is marked, and the distance between the two spots is measured. Normal diaphragmatic excursion is 5 to 6 cm but may increase to as much as 10 cm with maximal inspiration. It may be decreased when thoracic expansion is limited by pain or difficulty moving air.

Breath Sounds

Auscultation provides valuable clues to the functioning of the lungs and is one of the most frequently performed assessment techniques. Using the diaphragm of the stethoscope, auscultation detects air flow through the respiratory passages as well as the sounds of inspiration and expiration.

> Breath sounds are auscultated using the diaphragm of the stethoscope on bare skin. Normal breath sounds are: tracheal, vesicular, bronchial, and bronchovesicular. Abnormal breath sounds are crackles and wheezes.

Figure 2-13. Anatomic locations of different breath sounds.

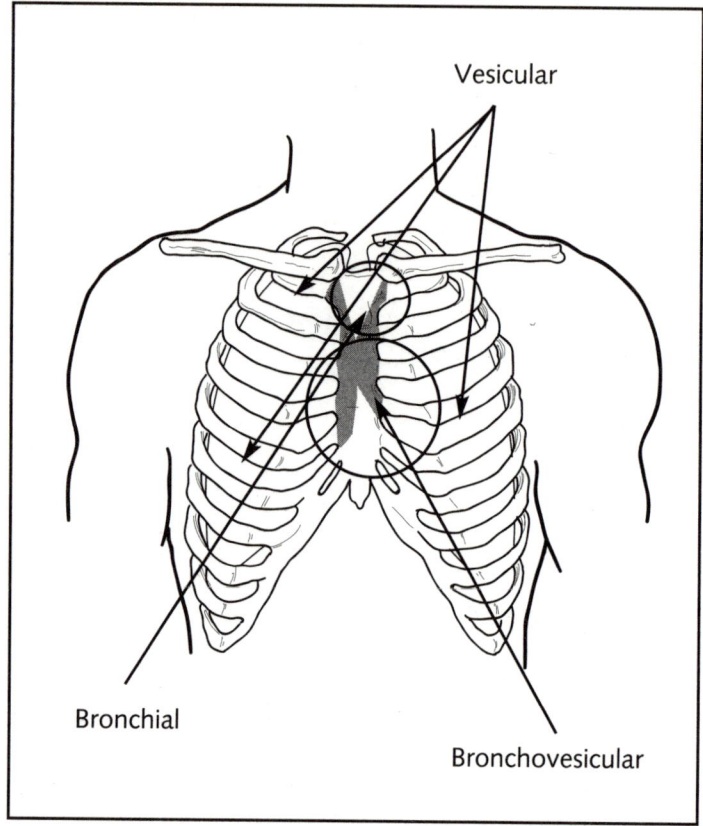

Vesicular

Bronchial

Bronchovesicular

Normal breath sounds vary over different parts of the lungs. A systematic approach helps to identify the appropriate breath sound in each anatomic area (Figure 2-13). Begin with the patient in a sitting position, breathing slowly and deeply through an open mouth. Breath sounds are best heard with the diaphragm of the stethoscope on bare skin. Drape the patient as necessary for warmth and privacy. If the patient is unable to sit up, seek assistance or roll the patient side to side, listening to the side that is upward.

Normal breath sounds are classified by their pitch, intensity, and duration in the respiratory cycle (Figures 2-14 and 2-15). The breath sounds normally heard are tracheal, vesicular, bronchial, and bronchovesicular.

- **Tracheal breath sounds** are loud and high pitched. Expiration may be heard slightly longer than inspiration.

- **Vesicular breath sounds** are heard over the majority of the lung fields. They are soft, low-pitched sounds that are heard longer during inspiration than expiration. Vesicular breath sounds are produced by air moving through the bronchioles and filling the alveoli. They are not heard over the sternum or between the scapulae.

- **Bronchial breath sounds**, which normally are heard over the trachea and mainstem bronchi, are high-pitched, hollow sounding, and loud, produced by air moving through the trachea and mainstem bronchi. Bronchial breath sounds are heard over the manubrium of the sternum and between the scapulae. They have a short inspiratory phase followed by a brief pause and then a longer expiratory phase. Expiration usually is twice as long as inspiration. Bronchial breath sounds heard over any other part of the lungs may indicate respiratory dysfunction and should be noted by their anatomic location.

Figure 2-14. Normal breath sounds—location, pitch, intensity, and timing.

Normal Breath Sounds	Description and Location
Tracheal 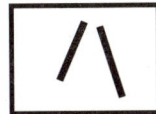	Highest pitched and loudest of normal breath sounds. Expiration may be heard slightly longer than inspiration. Heard over the trachea in the neck.
Bronchial 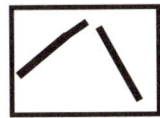	Hollow, high pitch, and loud—expiration is heard twice as long as inspiration, located over the manubrium of sternum and between the scapula.
Bronchovesicular 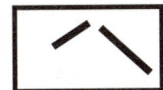	Medium pitch and intensity—inspiration is heard about the same length as expiration, located at the first and second intercostal spaces at the sternal border.
Vesicular 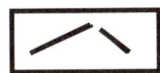	Low and soft pitch—inspiration is heard about twice as long as expiration over the normal lung fields.

Figure 2-15. Adventitious breath sounds—location, pitch, intensity, and timing.

Adventitious Breath Sounds	Description and Possible Conditions
Crackles (fine) 	Caused by air passing through moisture in alveoli and small airways. Not cleared by coughing; possible conditions: pneumonia, early congestive heart failure, pulmonary edema, and bronchiectasis in small airways.
Crackles (coarse) 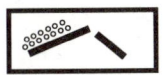	Inspiratory, soft, brief, popping sounds. Coarse crackles are lower in pitch and louder than fine crackles.
Sibilant wheezes 	Caused by air moving through narrowed tracheobronchial passages. They are loudest on expiration and are high-pitched, shrill, musical, and whistle-like. Conditions: bronchospasm and asthma.
Sonorous wheezes 	Formerly called "rhonchi;" they are low-pitched, snoring, or rumbling. Conditions: secretions or tumor in large airways.
Pleural friction rub 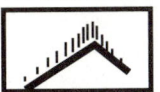	Caused by rubbing together of inflamed or roughened pleural surfaces during inspiration and expiration; loudest at the end of expiration. Conditions: pleurisy, pneumonia.

- **Bronchovesicular breath sounds** are intermediate in pitch and intensity with muted characteristics of both bronchial and vesicular breath sounds. They are produced by air moving through larger airways and are heard over the first and second inter-costal spaces along the sternal border and between the scapulae, if they are heard at all. The presence of bronchovesicular breath sounds in any other portion of the lungs is abnormal and indicates consolidation of the lung tissue, as in pneumonia, or the replacement of air-filled lung tissue by solid tissue, such as a tumor. Sometimes they are described as windy.

Transmitted voice sounds can be used to further assess portions of the lungs that have abnormal breath sounds. Bronchial or bronchovesicular breath sounds heard over parts of the lungs where vesicular breath sounds should be heard are considered abnormal. Increased transmission of voice sounds in the areas of abnormal breath sounds indicates consolidated lung tissue or the replacement of air-filled lung tissue with solid tissue. The patient is asked to produce sounds while the nurse listens with a stethoscope at the same sites used during percussion and auscultation. Comparing areas of abnormal breath sounds with areas of normal transmission identifies the anatomic location of abnormal transmitted sounds. The three types of transmitted voice sounds are:

- **Whispered petroliloquy.** The patient is asked to repeatedly whisper a phrase such as "ninety-nine." The transmission is louder over the area of consolidated lung tissue.
- **Bronchophony.** The patient is asked to repeat a phrase like "one-two-three." The transmission would normally be quiet and muffled; but in bronchophony, the words are louder and clearer.
- **Egophony (E-to-A change).** The patient is asked to say "eee." Normally this would be transmitted as "eee" but in areas of consolidated lung tissue it sounds like "ay."

Adventitious Lung Sounds

These sounds (see Figure 2-15) are heard in addition to normal breath sounds. They may be identified by their pitch, intensity, and duration during the respiratory cycle. There have been many terms for these sounds but there are now two classifications: crackles and wheezes. *Crackles* are brief, intermittent sounds that indicate the snapping open of collapsed or fluid-filled alveoli. They may be classified as fine crackles, sounding like hair rolled between the fingers close to the ear, or coarse crackles, sounding louder with more intermittent popping sounds. Crackles may occur in patients with respiratory disorders such as pneumonia, congestive heart failure, or bronchitis. Their presence should be noted and described by their anatomic location (eg, fine crackles, base of left lower lung, one-third of the way up). The timing of crackles in the respiratory cycle and whether they clear with coughing or changing of position should be noted. Crackles do not normally clear with coughing.

Wheezes (or *rhonchi*) are high-pitched, shrill, whistling sounds with a musical quality. They are caused by air moving through narrowed tracheobronchial airways. Wheezes may be heard in patients with asthma or bronchospasm. They may be more predominant on expiration but may be heard throughout the respiratory cycle.

Sonorous wheezes are low-pitched snoring sounds. They are usually produced by secretions in large airways and may clear with coughing.

A pleural friction rub is a harsh, loud, grating sound heard over an area of pleural inflammation. The roughened pleural surfaces grate over each other as the thorax expands in conditions like pleurisy or pneumonia. They are usually heard loudest at the end of inspiration.

The anterior chest is examined using the same steps as for the posterior chest. There are several anatomic differences of note. Inspection of the chest wall during normal breathing may reveal the use of abdominal muscles or retraction of the intercostal spaces during respiratory difficulty. Palpation of the anterior chest is useful for noting tender areas, particularly in costochondritis, which is inflammation at the juncture of the ribs and cartilage. Percussion of the anterior chest reveals dullness over the heart and liver, as well as a hollow note over the gastric bubble. Auscultation over the anterior chest proceeds in the same manner as for the posterior chest, progressing from the apices to the bases and moving from one side of the chest to the other while trying to envision the underlying anatomy. Tracheal breath sounds should be heard over the manubrium of the sternum. Bronchovesicular breath sounds may be heard over the first and second intercostal spaces at the sternal border. Vesicular breath sounds should be heard over the remaining lung fields. In women, the breasts may need to be displaced to hear the lower lung fields. In men, chest hair may produce sounds against the diaphragm of the stethoscope that need to be differentiated from adventitious breath sounds such as crackles.

DIAGNOSTIC TESTS OF THE RESPIRATORY SYSTEM

The functional ability of the lungs may be measured by a variety of pulmonary function tests (PFT) that measure air flow rates and calculate lung volumes and capacities. PFTs are performed to:
- Evaluate the function of the lungs.
- Confirm the presence of respiratory disorders.
- Differentiate between obstructive and restrictive disorders.
- Evaluate disease exacerbation or progression.
- Evaluate lung function prior to surgery.
- Evaluate response to bronchodilators.
- Evaluate the need for mechanical ventilation.

Some different types of PFTs include spirometry (which measures lung volumes and calculates lung capacities), measurement of airflow rates, estimation of diffusion capacities, bronchial provocation or inhalation tests, and exercise pulmonary stress testing. Arterial blood gases are another important measure of pulmonary functioning that will be discussed later in this chapter.

Lung Capacities and Volumes

Measurement of lung capacities and volumes is performed with spirometry. These are usually the first PFTs performed when a patient needs evaluation. Using a machine called a spirometer, the patient performs various breathing maneuvers. To get accurate measurements, a clip is placed on the nose, and the patient is asked to seal his mouth over the mouthpiece. The volume of air inspired or expired can be measured during breathing with a recording device called a kymograph. If the volumes are measured over time, then air flow rates can be calculated. Measurements of air flow rates are important when there is a question of obstruction or restriction. Normal values for volumes and air flow rates are predicted based on age, gender, height, weight, and race. Patient values greater than 80% of the predicted values are considered normal. Withholding bronchodilating or sedating medications for 4 hours prior to testing may be necessary to gain an accurate picture of the patient's respiratory status. These medications can be resumed immediately after the PFTs.

Five standard lung volumes are performed with the spirometer:

1. **Tidal volume (TV).** The TV is the amount of air inspired or exhaled during normal, quiet breathing. The amount is approximately 500 mL in a 70 kg person. It can range from 400 to 700 mL and reach 4500 mL during maximal exercise. Volume capacities are 20% to 25% lower in women. A decrease in TV without a decrease in respiratory rate indicates a restrictive disorder like pulmonary fibrosis. A decrease in TV with a decrease in respiratory rate indicates a neurological problem.

2. **Inspiratory reserve volume (IRV).** The IRV is the amount of air that can be inhaled after a normal or tidal inspiration (approximately 3300 mL).

3. **Expiratory reserve volume (ERV).** The ERV is the amount of air that can be forcibly exhaled after normal or tidal expiration (approximately 1100 mL).

4. **Residual volume (RV).** The RV is the amount of air remaining in the lungs after forced, maximal expiration (approximately 1000 mL).

5. **Minute ventilation (MV).** The MV is the volume of air inspired and expired during 1 minute of normal breathing.

Lung capacities also can be calculated during pulmonary function testing. They are determined by combining two (or more) lung volumes. Figure 2-16 shows the relationship of lung volumes and capacities.

- **Vital capacity (VC).** The VC is the maximal amount of air that can be exhaled after maximal inspiration (approximately 5000 mL). The VC is the total of the tidal volume, inspiratory reserve volume, and expiratory reserve volume.

- **Inspiratory capacity (IC).** The IC is the amount of air that can be inhaled with maximal effort after a normal exhalation (approximately 3000 mL).

- **Functional residual capacity (FRC).** The FRC is the amount of air remaining in the lungs at the end of normal exhalation (approximately 1200 mL).

- **Total lung capacity (TLC).** The TLC is the amount of air in the lungs at the end of maximal inspiration (approximately 6000 mL). It is also the total of the four lung volumes (TV + IRV + ERV + RV = TLC).

- **Forced vital capacity (FVC).** The FVC is the amount of air expelled with maximally forced exhalation.

Lung volumes and capacities also can be determined in special-equipped laboratories. Tests using tracer gases, such as helium or nitrogen, can be performed to determine the FRC. The FRC is the amount of air remaining in the lungs at the end of normal expiration.

There is always some air remaining in the lungs even after maximal expiration. This remaining air allows the alveoli to stay partially inflated and minimizes rapid fluctuations of the oxygen and carbon dioxide levels in the blood between breaths. Increased RV indicates that there is an abnormally large amount of air remaining in the lungs at the end of exhalation, as seen in conditions that cause air-trapping (eg, emphysema). The RV and FRC usually decrease together in restrictive conditions like pulmonary fibrosis.

Pulmonary mechanics, the measurements of air flow in the respiratory tract, are calculated by examining air flow versus volume. They can be graphically produced by specific machines or visibly produced by small devices that patients can use at home. Three measurements that are frequently used include:

- **Peak expiratory flow (PEF).** The PEF is the amount of air that can be forcibly exhaled after maximal inhalation. Small PEF devices for home use make this a quick and useful measure of disease exacerbation or response to medications such as bronchodilators.

- **Forced expiratory flow (FEF).** The FEF measures the rate of air flow during forced expiration on a flow-volume graph.

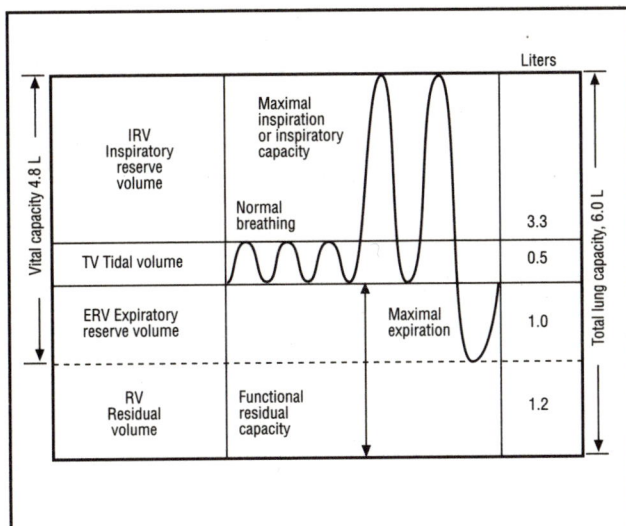

Figure 2-16. Relationship of lung volumes and capacities.

- **Forced expiratory volume (FEV).** The FEV measures the amount of air exhaled after full inhalation at various times during the exhalation (ie, 1 second, 2 seconds, 3 seconds). The FEV1 (volume expired at 1 second) is a good measure of airway resistance in disease exacerbations.

Another measurement of air flow in the lungs is the *airway resistance* (R_{aw}), which is performed to determine whether restrictive or obstructive disease is present. R_{aw} is the difference between the pressure in the mouth (atmospheric pressure) and the pressure in the alveoli. It is calculated from the airflow and changes in pressure in the respiratory tract (ie, the pressure gradient) during breathing. R_{aw} increases in obstructive diseases (eg, asthma) due to narrowing of the airways by secretions and edema.

Other PFTs include exercise pulmonary stress testing, diffusion capacities, and bronchial provocation tests. Exercise-induced changes in respiratory functioning can be monitored using spirometry and exercise machinery (eg, treadmill to help in the diagnosis of exercise-induced asthma).

Diffusion Capacities

Diffusion capacities measure the ability of gases to diffuse across the alveolar membrane. A given amount of carbon monoxide is inhaled by the patient and then exhaled. The exhaled amount is measured and compared to the amount in the blood. The difference represents the amount of gas that diffused across the alveolar membrane and into the blood. A decreased diffusion capacity occurs when defects in the alveoli, such as thickening of the alveolar wall (pulmonary fibrosis), inhibit gas diffusion.

Bronchial provocation tests are used to determine a cause-and-effect relationship between certain inhaled irritants and the reactivity of the patient's airways. Histamine or methacholine are inhaled by the patient. PFTs are then performed to assess for bronchial constriction. These tests are used to establish a diagnosis of hyperactive airway disease.

Arterial Blood Gases

Arterial blood gas (ABG) analysis is performed to evaluate respiratory functioning in a patient and determine the actual levels of carbon dioxide and oxygen in arterial blood. Three other values derived from the ABG analysis are the power of hydrogen (pH), the arterial oxygen saturation of the hemoglobin (SaO_2), and the bicarbonate (HCO_3^-) level. These provide information about the ventilation and diffusion of gases in the lungs and the acid-base balance of the blood.

An important concept used in measuring the levels of gas in the blood is *Dalton's law*, which states that each gas in the atmosphere contributes to the total pressure of all the gases in the atmosphere. Oxygen, carbon dioxide, nitrogen, and hydrogen each contribute a portion to the total pressure of the atmosphere, which is 760 mmHg. Room air is 20.8% oxygen, 78.6% nitrogen, and less than 1% other gases. The partial pressure of atmospheric oxygen is 160 mmHg and falls to about 100 mmHg in the alveoli after mixing with residual air in the lungs. The average arterial oxygen levels (PaO_2) at sea level is 95 to 100 mmHg (Table 2-2).

The partial pressure of oxygen (PO_2) can be determined from arterial, venous, or mixed samples of blood. The PaO_2 are useful for determining whether a patient is hypoxemic (ie, low levels of oxygen in the blood) or to determine the effectiveness of interventions such as supplemental oxygen. A sample is taken from the radial, brachial, or femoral arteries. Puncture of the radial artery requires that the patient has adequate arterial perfusion to the hand via the ulnar artery (Figure 2-17). The adequacy of the circulation can be evaluated by *Allen's test*, which is a simple compression of the radial artery to assess circulation to the hand by the ulnar artery. An arterial blood sample is obtained in a heparinized syringe, which is immediately placed on ice and taken to the laboratory for analysis. Care must be taken not to allow air bubbles in the syringe, as they might alter the gas analysis. The puncture site must be compressed for a full 5 minutes after the sample is drawn to prevent bleeding. The sample must be labeled with the time it was drawn, the patient's temperature, and the amount and method of supplemental oxygen (including mechanical ventilation).

The oxygen levels in the blood are an indicator of the ability of the lungs to match capillary blood flow to the ventilated alveoli. Oxygen levels also depend on the cardiac output, the amount of blood the heart is pumping, and the ability of the red blood cells to carry oxygen. Hypoxemia (low oxygen levels in the blood), exists when arterial oxygen levels fall below 75 mmHg. Hypoxia refers to inadequate oxygenation of the tissues. Of the oxygen carried in the blood, 98% is bound to hemoglobin as oxyhemoglobin. Only 2% is actually carried as dissolved gas, which is what is measured as a PaO_2.

P = partial pressure	HCO_3^- = Bicarbonate
O_2 = Oxygen	mmHg = mm of Hg
CO_2 = Carbon dioxide	(measurement of pressure)
A = alveolar	V = venous
a = arterial	Pa = Partial pressure in artery
PA = Partial pressure in alveoli	

When hypoxemia exists, the patient may develop signs of cyanosis, such as the bluish tinge or pallor of the mouth, lips, inner eyelids, and nail beds. The role of the cardiovascular and the hematologic systems in the process of oxygenation is discussed in more detail in later chapters.

The partial pressure of carbon dioxide in arterial blood ($PaCO_2$) fluctuates with the respiratory cycle. It is automatically calculated by the blood gas analyzer. The average $PaCO_2$ is 35 to 45 mmHg. The respiratory rate regulates the amount of carbon dioxide in the blood. In hyperventilation, more carbon dioxide is exhaled, decreasing the $PaCO_2$. The reverse is true in hypoventilation, although this is a less efficient system because a decreased respiratory rate also can cause hypoxemia, stimulating the medulla to increase the respiratory rate. An exception to this effect occurs in patients with COPD. The chron-

Table 2-2	
Arterial Blood Gas Ranges	
Value	*Normal*
pH	7.35 to 7.45
PaO_2	95 to 100 mmHg
$PaCO_2$	35 to 45 mmHg
HCO_3^-	22 to 24 mEq/L

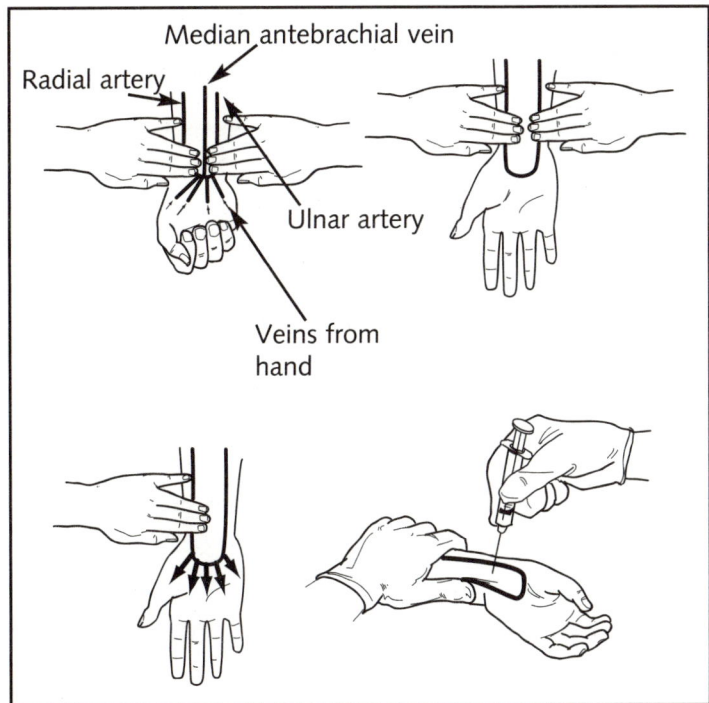

Figure 2-17. Arterial blood gas sampling.

ically elevated $PaCO_2$ levels no longer stimulate the respiratory centers in the medulla to increase the respiratory rate. The peripheral chemoreceptors take on the role of regulator of respiration based on the oxygen levels in the arterial blood. Blood gas analysis in patients with COPD allows supplemental oxygen levels to be adjusted to not only the PaO_2 but the $PaCO_2$ and pH.

Acid–Base Balance

The respiratory system participates in acid-base balance by altering the respiratory rate. The pH determines the alkalinity or acidity of the blood. A pH of 7.4 is considered neutral in blood, with a normal range being 7.35 to 7.45. When the pH is greater than 7.45, then the blood is considered alkalotic. Likewise, if the pH is lower than 7.35, then the blood is considered acidotic.

Table 2-3

Changes in Acid-Base Imbalances

	pH	PaCO$_2$	HCO$_3^-$	Compensation
Respiratory alkalosis	↑	↓	Normal until compensation	Kidneys increase HCO$_3^-$; 24 to 48 hrs
Metabolic alkalosis	↑	Normal unless lungs compensate	↑	Lungs increase PaCO$_2$ by decrease in respiratory rate; takes minutes
Respiratory acidosis	↓	↑	Normal until kidneys compensate	Kidneys keep more HCO$_3^-$; takes days
Metabolic acidosis	↓	Normal until lungs compensate	↓	Lungs decrease PaCO$_2$ by increase in respiratory rate; takes minutes

Alkalosis or acidosis may originate in the respiratory or metabolic systems or both. By examining the carbon dioxide levels and the bicarbonate levels, the origin(s) of an imbalance may be determined. Carbon dioxide levels reflect the role of the respiratory system in maintaining acid-base balance (Table 2-3). Carbon dioxide is carried in the blood as an acid, namely carbonic acid. Changing the respiratory rate can alter the amount of carbonic acid and the pH of the blood in minutes. When the respiratory rate increases, more carbon dioxide is exhaled, making the blood more alkaline (higher pH). Likewise, a decreased respiratory rate allows the levels of carbon dioxide to increase, making the blood more acidic (lower pH).

Metabolic changes to the acid-base balance are done by the kidneys. The levels of bicarbonate (HCO$_3^-$) in the blood are changed by the kidneys to normalize the blood's pH. This slower system requires 24 to 48 hours to alter the pH of the blood. Bicarbonate functions as a buffer in the blood to keep the pH within the normal range. The bicarbonate level is usually maintained in a 20:1 ratio with carbonic acid to keep the blood pH between 7.35 and 7.45. The normal values for serum bicarbonate are 24 to 30 mEq/L and are calculated by the blood gas analyzer. When the HCO$_3^-$ level increases, the pH increases and the blood becomes more alkaline. Likewise, when the HCO$_3^-$ level decreases, the blood becomes more acidic and the pH of the blood decreases. Generally, bicarbonate levels greater than 30 mEq/L indicate a metabolic alkalosis, and levels lower than 24 mEq/L indicate a metabolic acidosis. All components of arterial blood gas analysis must be examined in reference to each other and the patient's overall status to determine the nature of the acid-base disturbance.

Metabolic alkalosis (an increase in bicarbonate levels) is most commonly caused by the loss of gastric contents, such as prolonged nasogastric suction or excessive vomiting. It is also seen in patients with long-standing COPD because the increased bicarbonate levels buffer the chronically high PCO_2 levels. Metabolic acidosis (decreased serum bicarbonate level) is seen in patients with lower gastrointestinal losses (eg, prolonged diarrhea), and in diabetic acidosis, shock, dehydration, and after cardiopulmonary arrest.

There are also cases of acid-base imbalances that are mixed in origin when one system may compensate for the other, resulting in a compensated acidosis or alkalosis. For example, patients with COPD who have chronically elevated carbon dioxide levels and low pH may have increased bicarbonate levels because the kidneys have compensated for the respiratory acidosis by retaining bicarbonate. Because of the complex nature of acid-base balance, the patient's condition must be evaluated with the blood values.

Oxygen Saturation

Whereas the PaO_2 measures the amount of oxygen dissolved in the arterial blood, the oxygen saturation level (SaO_2) measures the amount of oxygen bound to hemoglobin as oxyhemoglobin. Pulse oximetry uses a spectrophotometer to determine the amount of light absorbed by hemoglobin in arterial blood. A clip placed on a finger or ear allows the oximeter to calculate the percentage of oxygenated hemoglobin as compared to the total capacity of hemoglobin available for binding. Because the clip relies on adequate perfusion of the tissue, conditions that decrease perfusion alter the reading. Hypothermia, hypotension, and drugs that cause vasoconstriction may result in decreased perfusion and a low reading.

A normal oxygenation saturation (O_2 Sat or SpO_2) is 96% to 100% but varies depending on the PO_2, the pH of the blood, the body temperature, and the structure of the hemoglobin. Oxygen saturation levels do not follow the PaO_2 proportionately. An O_2 Sat of 89% is equivalent to a PaO_2 of 60 mmHg, far below the level defined as hypoxemia. The pH of the blood affects the affinity of oxygen for hemoglobin (Figure 2-18). The oxyhemoglobin dissociation curve describes the changes in the oxygen binding and release from hemoglobin with the pH of the blood. If the blood is acidic (pH less than 7.35), then the curve is said to shift to the left with decreased O_2 Sat, increased oxygen release, and decreased oxygen binding. Conversely, if the blood is alkalotic (pH greater than 7.45), then the oxyhemoglobin desaturation curve shifts to the right with an increased O_2 Sat but increased O_2 binding and decreased O_2 release. In either case, the O_2 Sat needs to be assessed in relation to the patient's appearance, the vital signs, and, if necessary, arterial blood gases. Temperature increases allow more oxygen to be released from hemoglobin but also increase oxygen consumption by the tissues.

Hemoglobin is structured to combine with and release oxygen as oxyhemoglobin. Hemoglobin also may combine with 2,3-diphosphoglycerol (2,3-DPG), which is an intermediate product of glycolysis, the conversion of glycogen in liver stores to glucose. The levels of 2,3-DPG in the blood increase when there is decreased oxygen delivery to the tissues, increased altitude, or when glycolysis is occurring; also, 2,3-DPG causes oxyhemoglobin to more readily release oxygen.

Other Tests of Respiratory Function and Structure

There are a variety of tests that look at different aspects of respiratory functioning and anatomy. Some of the tests performed in the radiology department include radiographs, computerized axial tomography (CAT) scans, magnetic resonance imaging (MRI), lung scans, bronchography, and pulmonary angiography.

Figure 2-18. Oxygen-hemoglobin dissociation curve.

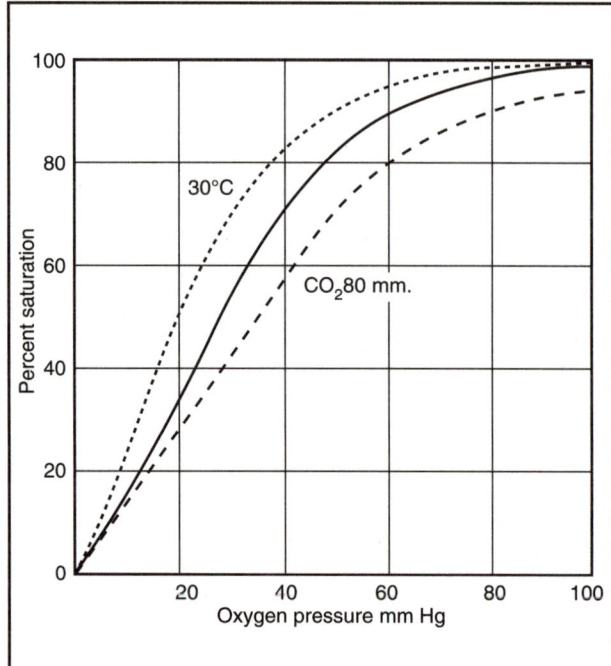

Radiologic examination or radiographs provide information about internal structures. The chest radiograph is performed from the posteroanterior view and the lateral view, where x-rays pass from one side through the other. They are useful for assessing pathophysiologic changes in the thorax, such as tumors, inflammation, fluid and air accumulation, integrity of bony structures, and diaphragmatic hernia. Chest radiographs are performed in the radiology department or at the bedside with a portable unit. They are completed in a few minutes and are painless. Radiographs also can be taken of the nose and sinuses to assess the integrity of the bony and cartilaginous structures and to detect fluid accumulation in the normally air-filled sinuses.

CAT Scans

These scans provide a different and more detailed view of internal structures than does traditional radiography. Using x-rays and a computer, a cross-section of the body through a horizontal plane can be constructed. This picture provides greater definition of internal structures and organs. Mediastinal tumors are best viewed by CAT scan. Needle biopsies can be performed with CAT scan guidance. The procedure takes 30 to 60 minutes and requires the patient to remain still in a horizontal position. Sedation may be required.

MRI

The MRI uses a powerful magnetic field and computer enhancement to create detailed, cross-sectional pictures of the human anatomy. It is useful for assessing normal internal structure, such as the pulmonary vasculature, lung tissue, and lymph nodes as well as abnormalities such as tumors, cysts, and pulmonary edema. MRI is a painless procedure that requires the patient to lie still for 30 to 60 minutes.

Lung Scans

These scans are performed to assess the perfusion of the lungs by the pulmonary arteries. They are used in diagnosing pulmonary embolism, lung malignancies, COPD, and pulmonary edema. Albumin tagged with radioactive technetium is injected into the patient's bloodstream. Then, radiographic images are taken of the lungs in the nuclear medicine department. The scintillation camera provides a picture of the pulmonary embolism, in which blood flow to part of the lung is blocked by an embolus. Simultaneous ventilation scans can be done to detect defects in ventilation as well as perfusion. Diminished or absent blood flow (ie, pulmonary embolism) is seen as a defect in perfusion on the scan. Defects in ventilation alone can be the result of an airway obstruction.

Bronchography

This is a test used to evaluate the structure of the trachea and bronchi. It is useful for identifying obstruction of the tracheobronchial tree caused by a tumor or foreign bodies, as well as for making the diagnosis of hyaline membrane disease in infants. A dye with radioactive iodine is injected through a catheter in the trachea. Radiographic films are taken with the patient in a variety of positions to move the dye around the structures and to improve visualization. Patients need to be encouraged to cough after the procedure to expel the dye.

Pulmonary Angiography

This test assesses the perfusion of the lungs by the pulmonary circulation. A radiopaque material is injected into a vein or artery and then radiographs are taken of the chest. These films provide a picture of the vasculature that can detect pulmonary embolism. Defects in filling of the vasculature indicate blockage of the blood vessel by an embolus or other obstruction such as a tumor.

Other tests to examine respiratory anatomy are performed by an endoscopic approach. These include laryngoscopy, bronchoscopy, and mediastinoscopy. Fiberoptic or rigid scopes allow direct visualization of the anatomy and may detect the presence of foreign bodies or tumors. The endoscope also can be used to cauterize bleeding vessels, biopsy tissue or remove a foreign body. Patients are at least locally anesthetized and sedated during laryngoscopy and bronchoscopy. Mediastinoscopy requires general anesthesia because an incision is made at the suprasternal notch, and the scope is passed into the mediastinum to visualize the anatomy of the mediastinum and identify possible growths.

Cultures

Laboratory cultures provide valuable information about diseases of the respiratory tract. Throat culture is one of the most commonly performed diagnostic tests. It is performed to detect and identify bacteria in the oropharynx. A swab is brushed along the back of the oropharynx and then sent to the laboratory to culture the growth and identify antibiotic sensitivity if needed. The most common reason to perform a throat culture is to rule out a streptococcal infection.

Sputum cultures identify infectious bacteria, check for malignancy, and detect the tubercle bacillus, the organism that causes tuberculosis. Sputum cultures are best obtained early in the morning and help to identify infecting organisms and the antibiotics to which they are sensitive. Malignant cells from the respiratory tract also may be shed into the sputum, in which case the sputum sample is sent to pathology for microscopic examination.

The sputum test for tuberculosis is called an acid-fast bacillus smear. It requires three consecutive early-morning sputum samples. Another test for tuberculosis is the tuberculin or Mantoux skin test. A small amount of purified protein (0.1 mL) is injected intradermally on the forearm. The area is then "read" 48 to 72 hours later to note any swelling and erythema. If the indurated or swollen area is greater than 10 mm wide, the test is considered positive for tuberculosis. Follow-up testing is required.

Other pathological tests that may be performed to assess the respiratory tract include pleural fluid analysis and blood cultures. Pleural fluid is obtained by inserting a needle into an area in which fluid has accumulated in the pleural space and withdrawing a sample to detect malignancy. Blood cultures are obtained by venipuncture at three successive times to identify blood infection caused by organisms in the respiratory tract.

There are many ways to evaluate the functioning of the respiratory tract. History taking, physical assessment, preparation of the patient for diagnostic testing, and education of the patient and family all are components of the nurse's role. But before the assessment forms are filled out and the numbers are analyzed, there is a person—a patient—who has the most important information. He can tell the nurse how he is feeling, what hurts, what he coughs up, and what makes him feel better. It is the nurse's role to listen to all the cues that the patient provides and let these guide her assessment of the patient's respiratory system.

The emergency department physician examines Mr. Z. and orders a portable chest radiograph, arterial blood gases, a sputum for culture and sensitivity, routine PFT, complete blood counts, and serum electrolyte tests. The nurse reassures Mr. Z. and his wife because they seem quite anxious. She tells them that the tests will help the medical team decide how best to treat the problem. The arterial blood gas is as follows: PO_2—65, PCO_2—58, pH—7.29, HCO_3^-—34. Mr. Z. is in a respiratory acidosis, but given his PO_2 and O_2 Sat, the physician orders oxygen at 4 L per minute via nasal prongs. The nurse watches for a decreased respiratory rate and signs of carbon dioxide narcosis. The FEV1 is markedly decreased, as is the tidal volume. Bronchodilators are ordered to help Mr. Z.'s breathing. The chest radiograph shows lobar consolidation in the right middle lobe. The tentative diagnosis is COPD and pneumonia. Mr. Z. states that he can breathe much better after the bronchodilator treatment, and he is admitted for antibiotic and respiratory therapy, as well as for re-evaluation of his antihypertensive medication.

The answers to the questions in the introduction are as follows:
- *Why is Mr. Z. sitting in the chair, and should he be on the stretcher?*

Mr. Z. is sitting in the chair with his elbows propped up because this position allows his rib cage to expand more easily, allowing more air in with each inhalation. Laying Mr. Z. down on the stretcher would make his breathing more difficult, unless he sat upright and propped his arms on an over-the-bed table.

- *What should be considered before starting oxygen therapy?*

If Mr. Z. has been smoking for a long time (1.5 packs per day x 35 years), COPD should be considered. His respiratory process may be driven by low oxygen levels in his blood because his central chemoreceptors no longer sense high carbon dioxide levels. Oxygen therapy should be initiated cautiously at 1 to 2 L per min. His respiratory rate and ABGs should be frequently checked to evaluate his response to therapy.

- *What changes might be seen on an arterial blood gas, given Mr. Z.'s smoking history and oxygen saturation?*

Given Mr. Z.'s smoking history, the arterial blood gas analysis will probably show a low oxygen level (PO_2), a high carbon dioxide level (PCO_2), and either a low pH with a normal bicarbonate or a normal pH with a high bicarbonate level.

- *What anatomic changes cause wheezes?*

Wheezes are caused by narrowing of the bronchi and bronchioles due to swelling, secretions, or bronchospasm of the smooth muscle around the bronchi.

- *What side effect of beta-blockers is making Mr. Z.'s breathing more difficult?*

Beta-blockers not only vasodilate the peripheral vasculature, which is therapeutic in patients with hypertension, but they also block the beta-2 sites in the lungs, causing constriction of the smooth muscle around the bronchioles in susceptible patients (eg, those with asthma or COPD).

BIBLIOGRAPHY

Ahrens T, Rutherford K. *Essentials of Oxygenation.* Boston, Mass: Jones and Bartlett Publishers; 1993.

Burrell LO, Gerlach MJ, Pless BS. Nursing management of adults with respiratory problems. In: Burrell LO, Gerlach MJ, Pless BS. *Adult Nursing: Acute and Community Care.* 2nd ed. Stamford, Conn: Appleton & Lange; 1997.

Corbett JV. *Laboratory Tests and Diagnostic Procedures with Nursing Diagnoses.* 4th ed. Stamford, Conn: Appleton & Lange; 1996.

Kee JL. *Laboratory and Diagnostic Tests with Nursing Implications.* 4th ed. Stamford, Conn: Appleton & Lange; 1995.

Leahy JM, Kizilay PE. *Foundations of Nursing Practice: A Nursing Process Approach.* Philadelphia, Pa: W.B. Saunders; 1998.

Levitsky MG. *Pulmonary Physiology.* 4th ed. New York, NY: McGraw-Hill; 1995.

Mahler DA. *Dyspnea.* New York, NY: Marcel Dekker, Inc; 1998.

Monahan FD, Neighbors M. *Medical-Surgical Nursing: Foundations for Clinical Practice.* Philadelphia, Pa: W.B. Saunders Co; 1998.

Pagana KD, Pagana TJ. *Manual of Diagnostic and Laboratory Tests.* St. Louis, Mo: Mosby, Inc; 1998.

Swearingen PL, Keen JH. *Manual of Critical Care Nursing.* St. Louis, Mo: Mosby, Inc; 2001.

Watson J, Jaffe MS. *Nurse's Manual of Laboratory and Diagnostic Tests.* 2nd ed. Philadelphia, Pa: F.A. Davis Co; 1995.

MULTIPLE-CHOICE QUESTIONS

1. Normal breath sounds heard over the mainstem bronchi are:
   A. Vesicular breath sounds
   B. Tracheal breath sounds
   C. Tord crackles
   D. Bronchovesicular breath sounds

2. The primary abnormality in respiratory acidosis is:
   A. Increased $PaCO_2$
   B. Decreased PaO_2
   C. Increased PaO_2
   D. Decreased HCO_3^-

3. The renal system responds to a respiratory acidosis by:
   A. Reabsorbing HCO_3^-
   B. Decreasing hydrogen secretion
   C. Increasing CO_2
   D. Increasing urine output

4. Vesicular breath sounds are best heard:
   A. Over the trachea
   B. At the first and second interspaces beside the sternum
   C. Over most of the lungs
   D. During expiration

5. Pulse oximetry measures:
   A. Carbon dioxide levels
   B. Dissolved oxygen in the plasma
   C. Amount of hemoglobin carrying oxygen
   D. PaO_2

CHAPTER 2 ANSWERS

1. D
2. A
3. A
4. C
5. C

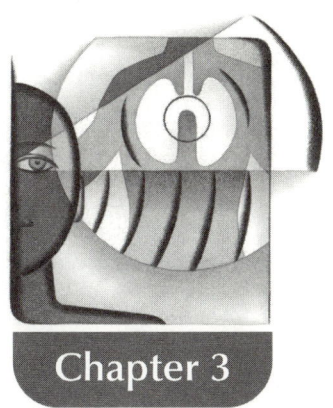

Chapter 3

Management of Adults With Respiratory Disorders

Mrs. A. is a 57-year-old woman who calls her physician's office because she cannot breathe. She has a history of asthma and hypertension. Yesterday, she helped her daughter clean out the basement. Mrs. A. found that her inhaler did not help her the previous night and she wants to know what to do. The triage nurse listening to her on the phone can hear her breathing rapidly and stopping between words to catch her breath. The triage nurse recommends that Mrs. A. have her husband drive her to the office immediately.

When she arrives, her vital signs are: temperature—100.5°F orally, respiration—32 breaths per minute, heart rate—96 beats per minute, and blood pressure 146/92 mmHg. Her oxygen saturation (O_2 Sat) is 90%. On examination, scattered wheezes are noted over both lung fields during inspiration and expiration. Pulmonary function tests show a 30% decrease in her normal peak expiratory flow rate (PEFR). She is visibly anxious and breathing in rapid, shallow breaths. The physician sees her and recommends a nebulizer treatment with albuterol.

- What physiologic changes cause wheezing?
- Why is her PEFR decreased during an asthma attack?
- What could have caused this asthma attack?

When oxygenation is disturbed, all tissues are affected. Oxygen is basic to the metabolism of every cell in the body. The process of supplying oxygen to the cells begins with ventilation, the moving of air into and out of the respiratory tract. It continues with the diffusion of gases across the alveolar membrane and into the circulation. The oxygen arrives at the cell by perfusion, the pumping of blood throughout the body. In this chapter, disorders of ventilation in the upper and lower respiratory tracts, as well as disorders of diffusion, are reviewed. Interventions to maximize oxygenation are discussed in Chapter 4.

RESPIRATORY TRACT DEFENSES

Ventilation is the movement of air between the atmosphere and the alveoli. The airways provide filtration of inspired air and protection of the respiratory tract, as well as humidification and temperature regulation. The respiratory tract has many methods of defense against the never-ending assault by the environment. The first line of defense is air filtration in the nose. The nasal hairs and mucus trap many foreign particles. Obviously, mouth breathing circumvents this system and reduces its effectiveness. The sneezing reflex is initiated in the nose when irritation or particles stimulate the trigeminal nerve. Further down the respiratory tract, the cough reflex also assists in expelling particles or mucus that is occluding or irritating the airways.

More sophisticated methods of defense involve the mucociliary blanket. Cilia are small hairs that line the respiratory tract and constantly beat to move particles and mucus up the respiratory passages to where they can be expelled by coughing, sneezing, or swallowing. Dehydration, smoking, and certain drugs (eg, atropine) can thicken sputum, rendering this defense mechanism less effective.

The mucus in the airways contains secretory immunoglobulins (IgA) that protect the respiratory tract against bacteria and viruses. Both B and T lymphocytes also protect the respiratory passages. Macrophages in the alveoli engulf and destroy foreign particles. Some particles, such as asbestos, may not be completely removed and can cause tissue changes, such as asbestosis or malignancy, over time. Smokers are particularly susceptible to lung damage because much of the debris from habitual smoking remains in the lung tissue.

The large airways of the lower respiratory tract also protect the lungs. The bronchi may constrict reflexively when irritants, such as dust and fumes, are inhaled. Overreaction to irritants occurs in diseases like asthma, causing prolonged narrowing of the airways and restricted ventilation. When the bronchi are irritated, mucus production increases to encase foreign particles. Excessive mucus production in diseases like chronic bronchitis may actually hinder ventilation because it narrows or occludes the airways.

Despite the elaborate protective mechanisms that exist in the respiratory tract, problems may occur. Assaults by the environment may be physical trauma, viral or bacterial infection, or altered cellular processes, such as emphysema or malignancy. The nurse's role in treating patients with respiratory disorders is to maintain the patient's oxygenation by optimizing ventilation, diffusion, and perfusion. Nursing care of patients with respiratory disorders requires:

- Understanding normal respiratory anatomy and physiology.
- Distinguishing different disorders of the upper and lower airways.
- Assessment of the patient based on the knowledge of different signs and symptoms of respiratory disorders and their impact on the patient's functioning.
- Developing nursing and collaborative care plans with appropriate long- and short-term goals for that patient.
- Implementing the principles of oxygenation into the care plans.
- Evaluating the effectiveness of the interventions.
- Revising the treatment plan as necessary.

Disorders of the upper and lower airways, their clinical findings, possible diagnostic studies, and collaborative treatment strategies to optimize ventilation and diffusion will be reviewed in this chapter.

Table 3-1

Symptoms of the Common Cold

1. Red, swollen nasal membranes.
2. Mucoid to thin nasal discharge.
3. Sneezing and coughing.
4. Malaise, headache, and possibly low-grade fever.
5. Decreased sense of taste and smell.

DISORDERS OF THE UPPER AIRWAYS

The nose, sinuses, and pharynx are the first passages through which air enters the respiratory tract. They provide many defenses against the environment, including air filtration, humidification, and warming. Unfortunately, the filtering abilities of the mucus membranes can lead to irritation and infection by the captured invaders.

Acute Rhinitis

The most frequent infection in human beings is *acute rhinitis*. It is usually caused by the common cold virus or rhinovirus (Table 3-1). There are more than 100 different rhinoviruses that can cause the annoying symptoms of a runny and stuffy nose (rhinorrhea), malaise, sore throat, coughing, and sneezing. Colds are most frequent between November and March, with most adults having two to three per year. The incubation period is usually 1 to 4 days after exposure to droplets containing the virus. During the assessment, the nurse should note the patient's breathing pattern, especially during speaking, noting any shortness of breath or change in breathing pattern. Clinical findings may include reddened nasal membranes and inferior turbinates, nasal discharge, and dry lips and mouth from mouth breathing. A complaint of sore throat should lead to an examination of the posterior pharynx and possible throat culture to rule out beta-hemolytic streptococcal ("strep") infection (Table 3-2). The patient's temperature and white blood cell count usually remain normal with a cold but may be elevated with a bacterial infection or influenza.

Assessment

Elderly patients and those with chronic respiratory disease are particularly prone to complications from the common cold, including sinusitis, bronchitis, and pneumonia. These conditions may lead to dyspnea, productive cough, fever, hypoxemia, and disorientation.

The nurse notes the type of nasal discharge in her assessment. Acute rhinitis from a cold virus initially produces clear, runny drainage followed by thicker, milky secretions.

Yellow or greenish nasal discharge may indicate a secondary infection of the sinuses. Allergic reactions usually produce thin, clear, or mucoid nasal secretions. Postnasal drip is drainage of nasal secretions down the posterior nasal pharynx causing repeated swallowing and irritation. Other causes of nasal discharge include sinusitis, drugs such as birth control pills and antihypertensives, as well as smoke and seasonal allergies.

Table 3-2

How to Obtain a Throat Culture

1. Assemble equipment: Tongue depressor, light source, sterile swab, and culture medium.
2. Explain procedure to patient and warn of gagging sensation when the swab is applied to back of throat.
3. In a seated position, have the patient tilt his head back slightly and open his mouth.
4. Depress tongue with a moistened tongue depressor. Avoid touching the walls of the mouth or throat.
5. Using a light source, visualize the posterior oropharynx, noting any areas of redness or exudate.
6. Put down the light source while maintaining the tongue depressor on the tongue and pick up the sterile swab. While the patient says "Ahhh" to elevate the soft palate, put the swab in the mouth without touching the tongue or walls of the mouth and brush the swab over the wall of the posterior pharynx and the tonsils, trying to reach areas of redness or exudate. Discard tongue depressor.
7. Put swab in appropriate culture medium per individual facility guidelines. Label specimen and send to appropriate laboratory. Wash hands. Document that a culture was obtained.
8. Tell patient that results will not be ready for 24 to 48 hours, depending on the lab and antibiotics that may be needed for treatment if the culture is positive. Some rapid strep tests may be ready in 10 minutes but are less accurate than a culture.

Treatment

Treatment of the common cold is directed at maintaining ventilation and minimizing symptoms (Table 3-3). Acute rhinitis is a self-limiting condition that usually resolves in 7 to 10 days. Because the nasal discharge may occlude the airways, interventions are directed toward liquefying secretions:

- Ensure adequate fluid intake (at least 2500 mL/day or one-half the body weight in pounds equals the total ounces per day).
- Avoid dairy products that may thicken secretions.
- Humidify the air with a vaporizer and use saline nasal drops to maintain moist nasal mucus membranes.
- Allow adequate rest.
- Take supplemental vitamin E, 400 international units (IU), selenium, and vitamin C (500 mg), which is thought to have antiviral and antihistiminic effects.
- Use over-the-counter medications like chlorpheniramine to decrease nasal discharge.

Unfortunately, antihistamines may also dry out the mucus, predisposing the patient to mucus stasis and a secondary bacterial infection. Over-the-counter sympathomimetics

Table 3-3

Cold Prevention

1.   Decrease droplet exposure by frequent hand washing, especially after blowing the nose or sneezing.
2.   Use a tissue for blowing the nose, sneezing, and coughing; discard after each use.
3.   Avoid using the drinking glasses and eating utensils of others with a cold.
4.   Take vitamin C supplementation for possible antiviral effects.

like pseudoephedrine may be used to decrease mucus production by constricting the vasculature of the mucus membranes. Nasal drops, such as phenylephrine, produce vasoconstriction but should be limited to less than 72 hours of use because of the risk of rebound congestion (rhinitis medicamentosa). Echinacea (coneflower), an herbal remedy, is thought to be effective as an antimicrobial, but this treatment is still being investigated. Zinc lozenges are advertised as useful in decreasing the length of cold symptoms, but studies about the effectiveness of zinc have provided inconsistent results.

Nursing management of acute rhinitis usually occurs in the outpatient setting. Along with an assessment and diagnostic testing, such as a throat culture, the nurse teaches the patient about symptom management. She instructs the patient to seek further health care if:

- Symptoms last more than 7 days.
- Temperature elevation exceeds 100.5°F.
- Nasal discharge becomes yellow to green or is accompanied by face pain or headache.
- The patient has frequently recurring colds.

Allergic Rhinitis

Another frequent cause of nasal discharge is *allergic rhinitis*. Unlike acute rhinitis where a virus causes the symptoms, allergic rhinitis, the result of environmental allergens, produces an antigen-antibody reaction in susceptible individuals. It affects 10% to 20% of adults, most of whom have a family history of allergies, atopic dermatitis, asthma, or eczema. In allergic rhinitis, inhaled substances (pollen, animal dander, or dust) cause a type I hypersensitivity reaction. This leads to the release of potent vasoactive and inflammatory substances by the mast cells in the nasal mucosa. These substances produce vasodilation and increased capillary permeability in the mucus membranes, causing sneezing, watery eyes, and hypersecretion of thin mucus.

Assessment

In allergic rhinitis, the assessment focuses on the patient's symptoms, their relation to possible causative agents, their clinical course, and seasonal variations. The patient should also be asked about occupation, smoke exposure, life stresses, alcoholic beverage intake, and drug exposure. The most common symptoms of allergic rhinitis are nasal congestion with thin, clear discharge, frequent sneezing, itchy eyes with increased tearing, and pruritus. The physical examination may show pale, swollen, nasal mucosa with swollen turbinates, watery nasal discharge, watery eyes with puffy eyelids, reddened conjunctiva, dark circles under the eyes (allergic shiners), and pharyngitis.

Table 3-4
Reducing Exposure to Pollen
1. Stay indoors during high pollen count times, especially in centrally air-conditioned homes where almost all pollen is filtered out by the system. Go outside only during or immediately after rainfall when the air has been cleared of pollen.
2. Avoid eating honey, which may contain pollen.
3. Drive with the windows closed.
4. Install an air filter in the house to capture pollen.

A diagnosis of allergic rhinitis may require further diagnostic tests, such as skin testing, serum immunologic studies, and nasal smear to identify the allergen and look at the number of eosinophils. A large number of eosinophils may indicate an allergic response; serum immunologic studies may also indicate an allergic response when the IgE is elevated. Skin testing involves the application of dilute allergen into needle scratches or pricks in the upper inner aspect of the arm or back. Normal saline is used as a control on the opposite side. Fifteen minutes later the sites are assessed for a response. A flare (reddened area) or a wheal (a raised area) over a site more than 5 mm larger than the control would indicate an allergic response. Identification of the allergen provides a direction for treatment.

Treatment

Seasonal rhinitis occurs only during specific times of the year and is usually related to pollen exposure ("hay fever"). The most common offenders are grasses, ragweed, and wind-pollinated trees. Despite the name, hay does not contribute. Skin testing is useful in identifying pollen allergies. Total avoidance of pollen would be difficult at best. Treatment focuses on teaching the patient strategies to avoid pollen exposure (Table 3-4).

Reduction of exposure to specific allergens can be difficult. Ingested substances like foods, food dyes, molds in cheese, wine, dried fruit, and some drugs may be identified with careful questioning of dietary patterns and possible skin testing. Once identified, foods and drugs can be avoided. Decreasing exposure to other allergens like animal dander may require getting the pet(s) out of the household. Sensitivity to house dust and mites is more involved and may require changing the environment (Table 3-5).

If the offending substance(s) cannot be completely avoided or symptoms continue despite measures to avoid allergens, then medications may be useful in minimizing symptoms. Antihistamines are the most frequently used treatment for allergic rhinitis. They help decrease the nasal stuffiness and runny nose, as well as the excessive tearing and pruritus. Tolerance to these drugs can occur, and patients should be taught to report changes in drug effectiveness so that another class of antihistamine may be initiated. They may be used in conjunction with decongestants to alleviate symptoms without the drowsiness which can occur with antihistamines alone. Both cromolyn and glucocorticoid nasal sprays are useful in relieving nasal congestion by stabilizing mast cells in the nasal mucosa. They may take 3 to 5 days to become effective. Prophylactic use of medications may be useful in seasonal allergies to minimize responses to a known allergen like pollen.

If medication and exposure reduction are not effective in decreasing symptoms, then immunotherapy may provide some relief. The desensitization process involves the subcutaneous injection of the known allergen in gradually increasing doses to increase the patient's tolerance to the substance. Because anaphylactic reactions can occur, desensiti-

Table 3-5

Reducing Exposure to Allergens

1. Remove wall-to-wall carpeting and use hard floors with washable throw rugs if desired.
2. Encase mattresses and pillows in airtight covers and change them yearly. Wash bedding three times a week.
3. Remove all feather-containing pillows and comforters. Use blankets and pillows made out of synthetic materials because they are less likely to harbor mites than feathers and wool.
4. Avoid sweeping. Dust gently with a damp cloth.
5. If possible, have someone else vacuum. Change the vacuum cleaner bag and filter regularly.
6. Remove dust-collecting furniture and draperies.
7. Reduce high humidity to decrease mite breeding. Do not use humidifiers or vaporizers.
8. Install a high-efficiency air filter.
9. Do not have pets. If that is not possible then do not allow pets in the bedroom and bathe them weekly.
10. Avoid cigarette smoke.

zation treatments are done in a physician's office where emergency supplies are immediately available. Although the treatment may be effective in many patients, it is lengthy and expensive, requiring 2 to 5 years of treatment. Patient compliance can be improved by teaching the patient about the treatment plan and possible side effects, and accommodating the patient's schedule into the treatment plan.

Nursing management of patients with allergic rhinitis usually occurs in the outpatient setting. Assessing symptoms and treatment effectiveness, observing for secondary complications, and encouraging compliance with treatment are important components of the nurse's role. The nurse teaches allergen avoidance and ways to minimize exposure. All these interventions help to maintain normal air passage through the nose, allowing the nasal passages to perform their important functions.

Sinusitis

An infection of the sinuses may be a primary infection or secondary to a viral infection. Bacteria, viruses, fungi, and an allergic reaction can all cause sinusitis. Acute sinusitis usually develops after a primary viral infection or the common cold. The normal drainage paths for the sinuses are blocked by swollen mucus membranes, and thick sputum and bacteria begin to grow. Fluid and white cells fill the sinus, causing pressure and pain.

Assessment

The most common presenting symptom is facial pain and headache. The area over the sinus may be swollen and tender to palpation. There may also be toothaches if the maxillary sinus is involved and a headache if the frontal or ethmoid sinuses are involved. The physical assessment will reveal reddened mucosa with yellow to green exudate. There is tenderness to gentle pressure over the involved sinuses.

Treatment

Most cases of sinusitis appear in the outpatient setting. The nurse will assess the patient, asking about recent colds and rhinitis, both viral and allergic. Fever and facial swelling may indicate more diffuse infection, requiring intravenous antibiotics. The treatment for acute sinusitis is humidification with a vaporizer to help drain the sinuses, oral antibiotics for 10 to 14 days, and topical vasoconstrictors like phenylephrine for, at most, 7 days. It is important to teach the patient about finishing the entire course of antibiotics even if he or she is feeling better. This will prevent reinfection by resistant organisms.

Chronic sinusitis may require more intervention. Antibiotics will be prescribed for 4 to 6 weeks. If the sinusitis does not respond to antibiotics, then surgical intervention may be required to open the sinus passages and improve ventilation and drainage of the sinus.

Other Disorders of the Nose

Normal ventilation through the nose may be interrupted by nasal fractures, septal deformities, nosebleeds (epistaxis), tumors, and polyps. Nasal fractures are the most common fracture of the facial bones. Refer to the section on facial trauma later in this chapter. Septal deformities may impede airflow. They may result from trauma or developmental deformities and are usually asymptomatic. Restricted airflow through one or both nasal passages or chronic sinusitis caused by the septum blocking the sinus opening may indicate the need for surgical correction.

Nosebleed or epistaxis occurs commonly and can result from trauma, including fracture and nose picking, from infections like sinusitis and rhinitis, drying of the mucus membranes, bleeding disorders, malignancies of the nose or paranasal sinuses, hypertension, and some systemic infections like scarlet fever. The diagnosis is obvious from the clinical exam. Treatment involves pinching the nose for 5 to 10 minutes while the patient remains seated with his head tilted forward to prevent aspiration of blood or clots. If this method does not stop the bleeding, topical medications like tetracaine should be applied to vasoconstrict the capillaries in the nasal mucosa. If the bleeding continues, the site needs to be located and cauterized chemically (silver nitrate) or electrically, or nasal packing may be needed to apply direct pressure. Chronic or recurrent nosebleeds may indicate a bleeding tendency and a need for further evaluation.

Nasal Polyps

Nasal polyps are grape-like masses of swollen nasal mucosa. They may block the nasal passages and promote sinusitis. Polyps are benign growths which occur in chronic sinusitis and allergic rhinitis. The treatment involves topical treatment with corticosteroids using a nasal inhaler. Nursing management involves teaching the patient about the medications and use of the nasal inhaler and follow-up appointments to evaluate the effectiveness of the treatment. Surgical treatment may be required to remove the polyps because they tend to recur.

Other growths in the nose may be benign or malignant. The most frequently seen benign growth is a papilloma. The most common carcinoma of the nose is a squamous cell tumor. Patients with intranasal growths show symptoms of a unilateral airway obstruction, bloody discharge, numbness, or swelling. Surgical excision may be required to determine the pathology of the growth and plan the treatment course.

Pharyngitis

Acute inflammation of the pharynx can be caused by viral or bacterial infections. Pharyngitis or a sore throat may cause pain, especially when swallowing, and tender lymph glands in the neck. Patients may also have a fever and malaise.

Clinical findings include mild to severe redness of the pharynx with or without swollen tonsils. Exudate may or may not be present. In viral infections, there is usually no exudate but the pharynx is reddened with a "cobblestone" appearance. In bacterial infections, the pharynx and tonsils are reddened, and a white to yellow exudate may be present over these areas. Cervical lymphadenopathy may also be present.

Assessment includes interviewing the patient about the onset and duration of symptoms, checking the vital signs for fever, and obtaining a throat culture to rule out beta-hemolytic streptococcal infection (see Table 3-2). "Strep" infections may have serious conse-

> Pharyngitis or "sore throat" is a common infection caused by viruses or bacteria. In viral infections, there is usually no exudate in the posterior oropharynx but rather a reddened or "cobblestone" appearance. Bacterial infections with organisms like streptococcus cause a reddened oropharynx with white to yellow exudate and cervical adenopathy.

quences like acute glomerulonephritis and rheumatic fever. Treatment of a "strep" infection includes antibiotic therapy, warm saline gargles, a soft diet, rest, analgesics for pain relief, throat lozenges, and plenty of fluids (2 to 4 L per day). Patients should be taught to finish the course of antibiotics, even though they may be feeling better, to prevent reinfection with antibiotic-resistant organisms. They should call if they are still having symptoms or fever after 3 days of treatment.

Oropharyngeal Cancer

Malignancies of the mouth, tongue, or pharynx often involve complex medical and nursing care. Screening for oral cancers should be done in those at high risk: individuals over 40 years who are smokers, those who use chewing tobacco, or drink alcohol regularly. Symptoms include a painless red or white lesion. The most common malignancy of the oropharynx is squamous cell carcinoma. Medical treatment often involves surgery, radiation therapy, and possibly chemotherapy. Surgery involves excision of the lesion, surrounding tissue, and perhaps the cervical lymph nodes. Nursing care includes maintaining the airway, ensuring adequate nutrition, teaching the patient about mouth care, controlling treatment side effects, providing methods of communication, and recognizing changes in body image and self-esteem that may occur after surgery.

All patients who will be receiving radiation therapy or chemotherapy should have a thorough dental examination prior to beginning their treatment. It will be difficult or even impossible to do certain dental procedures, such as extractions, after radiation treatment because it can destroy the blood vessels in the jawbone. Salivary glands may also be destroyed by radiation therapy, predisposing the patient with a dry mouth (xerostomia), accelerated tooth decay, difficulty chewing, swallowing, and speaking.

The dentist can work with the oncologist to prevent and treat mucositis, the breakdown, ulceration, and infection of the oral mucosa. This common side effect of cancer treatments can be so painful that patients may need a break during treatment. Mucositis develops because the cells that line the oral cavity have a rapid turnover rate like cancer cells. The cancer treatment affects rapidly dividing cells and can kill normal cells in the mucosa, as well as cancer cells. The damaged lining can ulcerate and become infected. A common infection is oral candidiasis or thrush. It creates distinctive whitish patches on the oral mucosa and is quite painful. Antifungal agents are used to treat these infections.

Treatment for mucositis involves preventative dental care, thorough mouth care by the patient before and during treatment, frequent assessment of the oral cavity, and treatment of mucositis. Current treatments include antibiotic (IB 367), antiulcer (misoprostol), and amino acid (glutamine) mouthwashes. Nurses can teach their patients how to care for

Table 3-6
Care of the Mouth During Cancer Treatment
1. Brush teeth gently after every meal and before bed with a soft toothbrush rinsed in warm water to further soften the bristles, or use a sponge toothbrush.
2. Do not use mouthwashes that contain alcohol as they can dry out the mucosa.
3. Eat soft foods that are warm, not too hot or too cold, and avoid spicy foods.
4. Avoid alcohol and all tobacco products.
5. Use a saliva substitute to keep the mouth moist if dryness is a problem.

their mouth prior to and during cancer treatment (Table 3-6). (Nursing care of the patient with cancer receiving chemotherapy and radiation therapy is reviewed in more detail in on page 93. Care of the patient with a tracheostomy will be discussed on page 117.)

Laryngitis

Laryngitis is the inflammation of the mucus membranes lining the larynx and sometimes the vocal cords themselves. It occurs most frequently as a result of viral infection but may also be related to other respiratory infections like bronchitis and influenza. Hoarseness and unnatural diminution of the voice may also occur due to overuse of the voice, exposure to inhaled irritants like cigarette smoke or volatile gases, allergic reactions, or endotracheal intubation.

Assessment of the patient with acute laryngitis focuses on the symptoms of hoarseness, difficulty swallowing (dysphagia), and any other symptoms of respiratory infections. Laryngeal examination is performed indirectly with a laryngeal mirror or directly with a fiber optic laryngoscope. When any disorder other than acute laryngitis is suspected or hoarseness lasts more than 2 weeks, patients are referred to an otolaryngologist. Treatment of acute laryngitis involves symptom relief and avoidance of irritants. Nursing management involves teaching the patient about voice rest, increased fluid intake (2 to 4 L per day), topical lozenges, and steam inhalation to relieve some of the symptoms. Voice rest involves not only the obvious but also refraining from whispering and heavy lifting, which strain the larynx. Antibiotics may be ordered if other respiratory infections like bronchitis are suspected. Inhaled irritants, such as cigarettes or noxious fumes, should be avoided. Recurrent bouts of laryngitis that do not respond to conventional treatment require further medical evaluation.

Vocal Cord Nodules and Polyps

Vocal cord nodules are frequently seen in people who use their voice frequently and loudly like singers and actors. Vocal cord polyps develop as a result of chronic voice abuse or inhalation of irritants like cigarette smoke (Figure 3-1). Symptoms in both cases include hoarseness and a breathy voice quality. Treatment involves surgical removal and voice therapy. Malignancy needs to be ruled out in both cases, especially in cases of chronic cigarette abuse. The nurse should focus on teaching the patient how to prevent voice abuse and methods of smoking cessation. If surgical removal is done, then complete voice rest will require the patient to use other methods of communication like picture, slate, and alphabet boards for 2 weeks. Preoperative education of the patient and family is important because most of these procedures are done on an ambulatory basis, putting the burden of the communication challenges on the family.

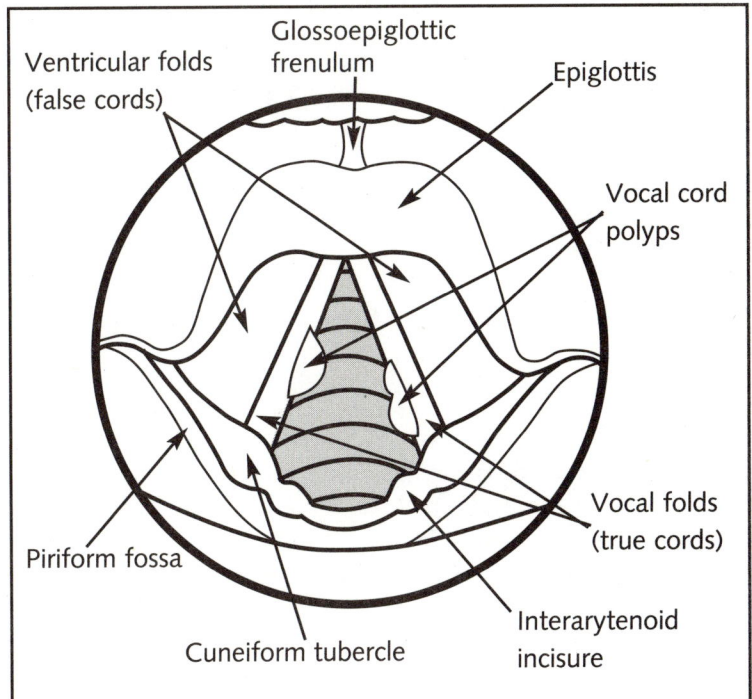

Ventricular folds (false cords)

Glossoepiglottic frenulum

Epiglottis

Vocal cord polyps

Vocal folds (true cords)

Piriform fossa

Cuneiform tubercle

Interarytenoid incisure

Figure 3-1. Vocal cord polyps.

Vocal Cord Paralysis

Vocal cord paralysis results from neck or chest lesions, central nervous system tumors, trauma, or viral illness. Other causes include prolonged intubation, total thyroidectomy, lung tumors, aortic aneurysms, and an enlarged right atrium. The patient has a diminished or hoarse voice and possibly difficulty breathing and swallowing. The cause must be sought and the airway protected. The diagnosis is made by direct laryngoscopy where the cords are visualized with a fiber optic scope. Nursing care focuses on airway protection by putting the patient in a high Fowler's position and suctioning as necessary to remove secretions. Stridor may indicate difficulty in moving air through the paralyzed cords and emergency intubation or tracheotomy may be necessary. The treatment focuses on maintaining the airway even at the expense of the voice. Patients are taught supraglottic swallowing (ie, taking a deep breath and holding it prior to swallowing). This maneuver allows the larynx to elevate and the epiglottis to close, preventing food and fluids from entering the lower respiratory tract during swallowing. Because these patients are at high risk for aspiration, they must be carefully watched and evaluated for aspiration pneumonia.

Laryngeal Trauma

Laryngeal trauma can occur from blunt force, fracture, or from prolonged endotracheal intubation. Symptoms may be an obvious laceration or hemoptysis, swelling and laceration, or symptoms of hoarseness, dyspnea, aphonia, and subcutaneous emphysema. Nursing care focuses on maintaining a patent airway, frequent evaluation of vital signs and pulse oximetry, and observation for symptoms of increased respiratory difficulty such as stridor, tachypnea, dyspnea, and restlessness. Respiratory distress may require emergency intubation. Prolonged intubation may result in laryngeal damage, and a tracheostomy may be created to bypass the larynx.

Facial Trauma

One of the most common injuries seen in emergency rooms is facial trauma. Whether from physical fights, automobile accidents, falls, or sports injuries, the bones in the face are susceptible to fracture. *Nasal fractures* are the most common facial injury. Patients complain of pain, tenderness, and swelling over the area and may have epistaxis and rhinorrhea. The nurse should quickly assess the adequacy of the airway and any other more serious trauma. A history of the event which caused the accident is important, including details about the patient's response to the injuries, especially any loss of consciousness. Blows to the head which were forceful enough to break bones can also cause head trauma. The nurse should be alert to signs of head trauma and increasing intracranial pressure.

Physical assessment may reveal ecchymosis, swelling, asymmetry, and bony fragments if a compound fracture occurred. Palpation of the area may reveal unusual mobility of the nasal bones or displacement, and crepitus (air in the subcutaneous tissues). Treatment of nasal fractures involves reducing the fracture if displacement occurred, ice packs, and analgesics. Closed reduction of a displaced nasal fracture usually returns the bones to their normal position, and packing may be inserted to stabilize the area. If there was not any displacement of the nasal bones, placement of a cast over the dorsum of the nose may protect it from further trauma.

Nursing management begins with evaluating the patient for serious injuries such as airway obstruction and head trauma that may have occurred with the nasal fracture. Care for the nasal fracture includes ice packs for 20 minutes of each hour for the first 24 hours. This will reduce swelling and hematoma formation. Patients are instructed not to blow their nose, as this could force air into the subcutaneous tissues, or to pinch the nostrils together. If bleeding recurs, this may cause further injury. The swelling and hematoma will resolve in 2 to 3 weeks. Patients should avoid situations where reinjury could occur, such as contact sports.

Maxillofacial Fractures

These fractures are more serious than nasal fractures. Rapid assessment of the patient is necessary. Hemorrhage and airway obstruction are the two most common life-threatening results. The nurse presumes that cervical injuries are present until x-rays are negative because the force that was required to cause the maxillofacial trauma is sufficient to cause a cervical spine injury. Bone chips may perforate the dura, causing cerebrospinal fluid (CSF) leaks. The patient may perceive this as a salty postnasal drip or rhinorrhea. The fluid can be checked for glucose by dipstick, which is present in CSF but not in nasal mucus.

Treatment of maxillofacial fractures involves maintaining a patent airway, controlling bleeding, protecting the cervical spine, and treating the head injuries. Nursing management involves trauma care: maintaining a patent airway with suctioning if needed, elevating the head of the bed if injuries allow to decrease bleeding, observing for head injuries and CSF leaks, assessing for orbital injuries and evaluating changes in vision and eye movement. Patients with jaw fractures who require intermaxillary fixation (the wiring together of the upper and lower jawbones by a series of stainless steel wires and elastics) need ongoing care after discharge to assess oral hygiene and nutritional status.

Cancer of the Head and Neck

Caring for the patient with head and neck cancer can be one of the greatest challenges for a nurse. The disease and its treatment may leave the patient with difficulty eating, swallowing, breathing, and speaking. Surgical excision may change the patient's body, altering his appearance and body image. Treatment depends on a multidisciplinary team

Table 3-7

Warning Signs of Head and Neck Cancer

1. Oral lesion or sore that does not heal in 2 weeks.
2. Persistent or unexplained oral bleeding.
3. Color changes (red, white, black, or brown) on the mouth or tongue.
4. Difficulty swallowing.
5. Persistent hoarseness or changes in voice quality.
6. Persistent or recurrent sore throat that does not respond to treatment.
7. A lump in the mouth, throat, or neck.
8. Pain in the mouth, lips, throat, neck, or under the dentures.

to identify the tumor, decide the appropriate treatment, and return the patient to his optimum functioning after treatment.

Squamous cell carcinomas account for 90% of head and neck tumors. The average patient is a male and over 50 years. Over 85% of all patients with head and neck cancer have a history of tobacco or alcohol use. Patients with these risk factors should have a careful oral exam annually. Head and neck tumors usually remain confined to the region and then spread in an orderly fashion along the associated lymphatic chains. Early detection of tumors while they are still relatively small and confined can greatly improve the prognosis. Even when the cancer has spread to the lymph nodes, cure is possible.

Head and neck tumors may present in a variety of ways. Oral cancers may be detected by a dentist, a health care provider during routine assessment, or by the patient (Table 3-7). Oral cancers usually begin with red patches (erythroplasia) or whitish patches (leukoplakia) on the mucus membrane. Nasal tumors may cause facial swelling, numbness, facial pain, and epistaxis. Patients with oropharyngeal cancer may complain of hoarseness, a lesion in the mouth, pain when swallowing, unilateral ear pain (from destruction of the glossopharyngeal nerve), and fullness in the face. Because of the variety of ways that head and neck cancers present, it is important for the nurse to understand the warning signs and assess patients who are at risk for developing any of these cancers.

The treatment course for head and neck cancers is determined by the stage of the disease. Tumors are biopsied to determine the histology, and follow-up CAT scans or MRIs are used to assess tumor size and local spread. Head and neck tumors are staged according to the TNM system. T indicates the size and site of the primary tumor, N denotes the number and size of local lymphatic spread, and M is used to indicate the presence of distant metastases.

The first contact that a nurse may have with a patient with head and neck cancer is during the history taking. Sensitive questioning about tobacco (all forms) and alcohol use is important. Calculate the number of packs per year of cigarette use with the formula in Chapter 2. Ask about other risk factors to potential carcinogens, such as occupational exposure (woodworkers, asbestos exposure, and petroleum workers). Review the course of the presenting symptoms and note their onset and duration.

The treatment course for head and neck cancers will vary depending on the location and stage of the disease, the physician's recommendation, and the patient's desires. Many tumors of the head and neck will require some surgery to biopsy and remove the tumor. More extensive surgery or radiation therapy will be required to treat the tumor bed and

Table 3-8

Potential Nursing Diagnoses for Patients With Laryngeal Cancer

1. Anxiety, preoperative and postoperative (related to diagnosis and treatments).
2. Knowledge deficit (related to surgery, radiation therapy, chemotherapy, and management of health care regimen).
3. Ineffective airway clearance (related to tracheostomy, management of secretions).
4. Altered nutrition: less than the body requires (related to pain and difficulty swallowing from surgery and radiation treatments).
5. Impaired verbal communication (related to surgery if laryngectomy is performed).
6. Impaired swallowing (related to tumor, surgery, and radiation treatments).
7. Pain (related to surgery and impaired tissue integrity).
8. Altered body image (related to surgery).

the associated lymph nodes that may have disease. Chemotherapy has an increasing role in advanced cancers. Because there are so many different tumors and treatments, this section will focus on the patient with laryngeal cancer.

Laryngeal cancer is the most common head and neck cancer, 95% of which are squamous cell carcinomas. The cancer may be in the true vocal cords, the epiglottis, the pyriform sinus, or the postcricoid area. Patients usually present symptoms of hoarseness, pain, a lump in the neck, or difficulty swallowing.

Early stages of cancer in the vocal cord and epiglottis are treated with radiation therapy. Daily radiation treatments for 6 to 7 weeks can be tiring for the patient. The treatments themselves are not painful, but the side effects can cause many difficulties for the patient as the treatment progresses. Because radiation affects all anatomic structures within the treatment field, the pharynx, larynx, and esophagus may all be affected. Side effects of radiation therapy appear as the treatment progresses and the total dose of radiation to the area increases. These include skin reaction, esophagitis, laryngitis, and pharyngitis. If the oropharynx is in the treatment field, then the patient may experience xerostomia (dry mouth), decreased taste, and possibly infections of the oropharynx. Mucositis, the inflammation of the mucus membranes, can be very painful and may make it difficult for the patient to eat and swallow. The challenge for nursing is maintaining optimum nutrition, controlling pain, and watching for treatment reactions (Table 3-8).

Surgical treatment of laryngeal cancer depends on the stage of the tumor. More advanced glottic cancers with cartilage invasion may require complete laryngectomy with a radical neck dissection to remove the associated lymph nodes. A complete laryngectomy is performed when previous treatment with radiation or chemoradiotherapy has failed (Figure 3-2). After the laryngectomy, the patient can no longer speak in the normal way. Later, a tracheoesophageal fistula may be surgically created into which a one-way valve can be inserted for speech. Other methods of creating speech are by eructation or esophageal speech and the use of an electrolarynx. When a tracheostomy is created, an opening is made from the trachea to the anterior neck to maintain the airway. The pharynx is sutured to the esophagus to allow for swallowing.

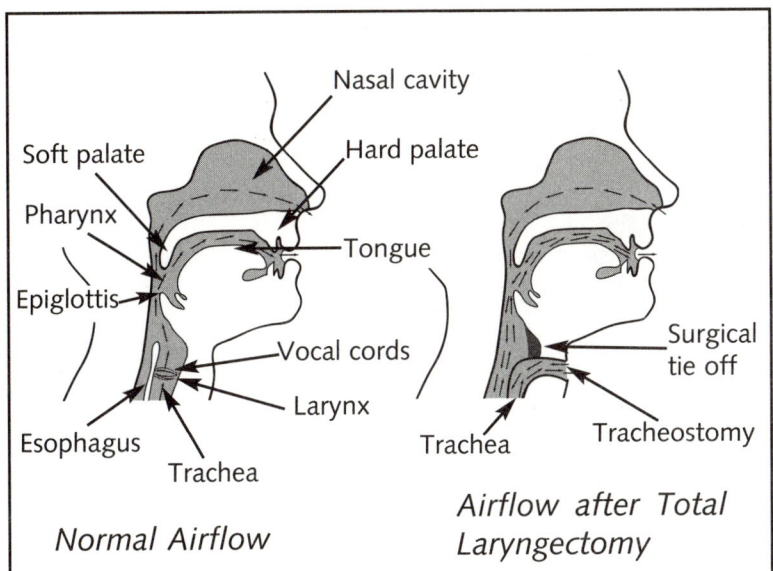

Figure 3-2. Altered airflow after total laryngectomy.

Soft palate
Pharynx
Epiglottis
Esophagus
Trachea
Nasal cavity
Hard palate
Tongue
Vocal cords
Larynx

Normal Airflow

Surgical tie off
Tracheostomy
Trachea

Airflow after Total Laryngectomy

Disorders of the Lower Airways

Disorders of the lower respiratory tract can be acute or chronic processes. Acute infectious processes can be brief but serious illnesses, such as pneumonia. Chronic conditions like asthma can have a course marked with remissions and exacerbations. The nursing care for acute and chronic respiratory disorders is a collaborative process with the nurse, the physician, and the respiratory therapist all contributing to the development of best care plan for the patient. In this section, acute infections (influenza, acute bronchitis, pneumonia, and tuberculosis) will be reviewed first. Next will be diseases of chronic airflow limitation (asthma, chronic bronchitis, and emphysema), acute respiratory failure, adult respiratory distress syndrome (ARDS), pulmonary vascular disorders (pulmonary embolus and pulmonary hypertension), pleural effusion, lung cancer, and chest trauma including pneumothorax. Specific interventions (ie, oxygen therapy, tracheostomy, mechanical ventilation, thoracentesis, and chest tube maintenance) and oro/endotracheal suctioning are reviewed in Chapter 5. Nursing diagnoses related to these groups of disorders will be reviewed at the end of each section.

Influenza

Influenza is caused by a viral infection of the respiratory tract. It usually occurs in epidemics during the fall and winter. Influenza can be lethal, particularly to people over 65 years of age, the immunocompromised, and those with chronic lung and heart disease. There are three types of the influenza virus: A, B, and C. The incubation period is 1 to 4 days after exposure to droplet nuclei that are spread by coughing or sneezing. The presenting symptoms fall into three syndromes: a *rhinotracheitis*, a *viral respiratory infection*, and a *viral pneumonia*. The presentation depends on the type of droplet exposure. Fine droplet exposure inhaled into the nasal passages may produce a rhinotracheitis. A larger exposure of viral-laden droplets directly into the lower airways may produce a viral pneumonia. Basic hygiene as used in common cold prevention (hand washing, covered sneezes, and coughs) may decrease the spread of influenza.

Assessment of the patient requires an understanding of the normal course of influenza versus other respiratory tract illnesses. The first symptoms are the abrupt onset of fever, chills, and malaise followed by a profusely runny nose, muscle aches, and headache. The symptoms of rhinotracheitis peak in 3 to 5 days and resolve spontaneously in 7 days. Secondary complications are related to bacterial infections including sinusitis, otitis media, bacterial pneumonia, and bronchitis. These secondary bacterial infections occur just as the patient is starting to feel better or when symptoms are prolonged after the normal influenza course.

The symptoms of influenza pneumonia are more severe and can rapidly progress to hypoxemia and even death. The symptoms of cough, fever, chills, and malaise come on abruptly and can be quite severe. Treatment should be sought early, especially in the elderly or otherwise compromised patients.

Treatment of patients with influenza includes rest, extra fluids, and acetaminophen for high temperatures (greater than 101°F). Acetaminophen is preferred over aspirin as an analgesic and antipyretic because of the risk of Reye's syndrome, a rare complication of influenza that causes liver failure and encephalitis. It is seen more often when aspirin is used during an influenzal illness, particularly in children.

Other treatments for influenza include antiviral therapy with ramantidine or amantidine. It is only effective against influenza A and must be used throughout the risk-of-infection period. Antiviral therapy may shorten the course of the illness and is useful in patients with chronic diseases or who are immunocompromised.

Influenzal infections can be prevented by use of a vaccine. At-risk individuals should be vaccinated annually in the fall. Populations at high risk are people over 65 years of age; residents of nursing homes and chronic care facilities; patients with chronic heart, lung, metabolic, or immunological problems; and children or adults receiving chronic aspirin therapy (because of the risk of Reye's syndrome). The vaccine is reformulated each year to include the most common strains of the influenza virus from the previous year's data. The vaccine should not be given to individuals with an allergy to egg whites. Side effects are infrequent and include redness and tenderness at the vaccination site and, rarely, malaise and fever.

Acute Bronchitis

Acute bronchitis is the inflammation of the large airways in the lower respiratory tract. It can be caused by bacteria, viruses, or exposure to inhaled irritants. Bronchitis can be classified as acute or chronic. Chronic bronchitis will be reviewed on page 71.

Acute bronchitis can result from a previous infection with a virus (ie, influenza) that predisposes the patient to a secondary bacterial infection. The most common infective agents are *Staphylococcus aureus*, *Pneumococcus*, and *Haemophilus* influenza. The bacteria are usually passed from the nasopharynx to the bronchi by small amounts of aspirant. The organisms cause an inflammatory response in the bronchi with swelling and excessive mucus production.

Symptoms of acute bronchitis include a productive cough, fever, malaise, substernal pain especially when coughing, and auscultatory crackles and wheezes. Wheezes indicate some degree of bronchoconstriction. The dry cough progresses to a productive cough with purulent to blood-streaked sputum. Acute bronchitis can progress to a severe illness with high fever, dyspnea, and cyanosis requiring hospitalization.

Treatment is usually based on the clinical findings and includes antibiotics, extra fluids, humidity, rest, and acetaminophen for fever and pain, and sometimes oxygen therapy. Cough suppressants should be used cautiously because excessive secretions need to be cleared from the lungs. Expectorants (like guaifenesin) may be useful in relieving chest congestion. Cigarette smokers are encouraged to quit smoking, as this further irritates the lining of the bronchi.

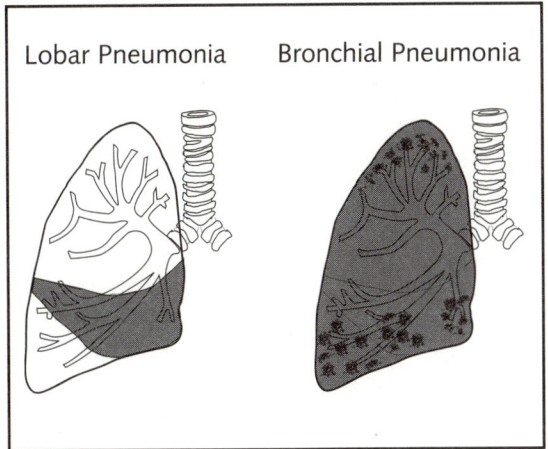

Figure 3-3. Lobar and bronchial pneumonia.

Pneumonia

Pneumonia is an inflammatory process of the parenchymal structures of the lung, such as the bronchioles and alveoli. Bacteria, viruses, fumes, and even gastric contents can cause pneumonia. Normally, respiratory defense mechanisms like the cough reflex and the mucociliary blanket protect the lower airways. Some factors that can impair the effectiveness of the defense mechanisms are immunodeficiency, smoking, viral diseases, and loss of the cough reflex due to neuromuscular disease or anesthesia. Although antibiotics have decreased the mortality associated with pneumonia, it is still a leading cause of death in adults in the United States.

Pneumonia is classified according to the anatomic distribution and the causative agent. Acute bacterial pneumonia has one of two anatomic patterns: either lobar or bronchial pneumonia (Figure 3-3). Lobar pneumonia is so named because a chest x-ray reveals inflammation of a large portion or an entire lobe of the lung. Approximately 90% of all forms of lobar pneumonia are caused by *Streptococcus pneumoniae*. The symptoms of lobar pneumonia are rapid onset of malaise, chills, high fever, and leukocytosis (eg, increased white blood cell count). Initially, the cough may produce watery sputum, and the breath sounds may be diminished due to congestion in the alveolar walls. Later, the sputum becomes rusty colored or purulent. Pleuritic pain, especially on deep respiratory movements, may be present.

Bronchial pneumonia differs from lobar pneumonia in both the presentation and the course of the illness. On chest radiography, a bronchial pneumonia appears as patchy consolidation in several lobules. It is usually the extension of a preexisting bronchitis or bronchiolitis. Bronchial pneumonia tends to be a disease of the very young, the very old, and the immunocompromised. It presents insidiously with a low-grade fever, cough, crackles, and leukocytosis. Many different organisms can cause bronchial pneumonia including the previously mentioned *Streptococcus pneumoniae*, as well as *Staphylococcus aureus*, *Haemophilus influenzae*, and *Pseudomonas aeruginosa*.

The treatment for either lobar or bronchial pneumonia is antibiotics, rest, extra fluids, and sometimes oxygen therapy. For debilitated patients, care should be taken to wash hands and use respiratory equipment between patients so as to prevent nosocomial spread of bacteria. Prevention of pneumococcal pneumonia can be achieved by means of a vaccination. A single dose usually confers immunity for 5 to 7 years. Pneumococcal vaccination is recommended for individuals with chronic respiratory, cardiac, and immunologic disorders; those with diabetes mellitus; and those with a history of alcoholism who

Figure 3-4. Tuberculosis.

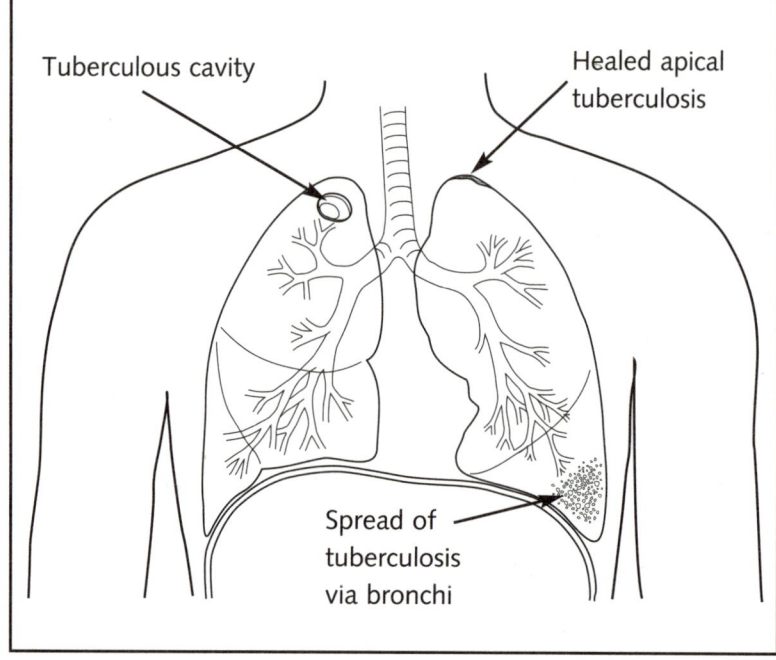

Tuberculous cavity

Healed apical tuberculosis

Spread of tuberculosis via bronchi

have increased morbidity due to respiratory infections. Healthy adults over 65 years of age may also benefit from being vaccinated.

Tuberculosis

Tuberculosis (TB) is a bacterial infection caused by the tubercle bacillus (*Mycobacterium tuberculi*), a distinctively rod-shaped bacterium. Once called consumption, its victims spent years isolated in sanatoriums until the disease was considered cured. TB is now better understood and treatment can be completed on an outpatient basis for most patients.

Tuberculosis occurs most commonly in the lungs but can affect other organs. TB is spread via airborne droplets from an infected person coughing, sneezing, or speaking. The tubercle bacillus is inhaled and lands in the alveoli, particularly in the upper lobes, and the body begins an inflammatory response. The response causes vasodilation and increased vascular permeability. Fluids, white blood cells (WBC), and macrophages leak into the area infected by the tubercle bacillus. Later, an immune response mediated by T-lymphocytes results in a walled-off area around the infection called a tubercle (Figure 3-4). This immune response can be detected 3 to 12 weeks after infection by a skin test (Mantoux or PPD test).

The walls of the tubercle are made of a cheesy white substance called *casein*. The bacteria within the tubercle begin to destroy the lung tissue, causing a *caseation necrosis*. The bacteria may stay within the tubercle, secluded from the rest of the lung and body, or the walls of the tubercle may liquefy and the bacteria will multiply and spread directly into other chest structures or indirectly, via lymphatic channels, to other parts of the body (miliary TB).

Many older people have walled-off lesions from earlier tuberculosis infections. Early in the 20th century, 80% of adults were infected with tuberculosis before the age of 30. While the tubercle may remain intact and the disease dormant for years, the TB may become active again if the host becomes immunocompromised (secondary or reactivated TB).

Since 1985, the incidence of tuberculosis has been increasing for the first time in 3 decades. Many factors are thought to be causing this alarming change, including an increased number of immigrants from countries with prevalent TB (Southeast Asia and Latin America), increasing poverty, crowded living conditions, especially in urban areas, people infected with HIV (human immunodeficiency virus), and an increase in alcohol and drug abuse. The public health implications are significant and nurses are active in community education programs, screening clinics, and treatment programs.

Nursing care of the patient with tuberculosis begins with an accurate assessment. There are numerous signs of tuberculosis. Symptoms may be present for months prior to the patient seeking health care. Persistent cough (usually productive), hemoptysis, and pleuritic chest pain are the most suggestive symptoms, but nonspecific changes in health like malaise, loss of appetite, weight loss, or just a loss of sense of well being may be present. Fever and

> Tuberculosis is caused by the tubercle bacillus when it is inhaled into the lungs, lands in the alveoli (particularly the upper lobes), and begins an inflammatory process. The response causes vasodilation and increased vascular permeability. Later, an immune response mediated by T-lymphocytes results in a walled-off area around the infection called a tubercle. The immune response can be detected 3 to 12 weeks after infection by a skin test (Mantoux or PPD test).

night sweats may also be present. At-risk populations should be carefully screened with questions regarding different presenting symptoms.

It is important to ask the patient if he or she has ever been tested for TB and what the results were at that time. The nurse should inquire about immediate members of the family or household who might have TB. The nurse should also ask the patient about recent travel to developing countries where TB is more common (eg, Asia, Africa, South America).

Diagnostic testing for TB is a standard skin test (Mantoux test) using purified protein derivative (PPD). The nurse injects 5 units (0.1 mL) intradermally (not subcutaneously) and has the patient return in 48 hours to have the area around the injection site read. A Mantoux induration is measured in millimeters at the greatest diameter. One practical method for reading the site is using a ball point pen and running it across the skin just before the area of induration until resistance is met and then lifting the pen off the skin. This motion is repeated on the opposite side and the distance between the pen marks is measured in millimeters. A positive reaction is considered 10 mm or greater at the site. Any reaction over 5 mm should be considered positive in patients with HIV, those patients who have close contacts with others with TB, or a previous chest x-ray which shows an old TB infection. All positive skin tests must be reported to the local or state health departments. It is important to tell patients that a positive skin test does not mean that they have tuberculosis but that they have been exposed to the bacillus.

Patients with positive TB skin tests are referred for further diagnosis and treatment. A chest x-ray, sputum cultures (three early morning samples), and blood tests are done. Patients with a diagnosis of active tuberculosis and those who have contact with others with active TB and are at risk for development of the disease are treated with antimicrobial medications. The most common medications for treating TB are isoniazid (INH), rifampin (RIF), pyrazinamide (PZA), ethambutol (EMB), and streptomycin (SM). One drug, INH, is used for prophylactic treatment.

At least two of these drugs are used during treatment of active TB to prevent the development of multiple drug resistant (MDR) strains of TB. MDR strains of tuberculosis have

Table 3-9

Potential Nursing Diagnoses for Patients With Tuberculosis

1. Knowledge Deficit or ineffective management of therapeutic regimen related to disease and treatment.
2. Ineffective Airway Clearance related to increased sputum from the tuberculin.
3. Diversional Activity Deficit related to respiratory isolation.

emerged recently in the HIV-positive population. Multiple drugs are used for extended treatment (12 months) in cases of known or suspected MDR TB.

If the patient had a positive skin test but no other manifestation of TB, he is put on a course of INH prophylaxis for 6 to 9 months. This long treatment may be more difficult to justify to asymptomatic patients. The lifetime chance of developing full-blown TB in an immunocompetent person is 10%. The issue becomes one of public health and safety, especially with the increasing numbers of multiple drug resistant TB strains and HIV-positive people. Individuals who are HIV positive and have a positive skin test have a 7% chance per year of developing full-blown TB. It is important to stress that compliance with the regimen is important because the patient may develop active TB and be contagious even though he or she does not have any symptoms. Common side effects of INH therapy are peripheral neuritis, hepatitis, and hypersensitivity. Patients are advised not to drink alcohol while taking INH.

For patients with active pulmonary TB, hospitalization and combined antimicrobial therapy are necessary. The patient should be in respiratory isolation with negative air pressure to minimize air (and bacillus) flow out of the room. If the patient leaves the room, a specialized mask should be worn. The door should be closed at all times. Isolation should be maintained for at least 2 weeks after initiating antimicrobial therapy and until the patient is showing clinical response to treatment (decreasing bacillus count in sputum). This may be difficult for the patient and his family, and alternative methods of socialization and recreation should be suggested. Some creativity on the part of the nurse and patient may yield interesting solutions to this problem: videotaped movies, computer games, telephones, etc. Nurses should encourage a healthy diet. Pyroxidine (B6) supplements may be added to prevent INH-induced peripheral neuropathies (Table 3-9).

Patients are followed periodically throughout their treatment to ensure compliance and to follow their response to treatment and monitor the side effects of treatment. Noncompliance is the cause of most treatment failures. If the patient and his family understand the disease and treatment, they are more apt to comply and complete the drug regimen. For patients where compliance is a concern, such as alcoholics, "observed therapy" may be a solution. With directly observed treatment (DOT), the patient makes regular appointments to take his medication as the nurse watches (usually a four-drug regimen three times a week). Patients are followed with regular sputum smears to evaluate the effectiveness of treatment as evidenced by decreasing numbers of bacilli in the sputum.

The term *chronic airflow limitation* is used to describe a group of disorders that impede airflow through the pulmonary airways. This group can be further broken down into the chronic obstructive pulmonary diseases (COPD) and asthma. COPD causes changes to the airways that do not improve over several months. Asthma, which was previously included in this group, is now considered separately because the changes to the airways are reversible. Chronic bronchitis and emphysema will be reviewed together because they share many of the same causative factors and treatments. The course of asthma and its treatment will be reviewed separately.

Chronic Obstructive Pulmonary Disease

COPD is increasing in prevalence in the United States and around the world. In the United States over 16 million people are afflicted with COPD and it is now the fourth leading cause of death (after cardiovascular diseases, cancer, and cerebrovascular disease). The cost in terms of direct health care and diminished quality of life is astronomical. COPD is characterized by obstruction of airflow out of the lungs with shortness of breath (dyspnea) as the most common symptom. Although the changes to the airways that are clumped together as COPD include several diseases, this section will review the two most common forms of COPD: chronic bronchitis and emphysema.

Chronic bronchitis is characterized by a hypersecretion of mucus and chronic cough. The productive cough is defined as being present for at least 3 months of the year for 2 years in a row. Infections develop secondarily as a result of mucus stasis. Most patients with chronic bronchitis are cigarette smokers and have a cough all year round. The changes associated with chronic bronchitis are not manifested until late middle age and occur most often in men.

Emphysema is characterized by loss of lung elasticity, narrowed bronchioles, and abnormal dilation of the terminal air spaces caused by the destruction of the alveolar walls (without evidence of fibrosis). Dilation of the air spaces results in hyperinflation of the lungs, air trapping, and increased total lung capacity. The physiologic changes associated with emphysema are thought to be due to the destruction of elastin in the alveolar walls by enzymes (elastases and proteases) released by neutrophils. Some alveoli deteriorate and form bullae (air-filled spaces), while others remain enlarged but lose their elasticity. Although the number-one cause of emphysema is cigarette

> COPD is increasing in prevalence and is now the fourth leading cause of death. COPD is characterized by obstruction of airflow out of the lungs. COPD is a group of disorders including chronic bronchitis, emphysema, and asthma. The most common symptoms are chronic cough, expectoration, and dyspnea.

smoking, certain genetic disorders like alpha-1-antitrypsin deficiency have been linked to the elastin destruction seen in this disease. Smoking may also decrease the amount of alpha-1-antitrypsin, resulting in increased destruction of elastin. Patients develop dyspnea after more than a third of their lung tissue is destroyed. Cough is rare and nonproductive.

Several risk factors are linked to the development of COPD. Without doubt, the number-one cause is cigarette smoking. Other established risk factors are occupational dust exposure (silica, cotton, chemical fumes) and congenital enzyme deficiencies. These other factors are only minor contributors compared to cigarette smoking. What smokers mistakenly call "smoker's cough" is related to the changes in COPD. Nurses can help to prevent COPD by teaching school-age children about the harmful effects of smoking, educating their patients about smoking cessation (Tables 3-10 and 3-11), and encouraging the use of masks for individuals who work in high-risk environments.

The physiological changes in chronic bronchitis start a cycle of airway obstruction and destruction. There is a hypertrophy of the mucus-secreting glands with excessive mucus

Table 3-10

Smoking Cessation

1. Ask your smoking patient about his smoking status and interest in quitting. It is more productive to find out his reasons for quitting (eg, health, family pressure, cost, and smoking-related illnesses in friends or family).

2. Boost his motivation by telling him about the harmful effects of smoking. Use his symptoms as a reason to quit. Explain that his symptoms (eg, cough, dyspnea, and sore throat) may be caused by cigarettes and that quitting may relieve them.

3. Make a plan with your smoking patient to quit smoking. Set a date for stopping. Enlist a smoking buddy to help the patient adhere to his goals. Use an informal contract signed by the patient and his buddy.

4. Follow-up with your patient, as most smokers need several attempts before they finally quit. Common withdrawal symptoms include cravings, irritability, insomnia, difficulty sleeping, and constipation. Explain that each attempt at quitting is a learning experience that will help the patient to successfully quit the next time.

5. Offer strategies for dealing with nicotine withdrawal symptoms:
    *   Cravings. These last 1 to 3 minutes. Chew a carrot or sugar-free gum, take slow, deep breaths, and engage in another activity.
    *   Irritability. Avoid stressful situations during quitting; use relaxation exercises or hypnosis.
    *   Temptation. Avoid smokers or tell them that you are trying to quit and to smoke elsewhere; throw away all cigarettes; change routine to avoid smoking.
    *   Pharmacology aids. These include nicotine gum, the patch, an inhaler, clonidine, and bupropion.

6. Help your patient stay on track with follow-up phone calls, posting honor rolls of quitters, and supplying patient education materials.

7. Refer your patient to established smoking cessation programs in his community (contact the local offices of the American Cancer Society and the American Lung Association for referrals).

production, a decrease in ciliated epithelial cells, and a decrease in mucociliary clearance. With excessive mucus and decreased effectiveness of the mucociliary blanket, there is mucus stasis, which invites inflammation and infection. Chronic inflammation causes scarring and ulceration of the epithelial lining of the pulmonary airways. It is also thought that the chemicals in cigarette smoke cause an inflammatory response that activates neutrophils. The neutrophils produce enzymes that break down elastin in the broncho-alveolar walls. Airways are stenosed or collapsed and fewer alveoli are ventilated. Air is trapped in the alveoli, resulting in decreased diffusion of oxygen and carbon dioxide. The PaO_2 declines and the $PaCO_2$ increases. The decreased PaO_2 results in pulmonary vasoconstriction and pulmonary hypertension. The increased pulmonary pressures put a strain on the right side of the heart and result in right-sided heart failure or pulmonary heart disease (cor pulmonale).

Table 3-11

Smoking Cessation Programs

1. Nicotine addiction. Nicotine replacement must be dosed accurately. Each cigarette is considered 1 mg. Nicotine replacement should be 1 mg per cigarette (ie, one pack per day equals 20 mg). In this case, the individual should begin with a 21 mg patch (or 10 pieces of 2g gum).

2. Psychological parameters. The following are helpful: stress management, hypnosis, relaxation techniques, massage, acupressure, imagery.

3. Breaking the "habit." Try changing routine. If morning routine is a cup of coffee and a cigarette, then take a shower first, brush teeth right away, and have orange juice instead. Changing the habit part is essential.

Assessment

The patient with COPD requires careful questioning about risk factors and an understanding of the physical changes that occur in COPD. The nurse should always ask about current and previous smoking habits and attempts to quit. She encourages honesty with a nonjudgmental attitude and matter-of-fact questions. The assessment should include questions about dyspnea, cough, sputum production, and recent colds. The nurse notes any postural changes in respiratory rate. The patient may be propping himself up on a table or elbows to increase the effectiveness of the accessory muscles used in breathing. The respiratory rate may be increased and expiration may be prolonged. The patient may use purse-lipped breathing to increase end-expiratory pressures and open distal airways. The chest may have an increased anterior-posterior diameter (barrel chest) with decreased chest movement and increased abdominal movement during breathing. The terms "blue bloater" and "pink puffer" were once used to differentiate between patients with chronic bronchitis and emphysema (Table 3-12). These mnemonics only partly describe the differences because many patients with COPD have components of both diseases. The physiologic changes cause a different responsiveness to hypoxia. Patients with chronic bronchitis were described as "blue bloaters" because the increased secretions and airway obstruction caused hypoxemia, cyanosis (blue), and peripheral edema from right-sided heart failure (bloater). Patients with emphysema have less surface area for ventilation and perfusion but are well compensated (pink) with hyperventilation (puffer).

Several tests are used to diagnose COPD. A thorough history and physical examination, pulmonary function tests, chest radiography, and laboratory tests are all used to diagnose COPD. Spirometry is the most frequently used pulmonary function test. It indicates whether an airway obstruction exists but does not discriminate between the different causes. The most specific spirometric test for airflow reduction is the forced expiratory volume in 1 second (FEV1). An FEV1 below 80% of expected without a significant decrease in forced vital capacity (FVC) is considered diagnostic of COPD. (See Chapter 2 for a description of spirometry.) In chronic bronchitis there may also be an increased residual air volume (RV) from air trapped within the alveoli. The total lung capacity (TLC) may be increased in emphysema.

Arterial blood gases may show changes in advanced disease. The PaO_2 will decrease and the $PaCO_2$ will increase with the kidneys compensating by retaining bicarbonate (HCO_3^-). The pH may be normal if the kidneys have sufficiently compensated for the acidosis caused by the high $PaCO_2$. The hypoxemia (decreased PaO_2) and hypercapnia

Table 3-12

Different Manifestations of Chronic Bronchitis and Emphysema

	Chronic Bronchitis	*Emphysema*
Onset of symptoms	>35	>50
Smoking history	Usually	Usually
Skin color	Pale to cyanotic	Pink
Respiratory rate	Increased	Increased
Dyspnea early	Predominant symptom	May be absent in stages
Cough	Chronic	Absent or mild
Sputum	Copious, mucopurulent	Absent or minimal
A-P diameter	Normal to slight increase	Increased
Auscultation	Wheezes, rhonchi	Diminished breath sounds, prolonged expiration, wheezes
Percussion	Normal	Hyperresonant
Blood gases	Hypoxemia, hypercapnia	May be normal until late stages
Other findings	Infections, right heart failure	Weight loss

(increased $PaCO_2$) seen in chronic bronchitis may not exist in emphysema because the increased respiratory rate compensates for the decrease in alveolar surface area. The hemoglobin may increase as a compensatory mechanism in chronic bronchitis to increase the oxygen-carrying capacity of the blood.

The course of COPD is one of increasing dyspnea and exacerbations of infections and respiratory insufficiency. Many patients with COPD have clinical features of both diseases. They may first seek medical attention later in life as their dyspnea increases or they have repeated respiratory infections. The increasing dyspnea makes eating difficult, with subsequent weight loss, malnutrition, and dehydration. Patients with chronic bronchitis may have a worsening cough particularly in the morning. As the disease progresses, patients may have decreased activity tolerance, increased dyspnea, weight loss, and declining mental acuity and, later, respiratory failure and heart failure.

Treatment

Treatment can facilitate the health and quality of life of patients with COPD. The goals of treatment are to alleviate the acute symptoms and prevent complications. The treatment of COPD includes:

- Bronchodilators (eg, ipratropium and albuterol or salmeterol via metered-dose inhalers) to improve airflow.
- Corticosteroids (to decrease inflammation) if bronchodilators are not sufficient.
- Low-flow oxygen if the PaO_2 is less than 55 mmHg or the SaO_2 is less than 88%. It can also be used during exercise or at night for patients with nocturnal hypoxemia.

Table 3-13

Nursing Diagnoses for Patients With COPD

1. Ineffective Breathing Pattern related to dyspnea, decreased chest wall expansion (Interventions from page 76: 1, 2, 3).

2. Ineffective Airway Clearance related to increased mucus production, mucus stasis, decreased mucociliary functioning, and inflammation of bronchial walls (Interventions: 2, 3, 4).

3. Impaired Gas Exchange related to decrease in alveolar surface, secretions, occluded airways, ventilation, or perfusion mismatches (Interventions: 1, 2, 3, 4).

4. Altered Nutrition: Less Than Body Requirements related to dyspnea, decreased intake, increased caloric expenditure with coughing, and increased respiratory rate, flattened diaphragm compressing the stomach (Intervention: 5).

5. Risk for Infection related to mucus stasis, poor nutrition (Interventions: 6, 8).

6. Activity Intolerance related to dyspnea on exertion, hypoxia (Interventions: 7, 10).

7. Altered Thought Processes related to cerebral hypoxia (Intervention: 8).

8. Altered Health Maintenance related to infection prevention, improving oxygenation, breathing techniques, smoking cessation (Interventions: 9, 11).

9. Sleep Pattern Disturbance related to excessive coughing, dyspnea (Intervention: 10).

10. Powerlessness related to disease progression, increasing dependence, alteration in roles (Interventions: 9, 11).

- Long-acting bronchodilator like theophylline if the patient does not improve with combination therapy. Theophylline serum levels and side effects must be monitored to prevent toxicity.
- Antibiotics to treat infections since most exacerbations are triggered by bacterial infections.

Nursing can facilitate the physical health and psychosocial functioning of these patients (Table 3-13). The nursing diagnoses focus on the impact of physiologic changes on the patient's functioning. The chronic dyspnea can influence activity tolerance and ability to care for the self. Coughing and shortness of breath can disturb sleep and contribute to chronic feelings of fatigue. The extra work of breathing can increase calorie requirements, but eating and swallowing may be limited by dyspnea. Certain medications like theophylline can cause nausea and vomiting contributing to decreased intake. Feelings of anxiety and suffocation can occur because of chronic hypoxia. The patient may also feel powerless as the disease progresses despite efforts to comply with the treatment regimen. Family members may have to take on new roles as the patient's activity tolerance declines. COPD is a chronic and progressive disease with many implications for the family as well as the patient.

COPD affects so many aspects of the patient's life, and nursing can help the patient and the family adjust to the changes. (See Bibliography on page 101 for sources of extensive care plans for patients with COPD). Nursing treatments begin with discouraging smoking because it will slow disease progression, decrease irritation and sputum production, and improve oxygenation. Nursing interventions for the patient with COPD might also include:

1. **Teach effective breathing patterns** such as purse-lipped and diaphragmatic breathing; use high-Fowler's position and tables to "prop" on. (Rationale: Improves ventilation of the alveoli by maintaining intrathoracic pressure at the end of exhalation.)

2. **Improve airway clearance** by encouraging the patient to cough or "huff" every 1 to 2 hours, humidify air, encourage 10 glasses of fluid per day, nebulizer treatments, bronchodilators, expectorants, and postural drainage therapy (PDT) as ordered. (Rationale: Removes mucus from airways allowing better ventilation.)

3. **Improve gas exchange** by using all the above interventions plus incentive spirometry every 1 to 2 hours, and low-flow oxygen therapy (1 to 2 L/min as ordered to maintain a PO_2 of 55 mmHg). Remember that many patients with COPD rely on the hypoxemic drive to stimulate respiration. Cautiously administer oxygen, watching for decreased respiratory rate and mental acuity or signs of respiratory failure. (Rationale: Low-flow oxygen therapy and incentive spirometry will help increase the tidal volume and available oxygen.)

4. **Take medications as ordered** by the health care provider. These may include an inhaled anticholinergic (eg, ipratropium), either alone or with an inhaled short-acting beta-agonist (eg, albuterol), or a long-acting beta-agonist (eg, salmeterol). (Rationale: Medications taken as directed can increase airway diameters, decrease mucus production, and decrease the incidence of exacerbation.)

5. **Encourage adequate nutritional intake** by monitoring meals and weight, serve easily chewed foods in small portions, and allow rest periods to minimize fatigue. (Rationale: Small eating periods and portions are not as fatiguing.)

6. **Prevent infections** with influenza (annually) and pneumococcal vaccines (one time, reassess in 5 years). Teach patient to watch for changes in sputum (yellow to green, more copious) or increased temperature, and report to health care provider. Avoid crowded areas, take antibiotics as ordered, and clean respiratory equipment properly. (Rationale: Patients with COPD are susceptible to infections, and prevention and early detection are essential components of nursing care.)

7. **Evaluate activity tolerance**, and help patient and family plan daily activities to minimize fatigue. Use breathing techniques and supplemental oxygen as needed. Activities should be spaced over the day and avoided for 30 minutes after eating when patients tend to be fatigued. Activities can be gradually increased as tolerated by the patient. Patient should coordinate activity with pursed-lipped breathing on exhalation during the work part of an activity. (Rationale: Paced activities allow the patient rest periods, minimizing dyspnea and fatigue.)

8. **Teach family to assess patient's orientation** and report changes like drowsiness and confusion to the health care provider. (Rationale: Disorientation may signal hypoxemia, and further assessment and intervention by the health care provider may be needed.)

9. **Teach patient and family about COPD; stress healthy behaviors, smoking cessation, and the signs of potential problems**. Encourage the patient to use local organizations like the American Lung Association. (Rationale: When patients and their families understand the disease and how they can actively participate in their care, they feel more in control and comply with treatment regimens.)

10. **Promote healthy sleep patterns** by evaluating sleep patterns, discouraging daytime naps and beverages with caffeine, and using techniques to optimize oxygenation, including position and supplemental oxygen as ordered. Evaluate patients for

obstructive sleep apnea syndrome (eg, snoring, choking, and gasping during sleep) as the incidence increases in COPD patients. (Rationale: Patients experience less fatigue and have more energy for their life activities.)

11. **Decrease feelings of powerlessness** by evaluating the patient's perceptions about heath, incorporating the patient in decisions about care, and explaining that exacerbations are part of COPD. (Rationale: Patients who feel more in control are less powerless to their disease process and are more compliant in their treatment plan.)

Asthma

Increasing numbers of Americans are suffering from asthma. Over 12 million people of all ages are afflicted with the airway obstruction and inflammation, which are the hallmarks of asthma. Over 5000 people a year die from asthma. It is more common in African-Americans and there seems to be a genetic component because it often runs in families. Asthma is characterized as a disease of increased responsiveness of the tracheobronchial tree to various stimuli with resulting bronchospasm and inflammation of the bronchial mucosa. Episodes are variable in severity and the changes in airflow are often reversible.

Asthma can be divided into two types: *intrinsic* and *extrinsic*. Intrinsic asthma is considered a nonallergic type of asthma where bronchospasm is the reaction to a virus in the upper respiratory tract to cold air or exercise. Extrinsic occurs as a response to an allergen or trigger to which the patient is hyperresponsive. It is thought that extrinsic asthma is mediated by immunoglobulin-E (IgE). Extrinsic asthma appears more often in children and may disappear during adolescence.

The classic wheezing and dyspnea of asthma are caused by a variety of cellular responses. Although the exact etiology of asthma is not known, there are many causative agents. Some of the more common triggers are:

- Air pollutants (cigarette smoke, industrial pollution, and formaldehyde)
- Perfumes
- Cold, dry air or abrupt weather changes
- Allergens (feathers, animal dander, dust mites, pollen)
- Foods, especially those with sulfites (wine, beer, salad, dried fruits, eggs)
- Viral infections
- Gastroesophageal reflux disease
- Stress
- Anxiety
- Exercise
- Wood and vegetable (flour) dust
- Assorted chemicals and enzymes (solvents, rubber and latex, paints, laundry detergents)
- Medications such as aspirin, other nonsteroidal anti-inflammatory drugs, and beta-blockers
- Food additives such as monosodium glutamate (MSG) and tartrazine (yellow dye)
- Endocrine factors (menses, pregnancy, and thyroid disease)

A trigger, whether intrinsic or extrinsic, causes a complex series of pathophysiologic responses during an asthma attack. An asthma attack can be divided into an early and late response. The early response is characterized by bronchospasm when the mast cells in the bronchial walls are stimulated and release histamine, which in turn triggers constriction of the smooth muscle in the bronchial walls, swelling of the mucus membranes, and increased mucus production. The early response lasts about 90 minutes.

The late response is the lung's immune system reacting to the trigger. This will occur 3 to 4 hours later and can last up to 12 hours. Eosinophils and mast cells produce a variety of chemical mediators such as prostaglandins, leukotrienes, bradykinin, and platelet activating factor. These mediators cause sustained inflammation of the bronchial walls with increased vascular permeability, edema, increased mucus production, and heightened responsiveness to the trigger. The next exposure to the trigger may cause a brisker response, beginning a vicious cycle of trigger and response. Prolonged inflammation may subsequently damage the pulmonary tissues, causing thickening of the membranes, destruction of the ciliated cells, and hypertrophy of the mucus glands (Figures 3-5 and 3-6).

Assessment

The classic symptoms of an asthma attack are dyspnea, wheezing, paroxysmal cough, and tightness in the chest. Patients are often very anxious and have increased respiratory and heart rates. In patients with severe asthma, the attacks may actually occur during sleep (nocturnal asthma). On auscultation, the patient may have wheezing and prolonged expiration. The severity of the attacks can be variable in the same patient. A severe asthma attack may be associated with loud wheezing, use of accessory muscles, and distant breath sounds on auscultation. The breathlessness may be so severe as to make the patient speak in one- or two-word responses. Asthma attacks can be fatal, and the mortality rate is increasing despite better understanding of the disease process. Ominous signs include decreased wheezing, inaudible breath sounds, cyanosis, fatigue, and inability to lie down. Nurses should be aware of these signs and the risk of respiratory and heart failure in these patients.

Diagnosis of asthma is based on clinical presentation, history, physical examination, pulmonary function tests, and pulse oximetry and/or arterial blood gas measurements. The nurse is often the first contact for the patient experiencing an asthma attack, and a calm attitude and reassuring manner will help decrease the patient's anxiety. The history should include the course of this attack, previous episodes of shortness of breath, age of onset, precipitating factors, and how the symptoms influence the patient's functioning. Conditions associated with asthma include atopic dermatitis, nasal polyps, rhinitis, and sinusitis.

Pulmonary function tests, particularly peak expiratory flow rate (PEFR), FVC, maximum mid-expiratory flow (MMEF), and FEV will show decreased values during an attack and improve after treatment. The PEFR measures the rate of airflow with a forced expiration. Small, inexpensive PEFR meters can be used at home by patients to measure treatment effectiveness and evaluate possible attacks. Following PEFR at home twice a day can aid in asthma management. A peak flow meter measures the highest expiratory flow volume (Figure 3-7). Arterial blood gas values and pulse oximetry are also used to reveal the extent of the hypoxemia and possible need for hospitalization. Typically, the ABGs will reveal hypoxemia and respiratory alkalosis as a result of the increased respiratory rate. If the asthma worsens, the acid-base balance will shift to respiratory acidosis from carbon dioxide retention as well as hypoxemia.

Other laboratory tests to diagnose asthma include the methacholine provocation tests, allergy testing, sputum stain for eosinophils, chest x-rays, possibly sinus x-rays, and rhinoscopy. The provocation tests are done in a hospital setting and a trigger such as methacholine (a beta-agonist) or cold air is used, and then pulmonary function tests meas-

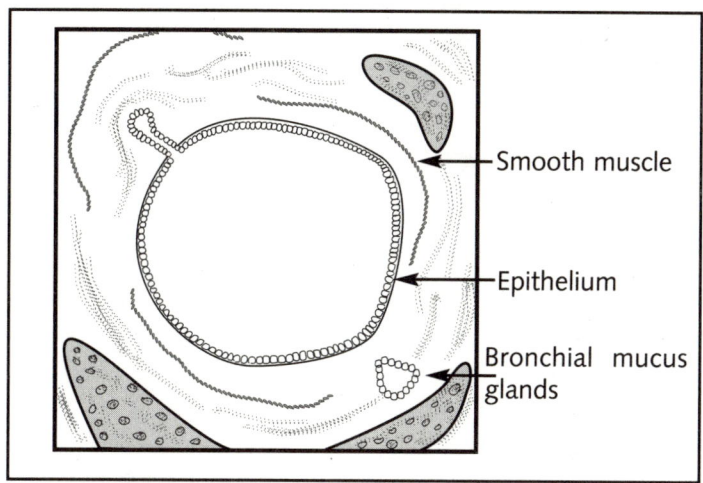

Figure 3-5. Normal bronchiole.

Smooth muscle

Epithelium

Bronchial mucus glands

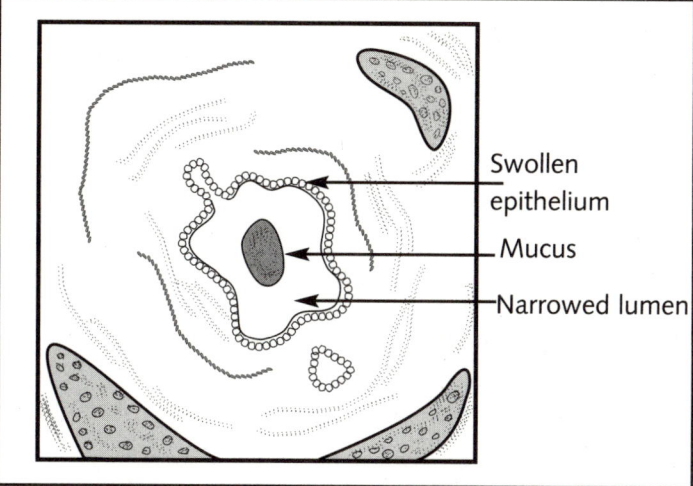

Figure 3-6. Bronchiole in asthma.

Swollen epithelium

Mucus

Narrowed lumen

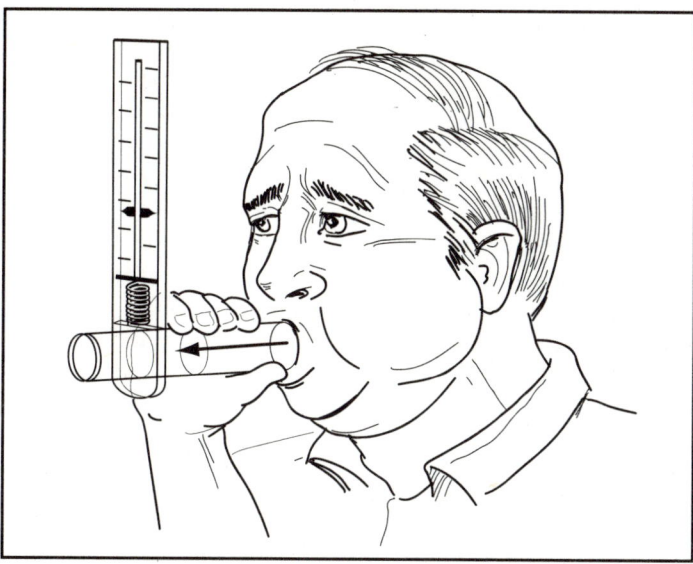

Figure 3-7. Peak flow meter.

ure the bronchial response to the trigger. The patient is then treated with a bronchodilator to relieve the bronchospasm.

Treatment

The guidelines for the treatment and management of asthma published by the National Heart, Lung and Blood Institute (NHLBI) in 1992 detail the primary objectives of therapy as the following:

1. Maintain normal activity levels (including exercise).
2. Maintain near normal pulmonary function rates.
3. Prevent chronic and troublesome symptoms.
4. Prevent recurrent exacerbations of asthma.
5. Avoid adverse effects from asthma medications.

Asthma is a reversible disease that is treated depending on the frequency and severity of the disease. The four stages are mild (episodic), moderate (one to two times a week), severe, and status asthmatic. Treatment of all stages involves nonpharmacological and pharmacological methods. Nonpharmacological methods are aimed at preventing attacks and intervening early during an attack. They include:

1. Patient education about disease.
2. Identification of triggers in the environment.
3. Eradication of triggers such as cigarette smoke, dust mites, and animal dander (see Table 3-5).
4. Relaxation techniques such as controlled breathing.
5. Immunotherapy through a desensitization program to block IgE response.

Pharmacological management of asthma includes bronchodilators and anti-inflammatory agents. Bronchodilators such as theophylline, beta2-agonists, and inhaled anticholinergics act primarily to relax bronchial smooth muscle and dilate the airways. Theophylline is administered orally or intravenously as aminophylline. Time-released oral formulations help to minimize toxicity and side effects and achieve more stable blood levels. Theophylline toxicity is fairly common and includes nausea, vomiting, dizziness, rapid pulse, twitching, insomnia, and seizures.

Beta$_2$-agonists are effective bronchodilators which do not affect the heart. Beta1-agonists, like epinephrine, are bronchodilators and cardiac stimulants. Beta$_2$-agonists are usually administered via inhalation with a metered-dose inhaler (MDI) but may also be administered subcutaneously and orally (Figure 3-8). Correct use of the MDI is essential for accurate administration of the medication into the lungs, and spacers are often used to make the coordination of inhalation and release of medication easier (Table 3-14).

Anticholinergics are used as bronchodilators in some patients. They are administered by inhalation and block acetylcholine, a chemical mediator involved in bronchoconstriction. Ipratropium bromide is an inhaled anticholinergic.

The anti-inflammatory drugs can be divided into the corticosteroids and cromolyn. Corticosteroids provide anti-inflammatory and immunosuppressive effects to relieve bronchial edema. They may be given orally, intravenously, intramuscularly, or by inhalation. Oral steroids like prednisone are given for severe asthma and should never be stopped abruptly, but tapered slowly. Some steroids are given by inhalation, like beclamethasone, because this route provides all the anti-inflammatory effects without the systemic side effects of steroids. An MDI with a spacer gives more direct steroid administration into the lungs without the residual drug in the mouth. Residual steroids on the oral mucosa can predispose the patient to thrush infections. In patients with moderate to

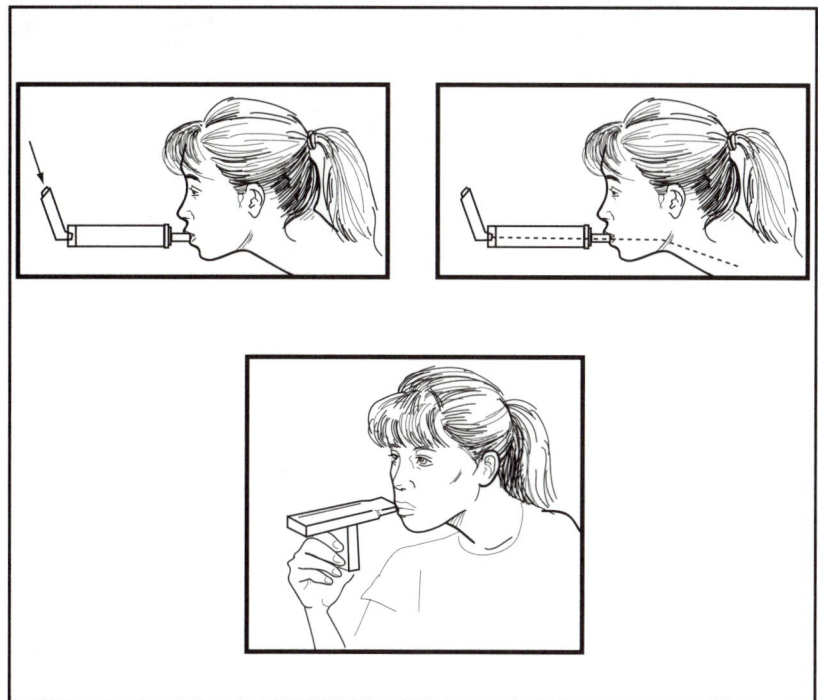

Figure 3-8. Metered dose inhaler.

Table 3-14

Correct Use of a Metered-Dose Inhaler (MDI)

1. Remove the cap from the MDI.
2. Shake MDI.
3. Place index finger on top of canister and thumb on bottom of mouthpiece.
4. Take a breath in and out slowly.
5. Place inhaler about 1 inch in front of open mouth.
6. At the beginning of inhalation, press down on the canister and, at the same time begin to inhale slowly and deeply.
7. Hold breath 5 to 10 seconds.
8. Wait 1 to 2 minutes and repeat as directed.
9. Rinse out mouth and spit out (if steroid inhaler is used).
10. If using a spacer, follow directions except place lips around spacer mouthpiece.
11. Rinse inhaler in warm water to clean.

severe asthma who require long-term steroid use, inhalation is the preferred route of administration.

Cromolyn is an anti-inflammatory drug in a different class from corticosteroids. Cromolyn stabilizes the mast cells, thereby preventing the release of histamine, a potent bronchoconstrictor. Cromolyn may be given by inhalation or in a nasal spray to stabilize the nasal mucosa in allergic rhinitis. It is used prophylactically before exposure to a known trigger. Cromolyn is never used during an acute asthma attack.

Table 3-15

Potential Nursing Diagnoses for Patients With Asthma

1. Impaired Gas Exchange (related to bronchoconstriction).
2. Fear (related to difficulty breathing).
3. Knowledge Deficit (related to health care management of asthma).
4. Ineffective Airway Clearance (related to increased mucus production).
5. Risk for Infection (related to airway changes).

Nursing management of the patient with asthma requires educating the patient and his significant others. For patients with mild to moderate asthma, education about asthma, environmental triggers, medications and their side effects, and treatment follow-up can control the disease and prevent attacks (Table 3-15). Patients also need to understand when to seek treatment if their medications are not relieving their symptoms. Nursing care for the patient with mild to moderate asthma includes:

- Monitor your PEFR per the NHBLI guidelines for 2 to 4 weeks to obtain a "personal best" average.
- Follow the "zone system" (green, yellow, red) for taking medications. Green for a PEFR 80% to 100% of personal best and no symptoms, use maintenance medications. Yellow for a PEFR of 50% to 80%, use rescue medication plan. Red for PEFR of < 50%, use bronchodilator and if no improvement in 10 to 15 minutes, call a health care provider or go to an emergency room.
- Take medications in the correct order: Beta-agonists first, followed by steroids. Use the MDI correctly. Use bronchodilator 30 minutes before exercise if this triggers asthma.
- Use beta$_2$-agonists like metaproterenol or albuterol to relieve wheezing during an attack. Do not use steroids or cromolyn during an attack (rescue medications). If the beta-agonist does not relieve symptoms in 10 to 15 minutes, go to the emergency room or contact your health care provider.
- Identify and eliminate environmental triggers, such as animal dander, dust mites, feather pillows and puffs, cigarette smoke. Clean regularly with a damp cloth. Clean furnace and air conditioners annually. Wash all bedding in hot water (see Table 3-5).
- Reduce stress and anxiety. Get enough sleep and rest. Try relaxation techniques.
- Avoid medications such as aspirin and NSAIDs that may precipitate attacks, and avoid antihypertensives that contain an angiotensin-converting enzyme (ACE) because these drugs may worsen a cough associated with bronchoconstriction.
- Try to avoid respiratory infections that may precipitate an attack by avoiding crowds and infected people and receiving the influenza vaccine annually.
- Continue activity at a normal level, avoiding possible triggers like cold air.
- Drink an adequate amount (2.5 to 3 L per day) to liquefy secretions.
- Seek emergency care if medications fail to control symptoms; nails or lips are gray or blue; difficulty breathing, walking, or talking; declining PEFR rates (falls into red zone < 50% of personal best).

Severe asthma and *status asthmaticus* are potentially life-threatening conditions that need close care and follow-up. Symptoms of severe asthma include frequent attacks with nocturnal awakenings that result in limited activity levels. Status asthmaticus is severe, prolonged asthma which does not respond to conventional treatment. Patients are seen in the emergency room for oxygen therapy, intravenous medications like aminophylline and epinephrine, inhaled beta-agonists, antibiotic therapy for presumed infection, and careful evaluation of respiratory function. They may be quite anxious and fatigued from the work of breathing. Pulse oximetry and arterial blood gases help to determine whether respiratory failure is imminent and whether endotracheal intubation with mechanical ventilation is necessary. Usually, the medications and oxygen reverse the wheezing and the patient recovers. In 1% to 3% of cases of status asthmaticus, respiratory failure, acidemia, and cardiac dysrhythmias result in death.

Asthma is a very treatable disease, and most patients do well with the appropriate medications and elimination of triggers. Thorough teaching about the disease and treatment plan gives patients and their families the ability to control the asthma. A caring health care team can give them the resources to call if home management is not working.

Acute Respiratory Failure

Patients with acute respiratory failure are seriously ill and require intensive care and support. There are many different causes of respiratory failure (Table 3-16). Acute respiratory failure is defined as gas exchange that is inadequate to meet the metabolic needs of the body. The signs of symptoms of acute respiratory failure depend on the underlying condition. The entire respiratory system (the lungs, the central nervous system, the heart, the respiratory muscles, and the airways) is involved in oxygenation. Disorders in any of these components of the respiratory system can lead to respiratory failure.

Assessment

The hallmark signs of respiratory failure are *hypoxemia* and *hypercapnia*. Hypoxemia is defined as an arterial oxygen concentration of less than 60 mmHg. Patients with hypoxemia are usually dyspneic and may be anxious, disoriented, confused, and delirious. Other signs of hypoxemia are central cyanosis, tachypnea, tachycardia, hypertension, and tremors. Hypercapnia is defined as an arterial carbon dioxide concentration ($PaCO_2$) greater than 50 mmHg. Patients are hypercapnic because they are hypoventilating. They may experience dyspnea and headache as well as changes to the sensorium: confusion and delirium. The only way to know for sure if respiratory failure is imminent is to obtain an arterial blood gas. Oxygen saturation (O_2 Sat) may be helpful, but it is wise to remember that an O_2 Sat of 90% approximates a PaO_2 of 60 mmHg.

The most common cause of hypoxemic respiratory failure is a ventilation/perfusion (V/Q) mismatch. In normal lungs, the areas of the alveoli that are aerated also have an adequate blood supply, allowing gas exchange to take place. The V/Q ratio is one way to compare the pulmonary ventilation to the pulmonary circulation. Ventilation without perfusion occurs when there is adequate ventilation but the circulation to alveoli is blocked (eg, pulmonary embolism). Perfusion without ventilation occurs when the oxygen does not reach the perfused alveolar membrane. This occurs when secretions and edema block ventilation and diffusion at the alveolar membrane (Figure 3-9).

Treatment

Treatment for respiratory failure revolves around maintaining an open airway and ensuring alveolar ventilation. Nurses constantly evaluate the patency of the airway and a patient's ability to clear secretions. The goal of treatment in hypoxemic respiratory failure

Table 3-16

Causes of Respiratory Failure

1. Disorders of chronic airflow limitation (asthma, chronic bronchitis, emphysema).
2. Acute respiratory distress syndrome (ARDS).
3. Congestive heart failure.
4. Pneumonia.
5. Pulmonary embolism (impairs pulmonary circulation).
6. Flail chest and pneumothorax.
7. Neuromuscular disorders (drug overdose, Guillain-Barré syndrome, spinal cord injury, stroke, and myasthenia gravis).
8. Airway obstructions (foreign bodies, secretions, tumors, infections).

Figure 3-9. Ventilation mismatch in pulmonary embolism.

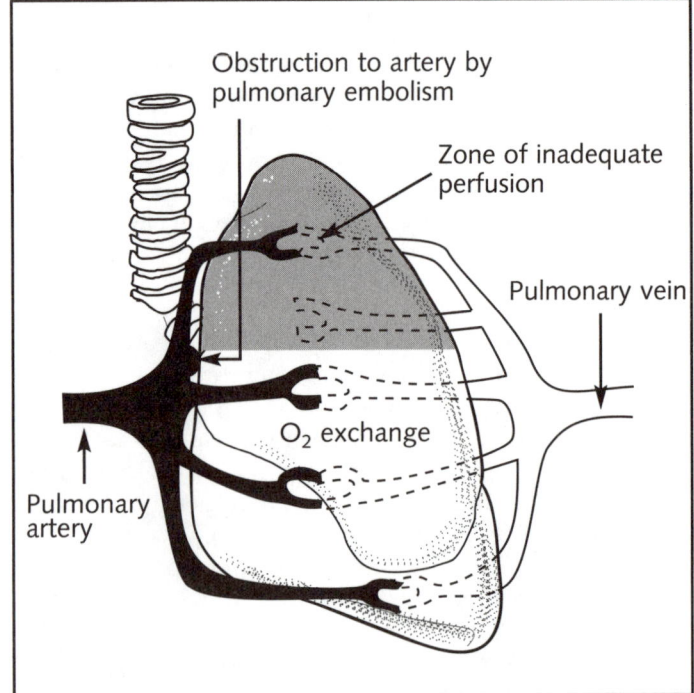

is to ensure adequate oxygenation to the vital organs (brain, heart, and lungs). Specific treatments are directed at the underlying disease process and symptoms. In the case of pulmonary embolism, treatment may include supplemental oxygen, V/Q scan, and TPA or heparin. The goal of oxygen supplementation is to maintain the O_2 Sat at or above 90% so that the patient's PaO_2 is about 60 mmHg. This will allow the organs to receive enough oxygen to remain viable. If more aggressive means are needed to maintain airway patency or ensure alveolar ventilation, endotracheal intubation and mechanical ventilation may be necessary. The care of the patient with an endotracheal tube and/or mechanical ventilation is discussed on page 128.

Table 3-17

Nursing Diagnoses for Patients With Acute Respiratory Failure

1. Impaired Gas Exchange (related to the underlying disease, secretions, COPD, air way obstruction, V/Q mismatch, etc).
2. Fear or Anxiety (related to dyspnea, worsening condition).
3. Ineffective Airway Clearance (related to secretions, neuromuscular weakness, and intubation).
4. Risk for Infection (actual as in pneumonia or potential due to interventions).
5. Potential Fluid Imbalance (related to heart failure, sodium retention, and inadequate fluid intake).

Patients with acute respiratory failure will have varying courses depending on the underlying disease. Nursing care of the patient with acute respiratory failure involves careful attention to vital sign changes, implementing respiratory interventions, and assessing the response to treatment (Table 3-17). The goals of treatment are to maintain adequate arterial oxygenation, pulmonary ventilation, and treating the underlying condition. Nursing interventions for each nursing diagnosis are as follows:

1. **Impaired Gas Exchange**
   - Monitor vital signs every 15 minutes.
     - Watch for tachypnea, tachycardia, and check temperature hourly, especially if infection in suspected. (Rationale: Increasing heart rate or respiratory rate could be indicative of increasing respiratory failure.)
     - Check for pulsus paradoxus. (A drop in systolic blood pressure greater than 10 mmHg during inspiration.)
   - Monitor arterial blood gases every 30 minutes or as ordered.
   - Watch for decreasing PaO_2, or increasing $PaCO_2$.
   - Watch for decreasing pH, or increasing pH if compensation by the kidneys has occurred with bicarbonate retention. (Rationale: Arterial blood gas values provide guidance to treatment and indicate patient response to interventions.)
   - Observe for restlessness or anxiety. (Rationale: This may signal falling O_2 levels.)
   - Encourage the patient to cough every 15 to 30 minutes. (Rationale: Secretions may block airways and prevent ventilation of the alveoli.)
   - If the patient with COPD is in acute distress, keep him awake and breathing deeply to keep his pH greater than 7.25. (Rationale: Patients with COPD may need hypoxemia to drive the respiratory rate and may not inhale deeply if their O_2 levels rise with supplemental oxygen.) As the patient improves he can be allowed short rest periods.
   - Auscultate breath sounds every hour or more often if vital signs change.
     - Notify physician if increasing crackles and dyspnea.
     - Notify physician if diminished breath sounds. (Rationale: Early changes in respiratory function will be detected and interventions altered.)

- Administer supplemental O_2 to maintain a PaO_2 above 60 mmHg and SaO_2 over 90%. Frequently assess the inspired oxygen (FiO_2) levels, ABGs, and pulse oximetry. Mechanical ventilation may be required if PaO_2 levels continue to fall below 60 mmHg despite reasonable oxygen concentrations. (Note: Cautiously administer oxygen at 1 to 2 L per min in patients with COPD, and increase as necessary based on the ABGs and pulse oximetry so as not to override the patient's hypoxic drive). (Rationale: Continuous assessment of respiratory status allows changes in interventions to maintain adequate oxygenation.)
- Use sedatives and hypnotics cautiously in patients who are in acute respiratory failure but not mechanically ventilated, as they may depress respiratory drive. Ventilated patients will require sedation and need support despite being sedated, as they may be conscious and frightened.

2. **Fear and Anxiety**
   - Allow for accepting environment for patient's feelings but be aware of the possibility that increasing anxiety and restlessness may indicate worsening hypoxia.
   - Stay with patient if he is dyspneic, as he may be frightened.
   - Reassure patient during episodes.
   - Gently remind him to take slow breaths.
   - Do not tell the patient to "relax," as this may provoke anger.
   - Allow visitors when appropriate for short visits so as not to make the patient tired. Make sure visitors do not have signs of colds or infections. (Rationale: Hypoxemia and dyspnea will both make the patient anxious and the nurse's support and reassurance are invaluable.)

3. **Ineffective Airway Clearance**
   - Remind the patient to cough every 15 to 30 minutes using whatever technique best clears the airway.
   - Elevate the head of the bed so the patient is in Fowler's or semi-Fowler's position and change position every 1 to 2 hours.
   - Use percussion or vibration and postural drainage to facilitate movement of mucus.
   - Increase fluid intake to keep secretions liquid.
   - Administer bronchodilators prior to percussion and vibration.
   - Provide humidified air to aid in liquefying secretions.
   - Obtain sputum for culture and sensitivity, if ordered.
   - Provide frequent mouth care and dispose of all secretions quickly. (Rationale: The lung injury that occurs in respiratory failure causes increased permeability in the alveolar membrane with leakage of fluid and proteins into the alveoli. Clearing the airways will increase alveolar ventilation and oxygenation.)

4. **Risk for Infection**
   - Monitor temperature every hour if fever is present.
   - Administer antibiotics as ordered.
   - Screen all visitors with colds or potential infections. (Rationale: Patients with respiratory failure often have infections that set off the chain of events that leads to respiratory failure. Careful monitoring of temperature and other signs of infection will direct treatment.)

5. **Potential Fluid Imbalance**
   - Monitor intake and output.
   - Follow hemoglobin and hematocrit for signs of fluid overload.
   - Watch for neck vein distention, tachycardia, and tachypnea as signs of right-sided heart failure.
   - Maintain nutritional status with small, frequent, high-protein meals; limit salt intake in patients with COPD as it could increase fluid retention and increase the risk of heart failure. (Rationale: The work of breathing greatly increases with respiratory failure and the patient may not be able to consume sufficient calories, requiring parenteral nutrition. Patients are at risk for fluid overload and heart failure due to increased pressure in the pulmonary vasculature.)

Adult Respiratory Distress Syndrome

Adult Respiratory Distress Syndrome (ARDS) is a severe, life-threatening condition that occurs as a complication of a variety of clinical disorders, from sepsis to trauma. ARDS is manifested by dyspnea, severe hypoxemia, decreased lung compliance, and noncardiac pulmonary edema. Despite the advancements in technology and the understanding of ARDS, this is a deadly syndrome with a mortality rate above 50%.

The onset of ARDS is often quite sudden and nursing care revolves around understanding the patients at risk and watching for early signs of respiratory failure. Certain disorders put patients at risk for developing ARDS, including:

1. Trauma—massive bodily injury, increased intracranial pressure from head trauma, tumor, or cerebral vascular accident.
2. Sepsis—infection, septicemia (particularly gram-negative sepsis), pneumonia.
3. Shock—hemorrhagic, septic, or anaphylactic shock.
4. Toxins—inhaled noxious gases and smoke, oxygen toxicity, drug overdose.
5. Hemolytic disorders—disseminated intravascular coagulation (DIC), multiple blood transfusions.
6. Complications of cardiopulmonary bypass.
7. Aspiration—gastric contents, near-drowning.
8. Fat and amniotic fluid emboli.
9. Pancreatitis.

ARDS develops as a result of damage to the lungs by chemical mediators. Many different mediators have been identified as causative agents, such as platelet-activating factor, histamines, and tumor necrosis factor (TNF). The process begins as an inflammatory reaction with increased capillary permeability and the release of neutrophils into the interstitium of the lung. The leakage from the capillaries results in massive fluid loss from the vascular space and into the alveoli. The flooded alveoli cannot participate in gas exchange, resulting in severe hypoxemia. With less alveolar surface area available for gas exchange, a ventilation-perfusion mismatch develops (the circulation is adequate but the ventilation is impaired). The terminal airways become compressed by the edema and lung compliance decreases. The chemical mediators cause damage to the alveolar epithelium. The cascade of events ends in fibrosis, scarring of the lungs, and refractory hypoxemia despite supplemental oxygen. ARDS can be fatal unless intensive interventions are initiated to maintain oxygenation.

Clinical presentations of ARDS vary depending on the precipitating event, but usually appear within 24 to 48 hours of the event. Nurses should be aware of patients who are at high risk for ARDS and should watch for the following signs and symptoms:

1. Rapid onset of tachypnea and dyspnea.
2. Tachycardia.
3. Increasing anxiety, restlessness, and agitation (due to worsening hypoxemia).

Early in the course of ARDS, the breath sounds and chest x-ray may be normal because the edema is in the interstitial spaces. As fluid begins to fill the intra-alveolar space, the breath sounds become diminished and there are diffuse fine crackles on auscultation. Initially, arterial blood gases show a low $PaCO_2$ due to compensatory hyperventilation. As the alveolar surface area available for gas exchange decreases, the $PaCO_2$ increases, PaO_2 decreases, and acidosis develops. The increasing fluid in the alveoli and lung interstitium soon becomes apparent on the chest x-ray as diffuse bilateral pulmonary infiltrates. Treatment of ARDS revolves around identification and treatment of the underlying cause and supportive respiratory care. Most patients with ARDS require endotracheal intubation and mechanical ventilation to support adequate oxygenation. Patients with ARDS respond poorly to increased concentrations of oxygen. The PaO_2 may not correspond to the amount of FiO_2. This is called the gradient between the alveolar and arterial oxygen content. Patients with ARDS need progressively higher concentrations of oxygen to maintain an adequate PaO_2.

Two methods of increasing the arterial oxygen levels are *positive end expiratory pressure* (PEEP) and *continuous positive airway pressure* (CPAP). PEEP can enhance oxygenation by keeping airways open at the end of expiration. CPAP may also be used to enhance oxygenation (discussion of these topics begins on page 126.) Pressures in the pulmonary vasculature are monitored with pulmonary artery catheters, such as a Swan-Ganz catheter.

> ARDS develops as a result of damage to the lungs by chemical mediators such as platelet-activating factor, histamines, and tumor necrosis factor (TNF). The syndrome begins with an inflammatory process with increased capillary permeability and leakage of fluid into the alveoli. The flooded alveoli can no longer participate in gas exchange, resulting in hypoxemia.

Antibiotics are used to treat any underlying infection that may have precipitated the ARDS. Blood transfusions and intravenous colloids are infused to maintain the circulating blood volume and improve the oxygen-carrying capacity of the blood.

Nursing management of the patient with ARDS begins with the identification of patients who are at risk and early detection of this syndrome (Table 3-18). Patients who are at risk for developing ARDS should be carefully monitored. Patients with ARDS are cared for in an intensive care unit. If changes in vital signs, arterial blood gases, or sensorium occur, then the physician should immediately be notified. Tachypnea and restlessness may be the earliest signs of impending ARDS. A minimal rise or a dropping PaO_2, despite treatment with a high flow rate (8 to 10 L per min) of oxygen, or a rise in the $PaCO_2$ may be early clinical signs of respiratory failure. A PaO_2 less than 55 to 60 mmHg in a patient without chronic lung disease is an indication of respiratory failure. Early treatment may prevent the development of full-blown ARDS.

The main objectives of nursing care for the patient with ARDS are to support the patient's vital signs and maintain the patient's oxygenation despite increasing demands for oxygen. Their care is similar to that of the patient with respiratory failure. Airway management with intubation and mechanical ventilation allows for greater control of ventilation and oxygenation if other noninvasive treatments fail to improve oxygenation. Techniques, such as coughing and suctioning, are used as necessary to maintain an open

Table 3-18

Potential Nursing Diagnoses for Patients With ARDS

1. Impaired Gas Exchange (related to ventilation failure, ARDS).
2. Inability to Maintain Spontaneous Ventilation (related to pulmonary edema, hypoxemia, head or chest trauma).
3. Fluid Volume Deficit (related to pulmonary edema, trauma).
4. Risk for Infection (related to artificial airway, retained secretions).

airway. Blood pressure, pulmonary capillary wedge pressure, and cardiac output are monitored to guide fluid replacement. Pulmonary capillary wedge pressures may increase during ARDS as a result of hypoxemia triggering pulmonary vasoconstriction. This vasoconstriction shunts blood to better-ventilated parts of the lungs. The goal of fluid replacement is to maintain an adequate circulating volume and maximize the oxygen-carrying capability of the blood. Different positions may be used to optimize oxygenation. The prone position or semi-Fowler's position may improve alveolar ventilation and oxygen diffusion. Antibiotics may be used to treat any infection.

The prognosis for patients with ARDS depends on the amount of lung and other organ damage and the precipitating event. The mortality rate exceeds 50%, but newer therapies such as monoclonal antibodies and surfactant may improve the outcome for patients with ARDS.

Lung Cancer

The incidence of lung cancer has increased steadily for men and women for several decades. While the rate for men has stabilized recently, the rate for women is now almost equal to men. The typical patient with lung cancer is a male, 55 to 60 years of age, with a smoking history. Most lung cancer results from chronic inhalation of carcinogens, particularly cigarette smoke. It is important to emphasize that cigarette smoking is the number-one cause of death and disability in the United States and the number-one cause of lung cancer. Occupational exposure to carcinogens can occur from sources such as asbestos, petroleum products, carbon-containing products, coal dust, and radiation exposure. Occupational exposure accounts for only a small proportion of lung cancer, and tobacco smoking is the overwhelming cause of most lung cancers.

Most patients are asymptomatic when their lung cancers are discovered, perhaps by a routine preoperative chest x-ray. They may present with hemoptysis, dyspnea, chest pain, or pleuritic pain. Patients with metastatic disease (ie, cancer that has spread from the original tumor to other parts of the body) may have more systemic symptoms like weight loss, fatigue, malaise, and anorexia. The prognosis is poor for patients with metastatic lung cancer. Regardless of the stage of the disease, less than 20% of all patients with lung cancer are cured of their disease.

The diagnosis is made by chest x-ray, lung biopsy, sputum cytology, bronchoscopy, mediastinoscopy, MRI, and/or CAT scan. There are four different classifications of lung cancer:
- Squamous cell carcinoma (25% to 35%)
- Adenocarcinoma (25% to 35%)
- Small cell or oat cell carcinoma (10% to 25%)
- Large cell or mixed carcinoma (5% to 20%)

Figure 3-10. Clinical features of lung cancer.

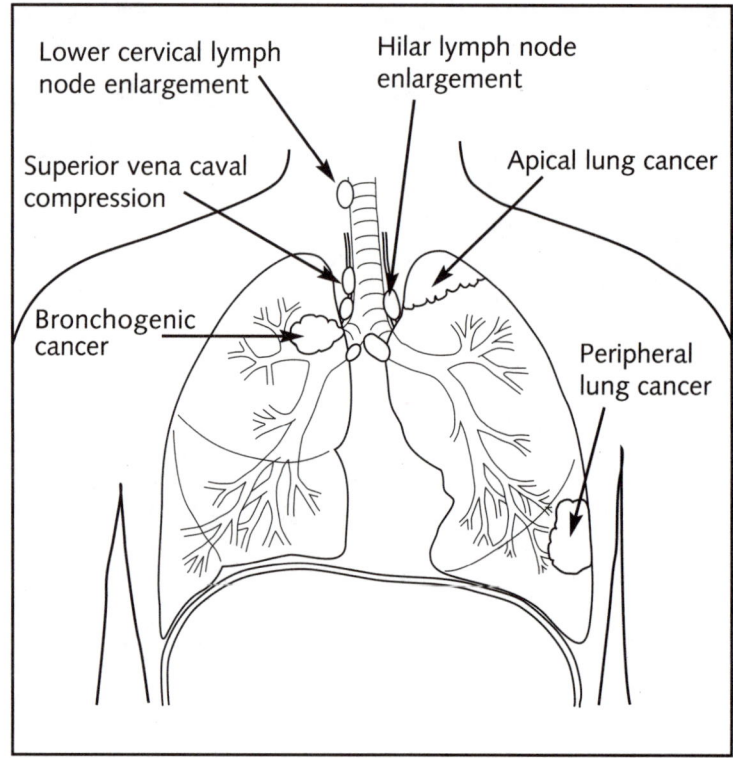

Small cell or oat cell carcinoma is considered separately because it is highly malignant and tends to metastasize early. Bronchogenic cancer can arise centrally at the hilar area (ie, where the mainstem bronchus splits into the right and left bronchi) or more peripherally in the bronchioles. The pathology of the tumor is useful in determining the appropriate treatment (Figure 3-10).

Staging of lung cancer is done with the TNM system (tumor, nodes, and metastases). There are four stages, with stage I being the smallest, most localized tumor and stage IV being advanced disease. Unfortunately, 80% of patients with lung cancer have advanced disease at the time of diagnosis. Lung cancer can grow quietly in the soft spongy tissue of the lungs, unnoticed for years. There are no pain receptors in lung tissue to signal tumor growth or invasion. The rich blood supply in the lungs feeds the tumor and provides a pathway for the tumor cells to spread throughout the body.

Advanced lung cancer shows a variety of symptoms that are far different from the tumor's pulmonary origins. The tumor can press against or destroy the recurrent laryngeal nerve, causing hoarseness. The lung cancer may have already metastasized to the bones, causing pain in distant sites. It may have spread to the bones in the vertebral column causing spinal cord compression with symptoms of weakness and numbness in the extremities. The bone metastases and altered renal function may cause symptoms of hypercalcemia (muscle weakness, anorexia, nausea, constipation, and lethargy). The superior vena cava may be compressed by a tumor, resulting in facial and arm swelling. In the syndrome of inappropriate antidiuretic hormone (SIADH), the tumor produces antidiuretic hormone (ADH), causing increased urine production and hypovolemia and hyponatremia. Advanced lung cancer does not always present respiratory symptoms.

The treatment is determined by the histology, location, and extent of the tumor; the lymph node involvement and the presence of metastases. Lung cancer metastasizes to other sites in the lungs and to the brain, bones, and liver. The patient's pulmonary and cardiac status also impact decisions about treatment, including surgery. Surgery is not curative in most cases of lung cancer.

Nonsmall-cell lung cancer in the earliest stages (I and II) may be treated surgically. If the patient has sufficient respiratory capacity, then the surgeon can perform a lobectomy (removal of the affected lobe) or pneumonectomy (removal of the lung). Surgery is not usually successful if the disease is advanced at the time of diagnosis. Chemotherapy and radiation therapy may be used together or separately to treat the disease. Small-cell cancer and stage III nonsmall-cell cancer are treated with chemotherapy, which may extend the patient's survival time. Radiation therapy is used to treat nonoperable cancers and also to treat metastases to the bone and brain.

The role of nursing in lung cancer treatment begins with prevention. Education programs in the schools are essential to preventing smoking in the young. Community programs can encourage smoking cessation in established smokers by teaching the effects of cigarette smoke and offering cessation programs (see Table 3-10). Nurses need to educate the public about the risks of smoking and the effects of secondhand smoke, especially on children. Increasingly, lung cancer has become a disease of former smokers. Smoking cessation greatly reduces the risk of developing lung cancer but does not eliminate it. Former smokers need to be carefully evaluated for symptoms of lung cancer.

Nursing care of the patient with a lung cancer diagnosis will vary depending on the treatment course and the progression of the disease. Patients undergoing surgical treatment, such as a thoracotomy for lobectomy or pneumonectomy, will need acute care before, during, and after their surgery (Tables 3-18 and 3-19).

Complications can occur after thoracic surgery. Potential problems during the postoperative period include atelectasis (collapse of alveoli) due to general anesthesia, poor cough effort, and stasis of secretions, pleural effusion related to the surgical disruption of normal pleural fluid drainage and malignant processes, and lung abscess related to infection and tumor necrosis.

Patients with lung cancer may require chemotherapy to improve their survival time, to treat symptoms of their disease, or to prevent complications. Cytotoxic drugs may be used alone or in conjunction with radiation therapy and surgery to shrink lung tumors and metastases. Multiple drugs are often used to increase the tumor cell kill. Some cytotoxic drugs are delivered intravenously and

> The role of nursing in lung cancer treatment begins with prevention. Education programs need to begin in schools to prevent smoking in children. Nurses need to educate the public about the dangers of secondhand smoke, especially for children.

others orally. The intravenous drugs may be delivered by different types of catheters, including central venous catheters and implanted infusion devices.

Cytotoxic drugs primarily affect the ability of the cell to replicate. This is a beneficial effect if the cell is malignant, but this same effect may be detrimental to normal cells. Since cytotoxic drugs can affect both normal and malignant cells, there are often side effects from chemotherapy. Specific drugs are known to cause side effects, such as vincristine, which sometimes has side effects related to neurotoxicity.

The drugs used in chemotherapy have their greatest effect on cells that are rapidly dividing (eg, in the hair follicles, bone marrow, skin and lining of the gastrointestinal tract and, of course, malignant cells). The most common side effects are hair loss (alopecia), bone marrow suppression with leukopenia (low white blood cell count), thrombocytope-

Table 3-18

Care of the Patient Undergoing a Thoracotomy

1. **Explain what the patient may experience during the perioperative period** (anesthesia, recovery room, chest tubes, incision, catheter, intravenous, etc). Describe preoperatively what the patient can do to facilitate healing and prevent complications (eg, deep breathing and coughing, using the incentive spirometer as indicated, asking for pain medication, ambulating with assist, splinting the incision, maintaining nutritional intake as soon as possible after surgery, increasing activity as allowed, balancing rest and activity, quitting smoking).

2. **Discuss the need for pain medication preoperatively, and try to reduce the anxiety related to the pain experience** (increased anxiety levels can increase pain). Administer pain medications or encourage patient to use patient-controlled analgesia (PCA) when uncomfortable so that he can cough effectively. Provide nonpharmacologic methods of pain relief (massage, position changes, diversional activities, relaxation techniques), teach patient how to splint the incision with a pillow during position changes and activity, secure drainage tubes, and report unrelieved pain to the physician.

3. **Decrease anxiety levels by working with the patient in a supportive, gentle manner.** Assess the patient's anxiety level and areas of concern, reassure him that you will do all you can to answer his questions and help him during the hospitalization, try to maintain the same caregivers on each shift, report excessive anxiety to the physician, and administer antianxiety medications as ordered.

4. **Promote solid respiratory recovery** with the following interventions: Assess the patient's airway, ventilation, and oxygenation; obtain vital signs every 15 minutes immediately postoperation; and then gradually decrease the frequency. Auscultate for breath sounds, encourage the patient to cough, deep breathe, and use the incentive spirometer every 1 to 2 hours. Assist the patient into the semi-Fowler's position when blood pressure is stable to improve the effectiveness of coughing and ventilation, help the patient splint the incision during activity including coughing, maintain patency of drainage tubes, use nursing interventions and medications to reduce pain, deliver oxygen therapy as ordered, monitor O_2 saturation and arterial blood gases as ordered, observe for complications such as increased drainage on the dressing, sudden increase in chest tube drainage, decreased or absent breath sounds, subcutaneous emphysema or any change in vital signs (tachypnea, hypotension, tachycardia), consult surgeon whenever the patient's status is questionable.

nia (low platelet count), nausea and vomiting, and mucositis (stomatitis), the breakdown of the lining of the gastrointestinal tract with oral ulcers and diarrhea.

The goals of nursing care for a patient receiving chemotherapy for lung cancer begin with educating the patient and family about the treatment and potential side effects. Nurses also administer cytotoxic agents in the hospital and in outpatient facilities. Prevention of complications, identification and treatment of side effects of chemotherapy, and maintenance of comfort are all part of nursing management. Some of the most challenging aspects of care are helping the patient to cope with changes in their body image, health, and lifestyle.

Table 3-19

Potential Nursing Diagnoses for the Patient Having a Thoracotomy

1. Knowledge Deficit related to the surgical course.
2. Pain related to the surgical incision.
3. Anxiety related to the diagnosis, surgery, and prognosis.
4. Ineffective Airway Clearance and Impaired Gas Exchange related to surgical pain, atelectasis, increased secretions, and removal of lung tissue.

Table 3-20

Potential Nursing Diagnoses for the Patient Receiving Chemotherapy for Lung Cancer

1. Anxiety related to diagnosis and chemotherapy.
2. Knowledge Deficit related to chemotherapy treatments and potential side effects.
3. Risk for Infection related to chemotherapy-induced bone marrow suppression, impaired immune system from cancer or long-term steroid treatment, mucositis, and invasive intravenous catheters.
4. Fatigue related to build-up of cellular degradation products, cytotoxic drugs, or the malignant process.
5. Altered Nutritional Intake: Less Than Body Requirements related to nausea and vomiting from cytotoxic drugs, mucositis causing difficulty eating and swallowing, or diarrhea impairing absorption of nutrients.
6. Pain related to mucositis or the malignant process invading bone and tissues.

Nursing interventions for diagnoses in the patient receiving chemotherapy (Table 3-20) are quite detailed, and the Bibliography at the end of the chapter will develop these diagnoses and interventions in more detail. Some interventions might include:

- Decrease anxiety by explaining the treatment plan and potential side effects with the patient and family; maintaining a calm and supportive manner; and assessing the patient's anxiety level, using relaxation techniques and medication if ordered to alleviate continuing anxiety.
- Teach patient about self-care during chemotherapy, including infection prevention (due to decreased white blood cell count), good oral hygiene, adequate fluid intake (10 glasses per day if not contraindicated), nausea control, adequate nutritional intake, ways to manage fatigue, and ways to minimize bleeding (due to decreased platelet count). Chemotherapy can affect the normal tissues to a degree that complications can occur and collaborative care will be needed to assess and treat the patient.
- Prevent infection by teaching the patient to avoid crowds and infected people, use good oral hygiene after meals and before bed, wash hands regularly, care for the skin

gently, use excellent sterile technique when caring for intravenous access devices, take axillary temperatures only, avoid sharing eating utensils, cook meat well and wash fruit and vegetables, report fever, bleeding, and changes in skin or mouth, cough, or urine to health care provider.

- Instruct patient on ways to manage fatigue, balance rest and activity, determine what activities are realistic in the present situation, modify daily activities, and avoid fatiguing situations.
- Assess nutritional intake by monitoring weight and intake, minimize nausea by teaching patient to eat cool, dry foods when nausea is present, eat small meals with liquids between meals, rest and allow a family member to prepare meals, avoid offensive odors, clean mouth regularly, use antiemetics as necessary.
- Assess patient's pain (location, intensity on a pain scale, aggravating factors), maintain comfort, and minimize pain using nonpharmacologic and pharmacologic methods as necessary (review nursing interventions for pain in Table 3-18). Care for mucositis with topical rinses and antifungal medications as necessary.

Potential complications of chemotherapy that the nurse should watch for are often related to the type of drug(s) used. Local tissue irritation and sloughing can develop at the site of intravenous infiltration of certain cytotoxic drugs (eg, doxorubicin, vinblastine, vincristine, and paclitaxel) called vesicants. Bleeding can occur more readily due to chemotherapy-induced thrombocytopenia (decreased platelet count). Kidney function can be impaired by certain drugs (eg, cisplatin, high-dose methotrexate, and streptozocin). Inflammation and fibrosis of lung tissue may be the direct result of cytotoxic drugs like bleomycin. Neurotoxicity is related to the toxic effects of drugs like cisplatin and paclitaxel. Cisplatin can also cause anaphylactic reactions.

Radiation therapy is commonly used to treat primary lung tumors and metastatic disease to the brain and bones. Radiation therapy may be used in conjunction with chemotherapy and before or after surgery. The treatments themselves are painless and are delivered to a specific site. The side effects of radiation therapy are mostly site specific (ie, only the treated area will have side effects). For example, if only a portion of the lung and thorax is treated, then the side effects will be skin reaction within the treatment portal and esophagitis if the stomach is in the field. Possible systemic side effects of radiation therapy are fatigue and anorexia.

The total dose of radiation needed to treat the tumor is too damaging to be delivered all at once so it is broken down into smaller doses. These smaller doses allow the normal tissue to recover, minimizing side effects. External radiation treatments to the tumor site are delivered on a daily basis for 2 to 6 weeks, depending on the site. Most treatments are done on an outpatient basis unless the patient's condition does not allow it. Each dose, which is measured in gray (Gy), increases the damage to the tissues in the treatment site or portal.

The type of side effects experienced by the patient will depend on the total dose delivered, the volume of tissue irradiated, and the cell's ability to repair damage. The radiation damages the DNA in both the malignant cells and the normal cells in the treatment field. Normal cells have more capacity to repair the damaged DNA, whereas malignant cells are less able to repair DNA breaks. The goal of radiation therapy is to maximize tumor cell kill and minimize damage to the normal tissues.

Nursing care of the patient undergoing radiation therapy for lung cancer focuses on educating the patient and family about radiation treatments and the potential side effects, teaching the patient how to care for the skin in the treatment field, promoting optimal nutrition, and maintaining comfort (Table 3-21). Nursing interventions are specific to the diagnosis and the etiology. The nurse has a major role in assisting the patient and his fam-

Table 3-21

Potential Nursing Diagnoses for Patients Undergoing Radiation Therapy

1. Anxiety related to the diagnosis of cancer and radiation treatments.
2. Pain related to surgery, bone metastases, skin irritation, or desquamation (shedding of the epidermal layer of the skin) in the treatment field, mucositis, or tumor invasion.
3. Potential for Impaired Skin Integrity related to radiation treatments, which can cause dryness, pruritus, and desquamation, or concommitant chemotherapy (ie, chemotherapy and radiation therapy being given at the same time).
4. Altered Nutrition: Less Than Body Requirements related to the malignant process, nausea if the stomach is in the treatment field and/or cytotoxic drugs, mucositis from chemotherapy making swallowing difficult, impaired sense of taste, and decreased saliva production if the salivary glands are in the treatment field.
5. Knowledge Deficit related to proper skin care, changing energy levels, and nutritional requirements during radiation therapy.

ily through the radiation treatments. Nursing interventions for patients receiving radiation therapy might include the following:

- Decrease anxiety by explaining the treatment schedule and clearing up misconceptions about radiation and its side effects. Tour the department to meet the staff and see the machinery; maintain a calm, supportive manner, and be available to the patient and his family for questions and concerns.
- Maintain comfort and diminish pain by assessing the patient's pain, administering medications as ordered, using nonpharmacologic methods (imagery, massage, diversion) to alleviate pain, treat mucositis with topical anesthetics and soothing gargles and antifungal medication as needed.
- Teach patient about skin care in the treatment area: Wash gently with mild soap and lukewarm water if tattoos are used (no washing if skin markings are used to mark the treatment area), pat dry, and hydrophilic moisturizers (no petroleum-based products, no deodorants or powders, cornstarch as needed to minimize friction, no scratching or rubbing skin, no tape, no bras, keep area open to air as much as possible, no sun, use electric shaver, treat skin reactions per facility protocol).
- Maintain optimum nutrition by monitoring patient's intake, appetite, and weight (use strategies in maintaining intake for patients undergoing chemotherapy).
- Instruct the patient about treatment, potential side effects, community resources for support and transportation to daily treatments, teach about skin care (as above), nutritional requirements for healing, and ways to manage fatigue. Complications of radiation therapy include a reduction in lung capacity, pneumonitis (inflammation of the lung tissue), and skin reactions. Bone marrow suppression can occur if the patient is receiving concommitant chemotherapy or if there is a large volume of bone marrow in the treatment field.

Pulmonary Embolism

When a thrombus (blood clot) detaches and travels through the venous circulation through the heart and into the pulmonary vasculature, it can occlude a pulmonary artery. The detached clot is called a pulmonary embolus and it can cause swelling and necrosis of lung tissue distal to the occluded artery. Pulmonary emboli can arise in the deep veins as a result of phlebitis in the extremities or less commonly in the right atrium of the heart. Atrial fibrillation, the heart arrhythmia that causes the atria to quiver erratically rather than contract, can predispose a patient to pulmonary embolism. The abrupt onset of chest pain, dyspnea, and sometimes cough is a common presentation. Hemoptysis is present in 20% to 30% of cases. Diagnosis is made by a ventilation/perfusion (V/Q) scan. Treatment is with anticoagulants (heparin followed by warfarin) and thrombolytics (streptokinase or tissue plasminogen activator, the so-called "clot-busters").

Because lung tissue may be destroyed by the lack of oxygenated blood distal to the embolus, nursing care involves assessing the patient's oxygenation. Interventions include frequent vital signs, O_2 saturation, and arterial blood gases as ordered. ABGs may show hypoxemia and respiratory alkalosis. A V/Q mismatch is caused by adequate ventilation but inadequate perfusion of the lung tissue distal to the pulmonary embolus. Oxygen is administered as ordered. The anticoagulant, heparin, is delivered intravenously for rapid anticoagulation, and partial thromboplastin (PTT) levels are monitored. Warfarin is an anticoagulant that is begun orally but can take up to 7 days to be fully effective in increasing the prothrombin (PT) levels. Precautions are taken to prevent excessive bleeding (eg, longer compression of venipuncture sites). Increasing dyspnea, tachypnea, or hemoptysis warrants notification of the physician.

Disorders of the Pleura

Pleurisy

Pleurisy is the inflammation of the pleural membrane. There are actually two pleural membranes: the parietal pleura, which lines the thoracic cage, and the visceral pleura, which covers the lungs. The potential space between the two membranes is filled with a thin layer of pleural fluid that allows smooth sliding of the lungs within the thorax. When either membrane becomes irritated, the roughened surfaces grate on each other, causing pain. Patients usually describe the pain as sharp and worse on deep inhalation. The pain is often low and unilateral. There is no diagnostic test for pleurisy and the diagnosis may be arrived at by clinical presentation. Treatment often includes antibiotics and pain medication. Nursing management of the patient with pleurisy involves ways to minimize pain. Besides pain medication, the patient is taught to splint the chest with a pillow during coughing or moving. Lozenges may decrease the urge to cough and moisten the throat.

Pleural Effusion

A pleural effusion is a collection of fluid in the pleural space. This potential space can fill with pleural fluid if the normal drainage routes are blocked or it can fill with pus or blood. Pleural effusions are caused by diseases that change the formation and absorption of pleural fluid, as in congestive heart failure (transudative pleural effusion), or when the pleural linings are diseased, as in lung cancer (exudative pleural effusion). A small pleural effusion (200 to 300 cc) may not cause any symptoms, but large amounts (up to 5000 cc) can cause dyspnea, cough, pleuritic chest pain, and even shifting of the trachea to one side. With large effusions, the chest exam may reveal dullness to percussion over the effusion and decreased or bronchial breath sounds on auscultation. Chest x-ray is often diagnostic but ultrasound, CAT scan, and MRIs may be useful in making the diagnosis.

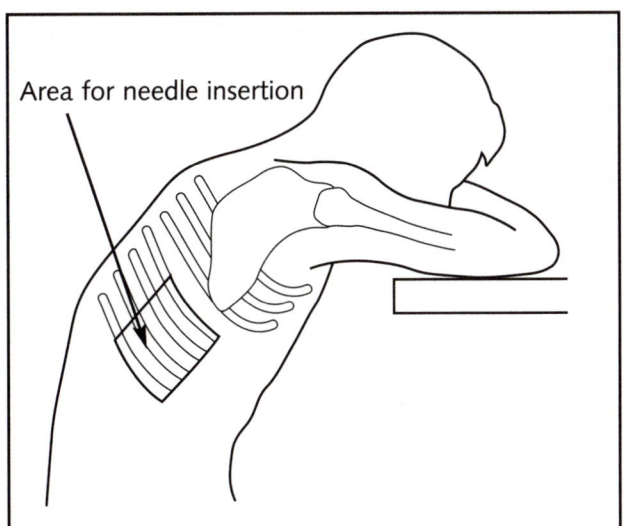

Figure 3-11. Thoracentesis area.

Area for needle insertion

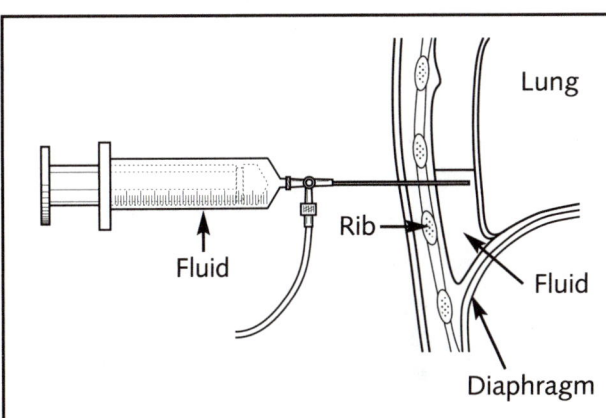

Figure 3-12. Thoracentesis insertion.

Lung

Fluid

Rib

Fluid

Diaphragm

The treatment depends on the underlying condition. Thoracentesis, the insertion of a needle into the pleural space to drain the fluid or air, often relieves the pressure and dyspnea (Figures 3-11 and 3-12). Laboratory analysis of the fluid may reveal the cause of the pleural effusion (eg, infection or malignancy). Antibiotics and chest tube drainage may be required to treat the pleural effusion (Table 3-22).

Pneumothorax

A pneumothorax is an accumulation of gas in the pleural space. The gas enters the space usually as the result of a break in the visceral pleura surrounding the lung (Figures 3-13 and 3-14). The break might be the result of a tuberculosis infection, a ruptured emphysematous bleb, trauma, or a surgical disruption. With a spontaneous pneumothorax, the onset is sudden with severe sticking pain and dyspnea. On examination, the chest may expand asymmetrically, and there might be fullness in the intercostal spaces. Subcutaneous emphysema (air in the subcutaneous tissues) follows puncture of the chest wall with air leaking out of the chest into the tissue.

Auscultation reveals absent breath sounds and tympanic resonance on percussion over the air-filled portion of the chest. Diagnosis is made by chest x-ray. A large pneumothorax

Table 3-22

Care of the Patient Undergoing Thoracentesis

1. Explain the procedure to the patient and obtain an informed consent. Let the patient know that a local anesthetic will be used to numb the area where the needle is inserted. The procedure takes a few minutes, and a chest x-ray will be obtained afterward (see Figure 3-12).

2. Assess the patient's vital signs and respiratory status before the procedure, including breath sounds and O_2 Sat.

3. Position the patient on the side of the bed with arms over a bedside table and a pillow for comfort.

4. Remind the patient not to talk or move during the procedure.

5. Stay with the patient and reassure him about the progress of the procedure. (Note: coughing is a common response to removal of pleural fluid.)

6. Place a dressing over the puncture site.

7. Send any specimens from the thoracentesis to the laboratory as ordered.

8. Reassess the patient's vital signs and breath sounds after the procedure.

9. Send the patient for a chest x-ray if ordered.

Figure 3-13. Pneumothorax.

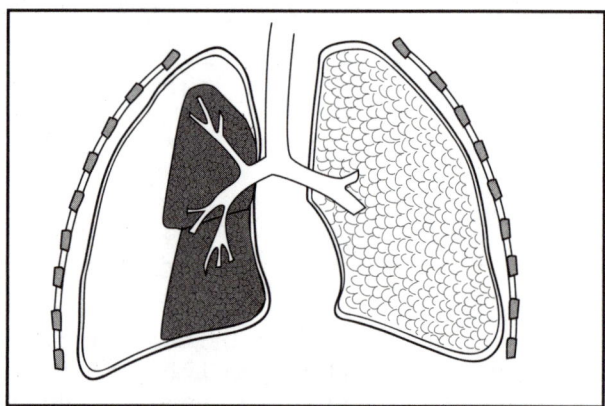

Figure 3-14. Tension pneumothorax with mediastinal shift.

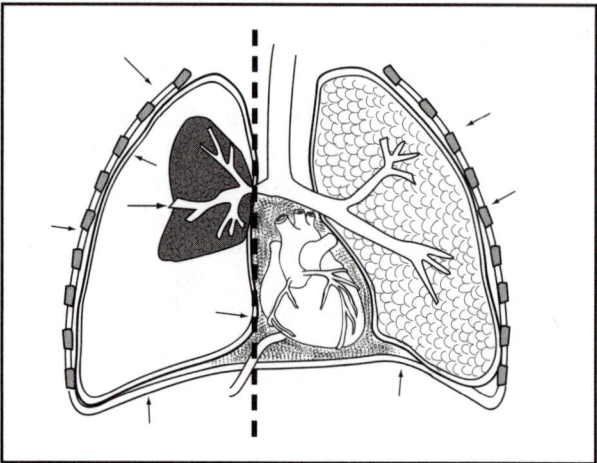

can be life-threatening if the air pressure continues to build, shifting the mediastinal contents to the opposite side with kinking of the great vessels and compression of the heart. Clinical signs of a mediastinal shift include deviation of the trachea away from the injured lung, distended neck veins, and progressive cyanosis.

One cause of a mediastinal shift is a tension pneumothorax where the damaged, visceral pleura allows air to escape into the pleural space during inspiration, but the air remains trapped in the space during expiration. Pressure can quickly build and can be life-threatening if not relieved by the insertion of a needle to decompress the pleural space. Chest tube placement with closed chest drainage is instituted to remove the remaining air coming from leaks in the visceral pleura.

Nursing management of the patient with a pneumothorax involves assessing the patient's vital signs, O_2 Sat, and breath sounds. Patients are often dyspneic, anxious, and need support while the pneumothorax is decompressed and the chest tube is placed. Oxygen should be administered as ordered to maintain adequate O_2 Sat while not decreasing CO_2 drive if the patient has COPD. Antibiotics are usually given to treat infection.

Chest Injuries

Chest injuries require rapid assessment of the patient and immediate treatment. Frequently, trauma to the head and abdomen may have occurred at the same time as the chest injury. Assessment of the patient with traumatic injuries follows the ABCs: airway, breathing, and circulation. Treatment is based upon the specific injuries. Common chest injuries include rib fractures, flail chest, pneumothorax, hemopneumothorax, and pulmonary contusion.

Rib fractures are the most common thoracic injuries. Causes of these fractures include trauma and those caused by sneezing or coughing. Severe coughing can fracture a rib in the elderly and those with osteoporosis or metastatic cancer. Simple fractures do not usually damage internal organs, like the heart and lungs, but more serious trauma can cause damage to the thoracic organs, such as cardiac contusion or hemopneumothorax (blood and air in the thorax) or to abdominal organs (eg, the liver, spleen, and kidneys). Treatment of a rib fracture includes analgesics to lessen pain, teaching the patient how to splint the area with a pillow during movement, and coughing and observation in case a pneumothorax develops later.

Flail chest occurs when multiple rib fractures result in paradoxical movement of the chest wall during breathing. If one rib has multiple fractures or several ribs in a row are broken, then the damaged chest wall retracts during inspiration and balloons out during expiration. Injury to the lung underneath the damaged chest wall (pulmonary contusion) is often present. Dyspnea and hypoxia can develop as a result of the paradoxical motion of the chest and the damaged lung tissue. Treatment involves stabilization of the flail chest and, if hypoxia worsens, intubation and mechanical ventilation with positive pressure ventilation. The patient would also be treated for any other complications like hemorrhage, pneumothorax, and shock. Antibiotics are used to treat possible infection.

Chest injuries can be caused by penetrating and nonpenetrating wounds. Nonpenetrating wounds, like blunt trauma, can injure tissues beneath the location of the force. Pulmonary contusion or bruising can occur if the lung is damaged. Pulmonary contusion can result in collapsed alveoli, interstitial hemorrhage, and atelectasis. The alveoli in that area may be ineffective in gas exchange. A leak may develop in the damaged lung, causing a closed pneumothorax. As described previously, a closed pneumothorax requires immediate thoracentesis to relieve accumulating air pressure.

Figure 3-15. Atelectasis due to obstruction.

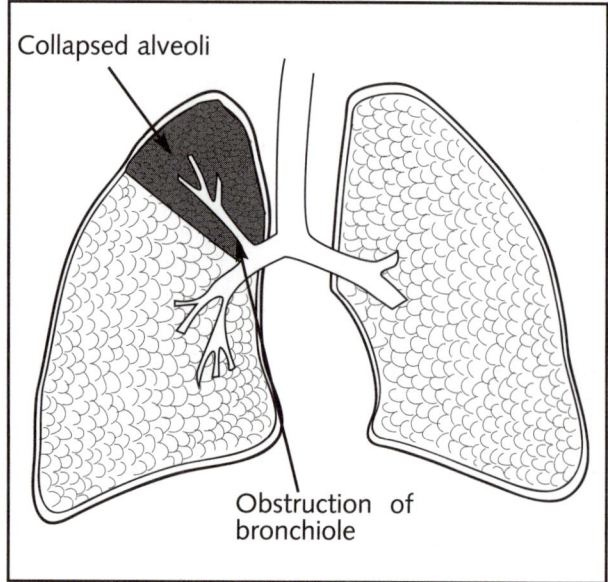

Collapsed alveoli

Obstruction of bronchiole

A penetrating chest wound (eg, knife or gunshot wound) may pierce the thorax and the lung. A "sucking" chest wound develops with air being noisily sucked into the chest through the wound during inspiration and blowing out of the wound during expiration.

The internal chest structures may also move back and forth during breathing with an open chest wound, causing a mediastinal flutter. Immediate treatment is necessary for mediastinal flutter before life-threatening hemodynamic changes develop.

Atelectasis

Atelectasis is a common complication of bronchial obstruction, compression of lung tissue, or loss of surfactant. It is the incomplete expansion of part or all of a lung distal to a blockage of the airways (Figure 3-15). It is a common complication of general anesthesia, but may also result from:

- Intrabronchial obstruction from secretions, foreign bodies, or bronchospasm.
- Extrabronchial obstruction from tumors and pleural effusion.
- Endobronchial disease, such as carcinoma.

The most common findings of atelectasis are decreased chest expansion and breath sounds over the affected area. There may be retraction of the intercostal spaces over the affected area. Symptoms may progress to hypoxia, dyspnea, and tachypnea if a large portion of the lung is compressed or collapsed. The patient may or may not complain of any symptoms depending on the degree and the cause of the obstruction.

Older patients are particularly prone to atelectasis because of decreased tidal volumes, lung capacity, lung elasticity, and chest expansion. Older patients undergoing general anesthesia require careful assessment of their pulmonary functioning and special attention to pulmonary hygiene after surgery.

The incidence of atelectasis increases after surgery. Pain, narcotics, and immobility can result in retention of thickened bronchial secretions, which can obstruct the airways. Nursing interventions to prevent and reverse atelectasis in all patients include:

- Turn the patient every 1 to 2 hours, especially when obtunded, immobilized, or on bedrest.

- Encourage the patient to use the incentive spirometer every 1 to 2 hours, holding the inspiration for 5 seconds before exhaling (to increase alveolar expansion).
- Promote thinning of secretions by encouraging good fluid intake (eight glasses or at least 2 L of fluid a day if not contraindicated) and humidification of oxygen or air.
- Encourage mobility and ambulation as soon as possible.
- Assist the patient with coughing and deep breathing every 1 to 2 hours and encourage the patient to use the incentive spirometer every 1 to 2 hours.
- Administer antibiotics as ordered to prevent or treat pneumonia.
- Administer narcotics carefully, as they can decrease tidal volumes and the cough reflex.

Mrs. A. responded well to the albuterol treatment with a decreased respiratory rate (22 breaths per minute) and diminished wheezing. Her O_2 Sat improved to 96%. Mrs. A. was given a prescription for antibiotics (clarithromycin) and an inhaled steroid (flunisolide) to use after her bronchodilator (metaproterenol). The nurse reviewed situations and substances to avoid (such as dust) and gave her a handout to take home. Mrs. A. went home with her husband.

The answers to the questions in the introduction are as follows:

- *What physiologic changes cause wheezing?*

Asthma is characterized by bronchoconstriction with inflammation and increased mucus production. As air travels through the narrowed respiratory passages, it makes the wheezing sound.

- *Why is her PEFR decreased during an asthma attack?*

The peak expiratory flow rate (PEFR) is decreased because the narrowed airways restrict the flow of air out of the lungs. Many patients with moderate to severe asthma use peak flow meters at home to monitor their lung function. Mrs. A's PEFR is at 70% of her personal best. Following the zone therapy guidelines, Mrs. A treats her asthma with her rescue medication plan.

- *What could have caused this asthma attack?*

Mrs. A. was cleaning her daughter's basement the day before the attack. Dust and mold can be sources of airway irritation for patients with asthma. The dust may have triggered the inflammatory response and a flare-up of her asthma. She also has a low-grade fever that could signal an infection.

BIBLIOGRAPHY

Agency for Health Care Policy and Research. *Smoking Cessation: Clinical Guidelines No. 18* (AHCPR Pub. No. 96-0692). Rockville, Md: US Department of Health and Human Services; 1996.

Barker LR, Buron JR, Zieve PD. *Principles of Ambulatory Medicine.* 4th ed. Baltimore, Md: Williams & Williams; 1995.

Burrell L, Gerlach M, Pless B. *Nursing Management of Adults with Respiratory Problems.* Stamford, Conn: Appleton & Lange; 1997.

Carpenito LJ. *Nursing Diagnose: Application to Clinical Practice.* 4th ed. Philadelphia, Pa: J.B. Lippincott Co; 1992.

Hoffman D. *The Herbal Handbook.* Rochester, Vt: Healing Arts Press; 1998.

Holleb AI, Fink DJ, Murphy GP. *American Cancer Society Textbook of Clinical Oncology.* Atlanta, Ga: The American Cancer Society Inc; 1991.

Ignatavius D, Workman M, Mishler M. *Medical-Surgical Nursing: A Nursing Process Approach.* Philadelphia, Pa: W.B. Saunders Co; 1995.

Kozier B, Erb G, Blais K, Wilkinson JM. *Fundamentals of Nursing: Concepts, Process, and Practice.* New York, NY: Addison-Wesley Publishing Co Inc; 1995.

National Heart, Lung and Blood Institute (NHLBI). National asthma education and prevention program. *Guidelines for the Diagnosis and Management of Asthma: Expert Panel Report II* (NIH Pub. No. 97-4051). Bethesda, Md: Author; 1997.

Porth CM. *Pathophysiology: Concepts of Altered Health States.* 4th ed. Philadelphia, Pa: J.B. Lippincott Co; 1994.

MULTILPLE-CHOICE QUESTIONS

1. All of the following would decrease exposure to allergens except:
   A. Encasing mattresses and pillows in airtight covers
   B. Installing wall-to-wall carpeting
   C. Avoid dusting and vacuuming
   D. Humidify air in the house

2. Individuals at high risk for oropharyngeal cancers are:
   A. Under 40 years old
   B. History of dental cavities
   C. Mouth breathers
   D. Tobacco and alcohol users

3. Tuberculosis can be detected by Mantoux or PPD:
   A. 3 to 12 weeks after infection
   B. After tubercle formation
   C. 1 week after inflammation
   D. 6 to 12 months after exposure

4. Emphysema differs from chronic bronchitis in the following way:
   A. In chronic bronchitis, the terminal airspaces are dilated
   B. In emphysema there is destruction of the alveolar walls
   C. Only patients with emphysema experience dyspnea and cough
   D Mucus production is less in chronic bronchitis

5. The pathophysiologic changes seen in adult respiratory distress syndrome (ARDS) are caused by:
   A. High levels of supplemental oxygen and mechanical ventilation
   B. Infection by virulent bacteria
   C. Inflammatory mediators in the lung
   D. Increased CO_2 levels and respiratory acidosis

CHAPTER 3 ANSWERS

1. B
2. D
3. A
4. B
5. C

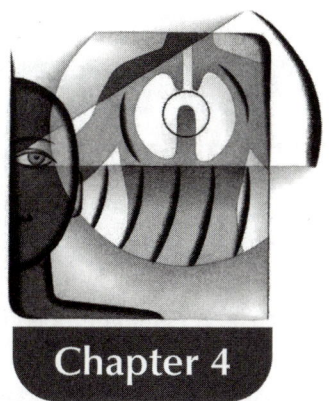

Chapter 4

Common Interventions to Improve Oxygenation

Mr. J. is a 47-year-old male who goes to the emergency room with a 10-day history of "flu-like" symptoms: fever, aches, loss of appetite, cough productive of yellowish green sputum, and increasing shortness of breath. His only significant past medical history is a 30-pack year of cigarette smoking. The physical exam reveals a slightly anxious, diaphoretic, pale, well-nourished appearing gentleman who is leaning forward in the tripod position breathing. Vital signs: temperature—102.4°F, apical pulse (AP)—112 and regular, BP—148/86 on the right and 152/90 on the left, respiration rate (RR)—28 breaths per min and slightly labored, and SaO_2 is 88% on room air. Lung sounds: scattered expiratory wheezing throughout both lung fields; crackles: anteriorly from the left sternal border fourth intercostal space (ICS) to the sixth ICS and to the fifth ICS at the midaxillary line, posteriorly from T5 down. Crackles decrease but do not disappear with coughing and deep breathing. The nurse practitioner examining the patient makes the decision to admit him and directs you to initiate oxygen therapy via nasal cannula to maintain an SaO_2 greater than or equal to 92%.

Improving oxygenation involves promoting ventilation, assisting diffusion of gases, and facilitating the perfusion of oxygen throughout the body. In this chapter, nursing interventions and collaborative strategies to enhance oxygenation will be reviewed with a special focus on incorporating interventions into the patient's nursing care plan. Some interventions are performed in the acute and intensive care settings, while others may be included in the patient's care at home. Because every person is unique, it is important to customize the interventions to the patient's abilities, lifestyle, and to the disease process.

Promoting healthy ventilation begins with promoting a healthy lifestyle. In healthy people, ventilation is maintained by exercise, clean air, and a competent cough reflex (Table 4-1). Exercise is an important part of promoting respiratory and cardiovascular health. During exercise, ventilation improves as the lungs expand more completely, and perfusion is enhanced by the increased cardiac output.

Table 4-1

Facilitating Respiratory Health

1. Exercise regularly—30 minutes, three to four times per week.
2. Do not smoke or use tobacco products.
3. Avoid secondhand smoke.
4. Support legislation to control and eliminate pollution.
5. Ensure adequate ventilation of wood stoves and furnaces.
6. Reduce exposure to noxious fumes at home and at work.

Part of promoting healthy ventilation is advocating for clean air in the environment, whether it is in the atmosphere or home and work environments. Of primary concern are the risks associated with cigarette smoking. Nurses need to teach their patients and the community about the hazards of cigarette smoking. Of particular concern is the rising number of adolescents who are smoking now. Education programs need to begin in the schools to educate children before adolescence and expand to adults in the community. The risks associated with secondhand smoke should also be emphasized to adults so they can protect their children.

Occupational hazards need to be evaluated in the nursing assessment. Interventions need to be geared toward reducing exposure to harmful chemicals and fumes by encouraging adequate ventilation in work sites and the use of protective gear.

When a patient's health is compromised by age, lifestyle, surgery, or disease, his or her respiratory functioning may be inadequate. Factors such as changes in pulmonary structure, pain, and immobility can cause shallow breathing and retained secretions. Mucus stasis can result in bacterial growth and possibly pneumonia. Nursing strategies to improve ventilation include basic interventions such as:

- Improving physical mobility and chest expansion by promoting comfort, encouraging exercise, or changing the patient's position if he is bedridden.
- Enhancing ventilation with exercise and breathing exercises.
- Mobilizing secretions with humidification and coughing exercises.

More advanced interventions require a collaborative approach. Nurses, physicians, and respiratory therapists work together to enhance ventilation and diffusion by:

- Maintaining a patent airway with appropriate positioning, removal of secretions and artificial airways if necessary (eg, oral or nasal airways, tracheotomy, endotracheal tubes).
- Improving oxygenation with oxygen delivery systems.
- Ventilating the patient mechanically to improve ventilation and diffusion.

In this chapter, these strategies for improving oxygenation will be reviewed.

IMPROVING PHYSICAL MOBILITY

When a patient's ability to move is compromised, an important nursing intervention is maintaining physical mobility. Pain, surgical incision, medications, and age may make it difficult for the patient to move. Chest expansion and alveolar inflation are diminished during immobility and can result in atelectasis, the collapse of alveoli, and possibly pneumonia.

The best position for maximum chest expansion is upright. Patients who are able should ambulate three times a day to enhance ventilation and maintain cardiovascular conditioning. Patients undergoing surgery should be ambulated postoperatively as soon as the surgeon allows and three times a day thereafter. Prior to walking after surgery, pre-medicate the patient with an analgesic (30 to 45 minutes before the activity) so he is more comfortable and less fearful while moving, and better able to deep breathe. For the bedridden patient, the semi-Fowler's or high-Fowler's position allows maximum chest expansion. In the patient with chronic airflow limitation, the "orthopnea position" or tri-pod position may provide relief from dyspnea and enhance ventilation. This position involves the patient sitting at the bedside with a table in front of him or her, allowing for propping of the elbows on the table while compressing the lower chest. If the patient is bedridden, he or she should be turned from side to side every 2 hours to allow improved chest expansion on the "upward side" and increased perfusion of the lung on the depend-ent side.

Patients with chronic respiratory disorders like emphysema may have their mobility limited by their impaired ability to oxygenate their blood. The structural changes to the lungs decrease their ability to ventilate adequately. The lungs' normal PaO_2 may be only 55 to 60 mmHg. With less oxygen in the blood, less is available for the cells when activity increases the oxygen demands of the tissues.

Chronic respiratory diseases like emphysema or chronic bronchitis change the struc-ture and the functioning of the respiratory tract. The diaphragm becomes flattened, reduc-ing the ability of the chest to expand. Air becomes trapped in distal alveoli and the bases of the lungs. Air trapping causes a ventilation-perfusion (V/Q) mismatch with hypox-emia. Oxygenation for these patients can be improved by reducing oxygen demand. Even normal activities, such as walking and eating, can be exhausting to a patient with a chron-ic respiratory disorder. Nursing care for these patients would include teaching ways to reduce oxygen demand, such as:

- Pace activities with rest periods.
- Eat frequent, light meals to decrease metabolic demands and gastric fullness, which might press the diaphragm upward.
- Avoid breath-holding during activities, which will further diminish the PO_2 and increase dyspnea.
- Avoid Valsalva's maneuver, which increases intrathoracic pressure and decreases blood return into the thorax, resulting in dizziness.
- Decrease temperature if febrile, as each degree (Fahrenheit) elevation results in a 7% increase in metabolic demand.
- Use energy conservation exercises such as performing the work part of an activity during exhalation and using pursed lip breathing during exertion.

BREATHING EXERCISES

Breathing exercises can help patients control their breathing, improve ventilation, decrease anxiety, and increase activity levels in patients with chronic respiratory disease. Some exercises are more suited to patients with chronic airflow limitations (CAL) and oth-ers to anxious patients or those with postoperative pain.

Diaphragmatic Breathing

Diaphragmatic breathing is indicated for patients with CAL or anxiety because it allows for slow, deep breaths:

- Explain to the patient about the breathing exercises.
- Place the patient in a sitting position on the side of the bed or in the high- or semi-Fowler's position.
- Have the patient place one hand on his chest and the other on his upper abdomen above the umbilicus. Another method that may be useful is to place a light object (eg, tissue box) on the patient's abdomen so he can see abdominal movement during diaphragmatic breathing.
- Teach the patient to inhale slowly through the nose, feeling the abdomen rise up under his hands but with little movement in the chest.
- Instruct the patient to exhale through pursed lips using the abdominal muscles (see next section on Pursed Lip Breathing).
- Assess the patient's response (eg, dizziness, lightheadedness).
- Repeat for three breaths and then rest for 1 minute.

Pursed Lip Breathing

The pursed lip breathing technique is especially useful in patients with diseases of CAL because it slows the collapse of the small airways by maintaining a higher bronchiole pressure and prolonging expiration. It can also be used to control breathing in the dyspneic patient, to prevent breath-holding during activity (a common problem in patients with CAL), and to reduce air-trapping in the alveoli.

- Assist the patient into a sitting or high semi-Fowler's position.
- Instruct the patient to purse his lips like he is about to whistle with his lips slightly open.
- Teach the patient to inhale through his nose to a count of two and slowly exhale through his pursed lips to a count of four or until he has completely exhaled.
- Repeat this technique for 10 minutes, increasing the frequency to four to five times a day.

Incentive Spirometry

Incentive spirometers or sustained maximal inspiration devices (SMIs) are tools that help visualize inhalation. They can be combined with breathing exercises to maximize ventilation. Incentive spirometers are usually plastic, disposable units which patients may take home after discharge from a facility. They are useful in patients who have the diminished ability to cough effectively and during the postoperative period, especially after thoracic or abdominal surgery. Pain during the postoperative period, general anesthesia, and narcotic medications all diminish alveolar inflation. The incentive spirometer provides visual cues of preoperative functioning and postoperative goals. The preoperative levels are marked on the spirometer and can be used to monitor recovery after surgery (Figure 4-1).

Mobilizing Secretions

Clearing respiratory secretions allows for an open airway, easier ventilation of the lungs, and prevention of mucus stasis. Secretions are easier to cough up if they are thin, rather than thick and tenacious. Therefore, adequate fluid intake, humidification of

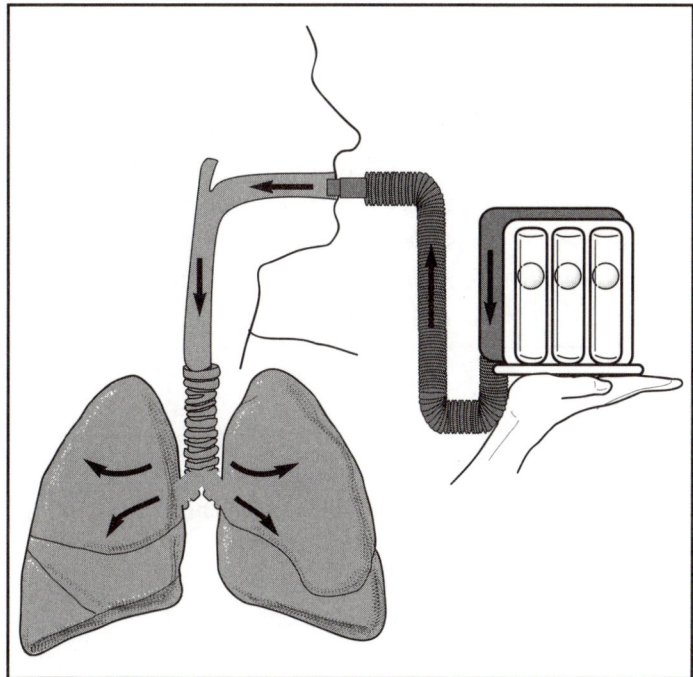

Figure 4-1. How to use an incentive spirometer.

inspired air, and possibly expectorant medication (eg, guaifenisen) are important interventions in mobilizing secretions. Other medications, which can be used before breathing exercises, are inhaled bronchodilators such as albuterol or systemic bronchodilators like theophylline (Table 4-2). These medications allow the airways to relax and dilate so that the breathing and coughing exercises are more effective.

Coughing is the most effective and natural way to clear the airways. A good coughing technique allows for adequate mobilization and expulsion of pulmonary secretions. Normally a cough is an involuntary response, but it can be controlled consciously. In healthy patients, a cough begins with inhalation, followed by glottic closure, and then the rapid opening of the glottis and rapid expulsion of the air. Sometimes the air is expelled at speeds up to 100 miles per hour. In patients with airway disease, the normal cough reflex may be diminished or there may be excessive secretions. Three techniques that can be used to help patients clear secretions are "cascade" coughing, "huff" coughing, and "quad" coughing.

Cascade Coughing

This technique is useful in the postoperative period and with patients who have CAL or neuromuscular diseases or those who are bedridden:
- Have the patient in a sitting or semi-Fowler's position.
- Teach the patient to inhale and exhale slowly and deeply.
- Have the patient inhale deeply and exhale, then close his throat and use small coughs without inhaling again, pause and then inhale again very slowly (to decrease the cough stimulus). If paroxysmal coughing starts, instruct the patient to use slow deep breaths or pursed lip breathing until the coughing urge passes.
- Rest and repeat for a total of three times.
- Assess secretions.
- Try to set up a coughing schedule to keep airways clear.

Table 4-2

Instructions for Patients Taking Theophylline

1. Take theophylline with food to reduce nausea and vomiting.
2. Take it on a regular schedule to maintain steady blood levels of the drug.
3. Report signs and symptoms, such as dizziness, nausea, and vomiting.
4. Have theophylline blood levels measured periodically according to physician's protocol.

Huff or Open Glottis Coughing

This technique is useful in patients with CAL:
- Have the patient in the sitting or semi-Fowler's position with his arms crossed below his rib cage (hugging a pillow may be more comfortable).
- Instruct the patient to inhale slowly, hold for 2 seconds, tighten the abdominal, leg, and gluteal muscles (to increase intrathoracic pressure), and then exhale in short "huffs," actually saying the word "huff."
- Repeat and try to cough on exhalation.
- Assess the patient response and secretions.

Quad Coughing

This technique is useful in patients with muscle weakness. Using a modified Heimlich maneuver, have the patient place the heels of both hands between the umbilicus and the xiphoid process and press inward and upward during coughing or huffing to clear secretions.

Chest Physical Therapy

Another method to mobilize secretions is *chest physical therapy* (CPT) or *pulmonary hygiene*. It is composed of three techniques that may be used individually or in combination. These techniques—percussion, vibration, and postural drainage—are performed by respiratory therapists or nurses. Percussion is performed by applying cupped hands in a rhythmic sequence over a part or the entire lung. A hollow sound is produced as the cupped hand creates an air pocket when applied to the chest wall. It is used to loosen secretions (Figure 4-2). Percussion may be combined with postural drainage positions to optimize drainage of particular lung segments (Figure 4-3). Percussion is contraindicated in patients with cardiac conditions, osteoporosis, pneumo/hemothorax, or pleural effusion.

Vibration is another technique of loosening secretions that usually follows percussion. It involves the placement of both hands pressing on the rib cage over the affected lung. The arm and shoulder muscles contract isometrically, producing a small vibration that is transmitted to the patient's chest wall and airways. This vibration is thought to increase the turbulence of the air in the lung and loosen secretions.

Postural drainage involves positioning the patient in such a way as to allow gravity to drain particular segments of the lungs (Figure 4-4). Several positions may not be tolerat-

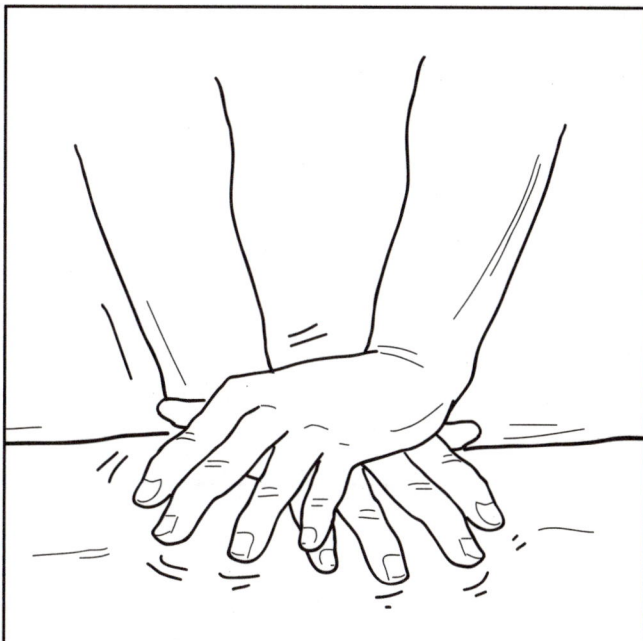

Figure 4-2. Hand position for vibration of the chest wall.

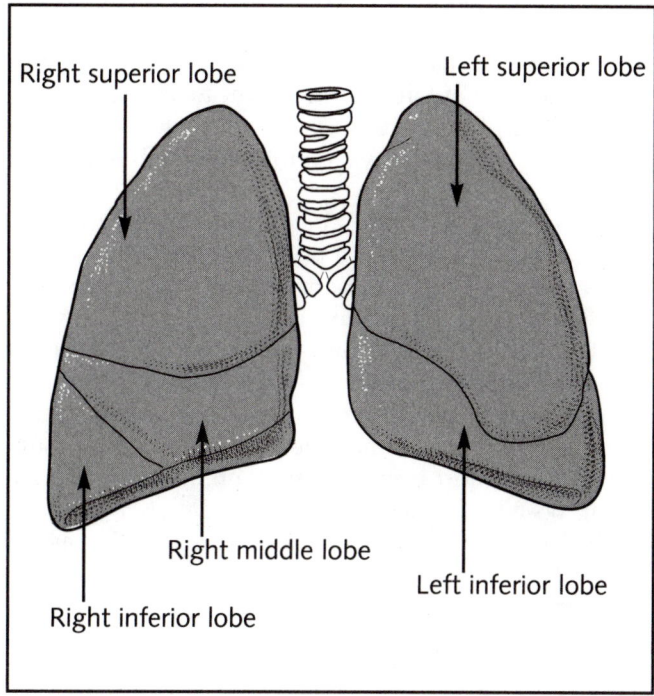

Right superior lobe

Left superior lobe

Right middle lobe

Left inferior lobe

Right inferior lobe

Figure 4-3. Lobes of the lungs.

ed by the patient because the head is lower than the torso. The positions can be adapted by raising the head of the bed so that the patient is comfortable and can breathe easily.

Postural drainage can be contraindicated if the patient has cardiac conditions or increased intracranial pressure. Particular positions can be combined with percussion and vibration to further mobilize secretions.

Figure 4-4. Postural drainage position.

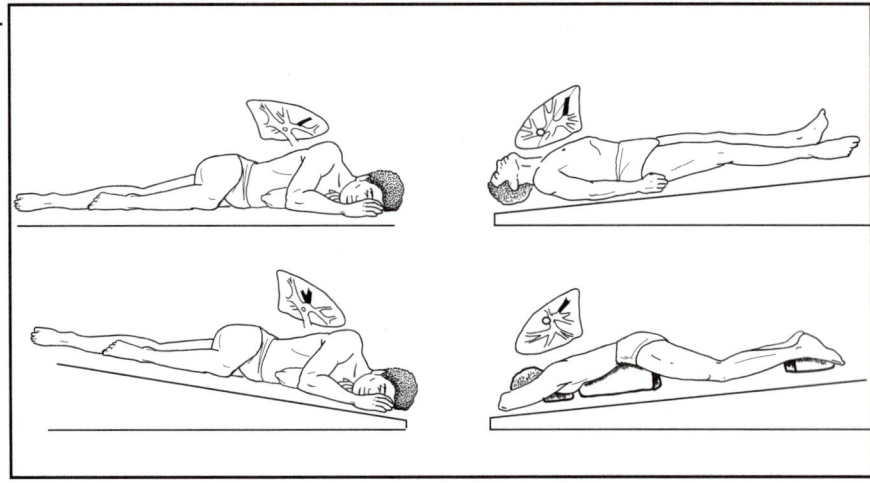

Maintaining a Patent Airway

In all patients, maintaining a patent airway is the most important intervention. It is especially important if the patient is unconscious, anesthetized, or obtunded. In these conditions, the airway may collapse and secretions can accumulate, not allowing air to pass into the lungs. For example, patients who are semiconscious after anesthesia may not be able to maintain an airway because the tongue falls back and can occlude the posterior oropharynx. Artificial airways can be placed to maintain patency of the airways, allow for suctioning of secretions, and permit mechanical ventilation. The most common types of artificial airways are oral airways, nasopharyngeal airways, endotracheal tubes, and tracheostomy tubes.

Oral airways are rigid, plastic devices (Figure 4-5 and Table 4-3) that can be used to maintain the normal structure of the oropharynx. They are used for short-term airway maintenance, such as in postanesthesia units while the patient recovers from anesthetic agents. Oral airways are curved to follow the form of the mouth from the lips, over the tongue, and into the posterior oropharynx. The opening allows for air passage through as well as around the airway and permits suctioning of secretions in the oropharynx. Once the patient is awake enough, the oral airway is removed because it can be very irritating.

Nasal or nasopharyngeal airways are soft rubber or latex tubes that are placed through one nares into the pharynx. They are used for short-term airway maintenance if the oral route is not amenable due to surgery or loose teeth (Table 4-4).

Endotracheal (ET) tubes are long tubes that are placed from the nose or mouth, past the glottis, and into the trachea. Endotracheal tubes are used when:

- Oral or nasal airways cannot maintain a patent airway.
- Effective suctioning cannot be performed with other airways.
- There has been trauma to the upper airways.
- The patient needs assisted or mechanical ventilation.

Endotracheal tubes (ET) are long (240 to 360 mm in length) and 5 to 10 mm in internal diameter. Most ET tubes have a cuff at the distal end, which can be inflated with air via an external catheter to create a seal between the tube and the patient's trachea. The seal may be complete with "no leak" or incomplete with a "minimal leak" or "minimal occlusive pressure." The difference between these two depends on the patient's ventilatory requirements. The "no leak" seal ensures that all air exchange takes place only through

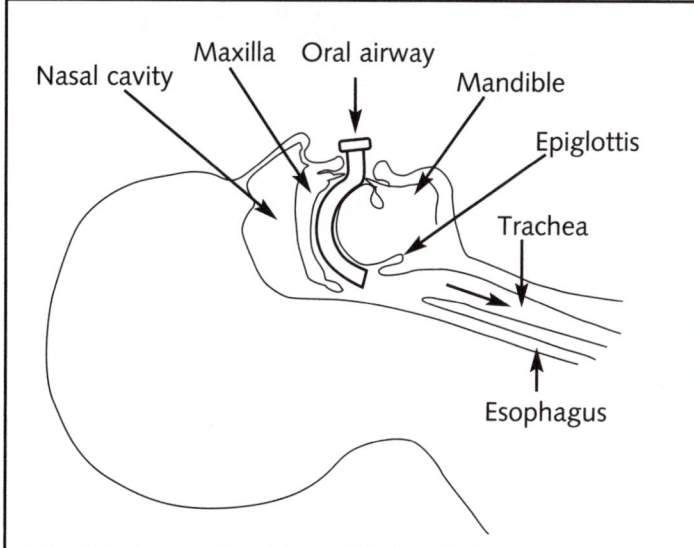

Figure 4-5. Oral airway.

Table 4-3

Insertion of an Oral Airway

1. Measure the oral airway along the patient's jaw with the open end of the curve facing the patient's neck to ensure that the airway is the correct size. The curve of the airway should follow the angle of the patient's jawline.

2. Check that dentures are removed and that there are no loose teeth before inserting the airway.

3. Place the patient in the supine position and open the mouth using the "crossfinger technique," using the thumb and forefinger on the upper and lower teeth to open the mouth.

4. Gently put the airway in upside down until past the teeth and then rotate it over the tongue to follow the curve of the oropharynx.

5. Tape the airway in place and position the patient on his side to prevent aspiration of secretions or vomitus.

6. Suction at least hourly to remove secretions.

7. Evaluate respiration and adequacy of the airway frequently.

the tube. This is especially important when positive end expiratory pressure (PEEP) is used in mechanical ventilation or if a feeding tube is in place (Figure 4-6). The seal prevents aspiration of secretions or gastric contents. Other conditions may allow for a minimal leak to exist between the trachea and the cuff when the patient's condition does not require complete ventilatory support. The "minimal leak" seal also minimizes damage to the tracheal wall, such as irritation and necrosis, because microcirculation in the trachea is preserved. The cuff is inflated using a cuffalator and the pressure is measured. The normal pressure in the cuff is approximately 25 mmHg. The amount of leak around the endotracheal tube cuff can also be auscultated by placing the stethoscope on the patient's trachea and slowly inflating the cuff or balloon with air. When there is no sound during the

Table 4-4

Insertion of a Nasal Airway

1. Measure the nasal airway following along the patient's cheek, starting at the nose and down the cheek past the jaw to ensure the tube is long enough to maintain an airway past the posterior oropharynx. The tube should be slightly wider than the patient's nares.
2. Using a water-soluble gel, lubricate the distal end of the airway.
3. Hyperextend the patient's neck, if allowable, and gently insert the airway in the nares. If any resistance is felt, stop and try the other nares.
4. Assess adequacy of respiration and air exchange and suction as necessary.
5. Examine the posterior oropharynx to ensure the tube is present and tape is in place.

Figure 4-6. Positive end expiratory pressure (PEEP).

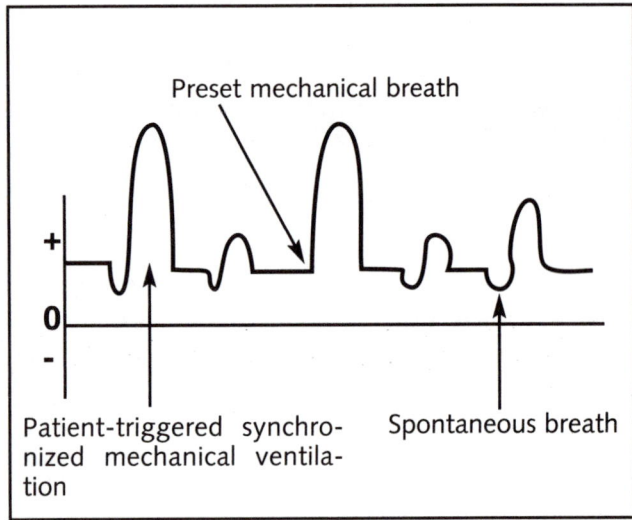

highest pressure phase of the ventilatory cycle, then there is "no leak." When only a small rush of air is heard at peak inspiratory pressure, then there is a minimal leak. A minimal leak is acceptable if there is no significant volume loss on exhalation.

Patients with endotracheal tubes are cared for in the intensive care setting and require a great deal of nursing care. Because their ability to maintain an airway, to mobilize secretions, and to oxygenate adequately are all compromised, the team must work together to ensure the best outcome for the patient. Nurses,

> Endotracheal tubes are used to maintain a patent airway, to perform effective suctioning, and allow mechanical ventilation. They are 240 to 360 mm long and 5 to 10 mm in internal diameter. A cuff at the distal end can be inflated to create a seal between the tube and the patient's trachea.

physicians, and respiratory therapists are all part of the team that plans the appropriate interventions for these patients.

Tracheostomy tubes, another type of airway, are placed into a surgically created opening in the trachea (Figure 4-7). A tracheostomy stoma is created either electively or emer-

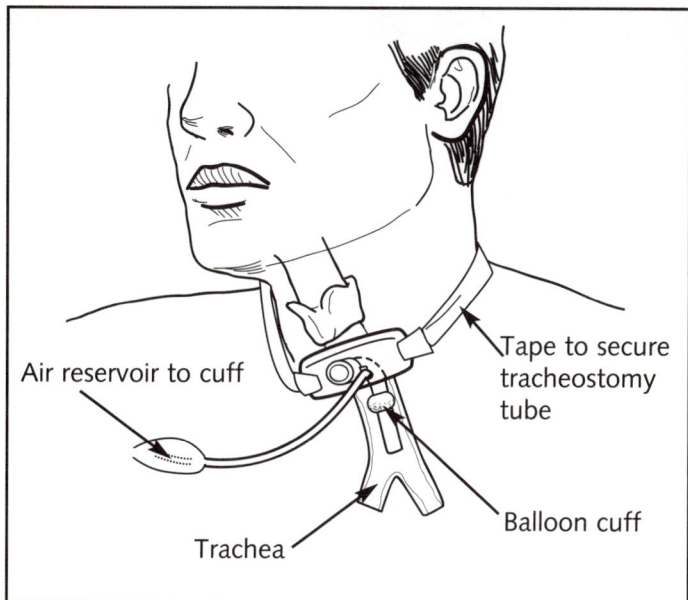

Figure 4-7. Tracheostomy tube.

Air reservoir to cuff

Tape to secure tracheostomy tube

Balloon cuff

Trachea

gently through the third or fourth ring of the trachea. It is created after total laryngecto-my for cancers of the vocal cords or larynx. It may also be created if the patient has a severe airway obstruction, difficulty expelling pulmonary secretion (as in some chronic airway diseases), as part of the care of a patient who requires long-term ventilation, or as a means of delivering oxygen to the distal tracheobronchial tree.

Tracheostomy tubes are inserted through the tracheostomy stoma and down into the trachea. They are made of two types of materials: plastic and metal. Metal ones are used less frequently because the plastic types are found to be less irritating to the trachea. Metal tubes may be composed of an outer and inner cannula. The outer cannula is inserted into the trachea with a soft-ended guide called an obturator. The obturator is removed once the catheter is in place and an inner cannula is inserted. The inner cannula is removable for cleaning of dried secretions.

The tracheostomy tube may be either cuffed (having a balloon at the inner end, which may be inflated) or uncuffed (no balloon cuff or a metal cuff). The outer cannula of a metal tube or the outer portion of a plastic tube has a wider flange that allows the tube to be anchored and secured with sutures or taped around the neck. Fenestrated tubes have an opening in the outer cannula which when plugged allows the patient to phonate. Otherwise, when a tracheostomy tube is in place, the patient cannot speak.

Tracheostomies require very careful care in order to maintain the airway and prevent complications. Because the tube is a direct opening into the lower respiratory tract, all the protective mechanisms of the upper airways have been bypassed. Air is no longer filtered, warmed, or humidified. The ability to cough effectively is diminished because it is diffi-cult to build up sufficient intrathoracic pressure with an opening in the trachea. Bacteria can easily access the lungs, and patients are at risk for infection.

To maintain the airway, nursing care involves humidifying and warming the inspired air and suctioning the secretions (Table 4-5). A tracheostomy collar is a specially designed oxygen delivery mask that fits over the tracheostomy to deliver humidified air or oxygen. Sterile water is always used when humidifying inspired air.

Table 4-5

Suctioning a Tracheostomy Tube

1. Assess the patient's breath sounds and breathing patterns. Loud, noisy respiration, an increased respiratory rate, crackles, wheezes, or rhonchi on auscultation may indicate the need for suctioning or the patient himself may request it.

2. Prepare the needed equipment and always have suctioning equipment in the room of a patient with a tracheostomy (some prepackaged suctioning kits are available):
   - Sterile and nonsterile gloves
   - Sterile saline or water and a container for it
   - Manual resuscitation bag
   - Suction catheters
   - Syringe (5 mL)
   - Suction machine (at 60 to 80 mm suction) or wall-suction

3. Wash your hands.

4. Explain the procedure to the patient. Be calm and reassuring because the patient may be concerned about choking and being unable to communicate.

5. Ventilate the patient with 100% oxygen using the manual resuscitation bag for 5 breaths. If there are superficial secretions, suction them first before manually inflating the lungs.

6. Fill the container with saline or sterile water.

7. Place a sterile glove on the dominant hand that will hold the sterile catheter and a nonsterile glove on the nondominant hand that will control the suction.

8. Insert the sterile catheter into the tracheostomy and down into the bronchus about 6 to 12 inches or until resistance is felt. (Do not use suction during insertion.)

9. Withdraw the catheter slowly, rotating it and applying suction only intermittently so as not to damage the airway walls. (Suction for no more than 10 seconds.)

10. Return the tracheostomy collar (oxygen) and assess the patient's status. If the patient requires more suctioning, wait at least 2 minutes before performing it again.

11. Clear the suction catheter when finished by suctioning the sterile water or saline from the container until the tubing is clear. Discard the suction catheter.

12. Document the color, type, amount, consistency, and any odor of the secretions.

The tracheostomy site and tube also requires careful cleaning to prevent infection. The tracheostomy stoma needs to be cleaned daily and more often if there are signs of infection (ie, redness, drainage, or swelling). If an inner cannula is present, then it should be cleaned every 8 hours (Table 4-6). Complications of tracheostomy tubes include both immediate problems and long-term risks. Postoperatively, patients with newly created tracheostomies are at risk for hemorrhage, pneumomediastinum (air in the mediastinum), subcutaneous emphysema (air in the tissues around the tracheostomy), and tracheoesophageal (T-E) fistula. T-E fistula can occur at any time after tracheostomy creation. They develop because of necrosis of the posterior wall of the larynx from prolonged pressure (from the cuff) or malposition of the tube. Long-term problems include dislodgment of the tube, expelled tubes, and infection. Patients with permanent tracheostomies need to be

Table 4-6

Care of the Tracheostomy Site

1. Gather the needed equipment or a prepackaged kit. Supplies include:
   - Sterile hydrogen peroxide
   - Sterile saline
   - Sterile plastic forceps or swabs
   - Sterile tracheostomy dressing
   - Sterile bowl for soaking inner cannula if present
2. Explain to the patient what you are going to do.
3. Suction the patient as described in Table 4-5 before removing the cannula.
4. Use gloves to remove and discard the old tracheostomy dressing. Assess the drainage on the dressing and the site.
5. Pour sterile saline into one bowl and sterile hydrogen peroxide into the other bowl.
6. Put on sterile gloves.
7. Hold the tracheostomy tube with one hand to keep it from moving (which could stimulate coughing) and use the other hand to gently clean around the tube with sterile saline (or half-strength saline and peroxide depending on the institution's guidelines).
8. Soak the inner cannula, if present, in the peroxide for 1 minute and rinse it in the saline. Allow it to drip dry on the sterile field or gauze.
9. If you are changing the tapes that anchor the tube (usually done every 48 hours or more often if soiled), have another nurse help you keep the tube secure while changing them. Check the tension on the ties frequently to make sure that they are not too tight. They should be snug enough to prevent slippage but loose enough to allow circulation.
10. Keep a spare tracheostomy tube with its obturator of the patient's size taped over his bed at all times in case the tube should become dislodged during cleaning.

taught the signs of infection (fever, painful cough, increased sputum, and chest pain) so that they can receive early treatment.

One of the more emergent situations is an obstructed airway. The airway at any level can become blocked by food, mucus, or foreign material, causing partial or complete obstruction of the airways. When this emergency occurs, immediate action must be taken to remove the obstruction.

CLOSED CHEST DRAINAGE

Many disease processes and surgeries can result in the accumulation of air and fluid in the pleural space. Irritation of the pleural lining from malignancy or infection can produce fluid. Chest surgery like a thoracotomy for lung cancer can produce excess fluid and air leaks that fill the pleural cavity and prevent lung re-expansion. The pleural space is a potential space where the pressure is subatmospheric (lower than atmospheric pressure). This negative pressure allows the lungs to remain expanded. When the pleural space is opened, air rushes into the pleural space and the lung collapses. Increased pressure in the

Figure 4-8. Closed chest drainage.

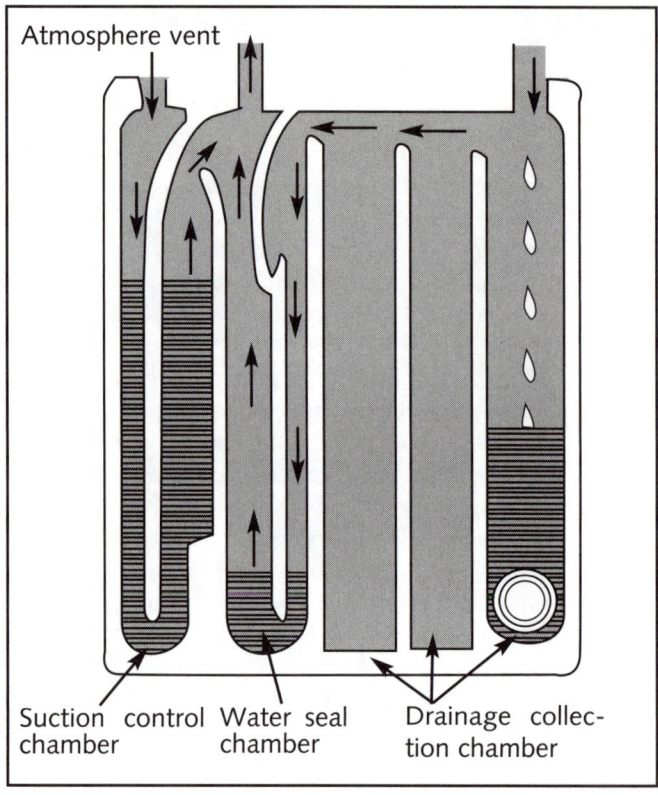

Atmosphere vent

Suction control chamber   Water seal chamber   Drainage collection chamber

pleural space can result in complete collapse of the lung on the affected side and shifting of the mediastinal contents to the opposite side of the chest. This dangerous condition, a mediastinal shift, can kink the great vessels and compromise cardiac and respiratory function. It must be treated immediately.

Closed chest drainage (ie, chest drainage that is closed to atmospheric pressure) allows a system for drainage of fluid and air and reexpansion of the lung. Closed chest drainage systems were historically made of three glass bottles: one to collect drainage, one to maintain a seal to atmospheric pressure, and one for suction control. Now, disposable single unit systems are used in most health care facilities (Figure 4-8). The closed chest drainage system is used to:

- Collect drainage and evacuate air from the pleural space.
- Reestablish negative intrapleural pressure to promote lung reexpansion.
- Equalize pressure in the thoracic cavity to prevent mediastinal shift.

Each component of the chest drainage system must be frequently assessed. The chest tubes that run from the patient to the unit must be free of kinks and clots. The unit itself must always be lower than the patient to allow gravity to assist in draining fluid from the chest. The unit usually has hooks for hanging on the end of the bed or feet to permit standing it on the floor. It should always be upright. If it tips over it must be replaced. The amount of drainage should be marked on the container every hour immediately postoperatively to assess the flow rate and the amount of blood loss. The surgeon should be notified if the drainage exceeds specific parameters.

The water seal compartment allows for a one-way valve between the intrapleural space and atmospheric pressure. Air and fluid can leave the cavity but atmospheric air cannot enter the pleural cavity. The air bubbles out of the water seal chamber and the fluid drains into the drainage compartment. An air vent at the top of the water seal chamber allows the air to escape the unit. Intermittent bubbling in the water seal chamber is normal and indicates that air is leaking into the pleural space and out into the unit.

> Closed chest drainage (ie, chest drainage that is closed to atmospheric pressure) allows a system for fluid and air drainage and reexpansion of the lung. A closed chest drainage system is a single unit used to collect drainage and air from the pleural space, reestablish negative intrapleural pressure, and equalize pressure in the thoracic cavity to prevent mediastinal shift.

Continuous bubbling means that there is an air leak in the system and it needs to be found and corrected. The water level in this chamber fluctuates (tidaling) during inspiration and expiration.

The suction chamber allows for suction to be applied to the intrapleural space in a regulated manner. Depending on the amount of sterile water instilled in the chamber, the suction may be 10 to 20 cm H_2O. The more water in the chamber means that there is more to suction. Continuous bubbling in the suction chamber indicates that the unit is working properly. Newer systems apply "dry" suction, using a spring or dial mechanism in place of a water column. Suction allows for more rapid evacuation of air and drainage.

Nursing care of the patient with a closed chest drainage system involves frequent assessment of the patient's status and the functioning of the unit.

1. Keep the chest tubes free of kinks or bends. Patients may compress the tubes if they are lying on them, so follow positioning orders carefully. Clots may block the tubes postoperatively, and "milking" the tube may be necessary to clear the clots (Figure 4-9). This is a controversial practice because it greatly increases the suction into the pleural space, so check the surgeon's orders before performing this technique.
2. Place the chest drainage unit lower than the patient and always in the upright position.
3. Check the suction chamber to make sure that it is bubbling continuously.
4. Encourage the patient to cough and deep breathe not only to clear secretions but to help reexpand the lung.
5. Check the water seal chamber for tidaling during breathing. Lack of fluctuation in the water seal chamber may indicate a blocked tube or the lung has reexpanded.
6. Never clamp a chest tube without a physician's order. When necessary, this may be done to assess lung expansion and pleural leaks.
7. Medicate the patient 30 minutes before chest tube removal, as it is moderately painful.

Oxygen Therapy

The purpose of oxygen therapy is to deliver more oxygen than is present in room air (21%). It is the most common treatment for patients with respiratory problems, such as chronic bronchitis, emphysema, arterial hypoxemia, and adult respiratory distress syndrome. Although it does not cure any diseases, it can reduce the cardiac workload and decrease tissue hypoxia.

Oxygen is prescribed by a physician specifying the technique, amount, and route. The prescription for oxygen is written in liters per minute or the FiO_2, the fraction of inspired oxygen (eg, 40% or 0.4). The safest way to administer oxygen is to titrate it to achieve a certain O_2 Sat or PaO_2. In patients without chronic respiratory diseases, a PaO_2 of 70 to 100 mmHg would be acceptable. But in those with chronic respiratory disease,

Figure 4-9. Milking (or "stripping") chest tubes to remove blood clots.

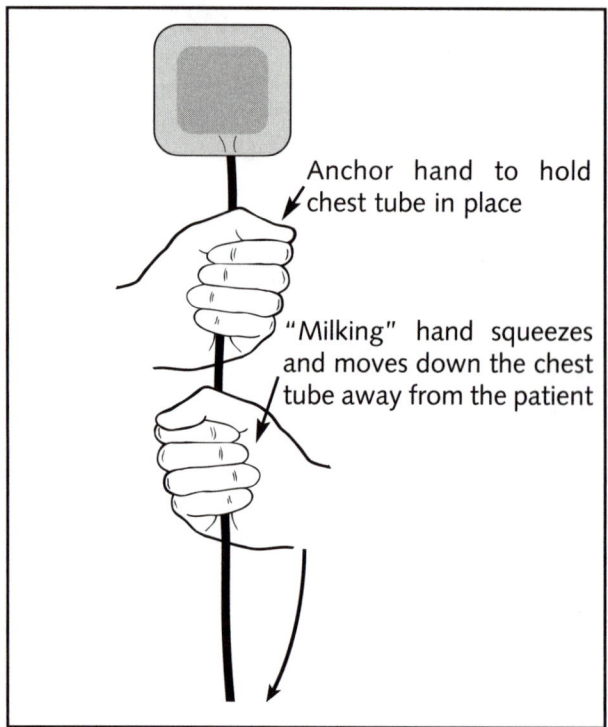

Anchor hand to hold chest tube in place

"Milking" hand squeezes and moves down the chest tube away from the patient

whose stimulus to breathe may be their hypoxic drive, the goal of O_2 therapy can be 55 to 60 mmHg. The order for oxygen has to be customized for each patient and his or her condition.

Oxygen can be delivered by several routes. It is available in canisters (green is the universal color for oxygen-carrying containers) or in wall sockets in health care facilities. The least invasive method is the nasal cannula (Figure 4-10). Oxygen may also be delivered by a variety of masks, as well as by tracheostomy and endotracheal tubes. Newer routes include the transtracheal catheter, where it is delivered via an implanted tracheal catheter to allow greater mobility, less oxygen, and more discretion. Hyperbaric oxygen is the use of higher percentages of oxygen at pressures greater than atmospheric pressure to increase the amount of oxygen dissolved in the blood. It is useful in healing skin grafts and ischemic or gangrene tissue, and treating carbon monoxide poisoning. Hyperbaric oxygen chambers can hold the entire body.

Oxygen should be viewed as a drug with concerns about potential complications. The most common side effect is drying of the mucus membranes. Normally, inspired air passes over the nasal mucosa where it is humidified before it reaches the lower respiratory tract. When supplemental oxygen is delivered at greater than 4 L per min, it should be humidified. This is accomplished by passing the oxygen through a container of sterile water before it enters the patient.

Preoperative Care of the Patient Undergoing Surgery

A special note needs to be made about the patient undergoing surgery. Preoperatively, every patient needs thorough assessment and comprehensive teaching about the operative experience. The assessment should identify patients at risk for problems with oxygenation (eg, smokers, those with preexisting lung disease like COPD or asthma, the elderly, and those with circulatory problems like varicose veins). Varicosities can predispose

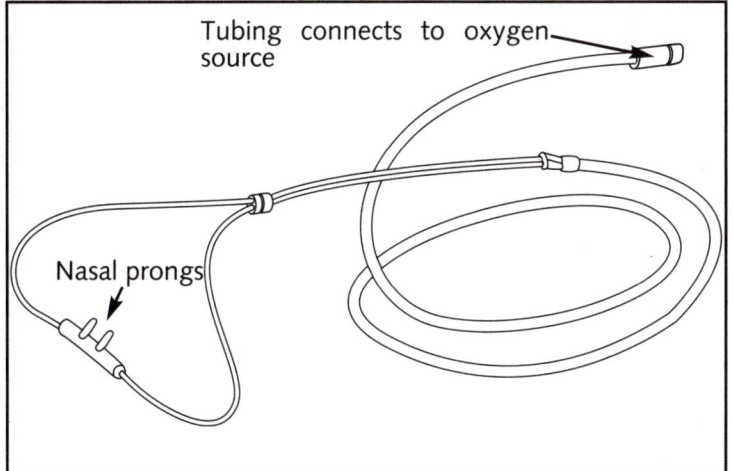

Figure 4-10. Nasal cannula (prongs).

patients to venous stasis in the extremities with the potential for the development of deep vein phlebitis and pulmonary embolus. Some of the most common postoperative complications are atelectasis, pneumonia, and pulmonary emboli.

Preoperative teaching about the operative experience is an important part of nursing care. It involves teaching the patient about what to expect around the perioperative period and what the patient can do to facilitate his recovery from the anesthesia and surgery (Table 4-7). Preoperative teaching not only allays anxiety in the patient but it also shortens the recovery time and prevents complications in many patients. Try to enlist the patient as a partner in his recovery.

OXYGEN THERAPY

Oxygen therapy delivers to the patient a greater concentration of oxygen than is available in room air (21%). The goals of oxygen therapy are the prevention or treatment of hypoxemia. The correction of hypoxemia will decrease the work of breathing and facilitate myocardial and tissue oxygen supply. There exists a wide variety of oxygen delivery devices. All oxygen delivery systems consist of an oxygen source: cylinder or piped-in wall; valve handles to open the cylinder/system; flow meter to regulate the control of oxygen flow in liters per minute; tubing that connects the oxygen supply source to the patient's oxygen administration device; and a humidifier to counteract the drying effects of oxygen flowing over mucus membranes (some institutions do not use humidifiers with very low-flow oxygen systems unless requested by the patient). Oxygen delivery systems can be classified as either low-flow systems, which are designed to provide supplemental oxygen to an inspired tidal volume; or high-flow systems, which are designed to provide oxygen sufficient to supply an entire inspired tidal volume. Examples of a low-flow system include nasal cannula, simple mask, and partial nonbreathing and nonrebreathing masks with reservoir bags (Table 4-8). Examples of high-flow systems include the Venturi mask and mechanical ventilation (Table 4-9). Selection of the appropriate device is contingent upon the clinical condition, desired fraction of inspired oxygen, patient compliance or tolerance of the device, and the cost.

Table 4-7

What You Can Do to Help Your Recovery

1. Take deep breaths every few minutes or when the nurses remind you. Inhale filling the lower chest, then the midchest, and finally the upper chest, holding for 5 seconds and then slowly exhaling for 6 to 8 seconds.
2. Cough every 1 to 2 hours if you have secretions. Remember to splint the incision with a pillow or your hands to decrease the pain.
3. Use your incentive spirometer as directed or every 1 to 2 hours. Remember that slow breaths and holding the deep breath for 2 to 5 seconds help open the airways.
4. Ask for pain medication when you start to get uncomfortable. Do not wait until the pain is severe.
5. Remember to move from side to side if your surgeon allows this to allow your lungs to expand.
6. Start ambulating with assistance as soon as your surgeon says that it is all right. Take pain medication before you start walking.
7. Perform leg exercises as allowed by the surgeon to facilitate blood flow in the legs.
8. Remember that the staff is here to help your recovery—call them if you are having any problems or questions.

Table 4-8

Low-Flow Systems

Device	Flow Rate (L/min)	FiO$_2$ (%)*
Nasal cannula	1	22-24
	2	26-28
	3	28-32
	4	32-36
	5	36-40
	6	40-44
Simple mask	5-6	40
	6-7	50
	7-8	60
Partial rebreather mask	7	65
	8-15	70-80
	12-15	85-100
Nonrebreather	Set to prevent collapse of oxygen reservoir	

*FiO$_2$ will vary with respiratory pattern, rate, and tidal volume

Table 4-9	
Venturi Devices	
Flow Rate (L/min)	*FiO_2 (%)**
4	24
6	28
8	35
8	40
12	60

*Color-coded adapters for each desired FiO_2

Low-Flow Devices

Nasal Cannula

This device (see Figure 4-10) is utilized when the patient requires low to medium concentrations of oxygen. Because the cannula is a low-flow system, a large part of the tidal volume inspired by the patient will be ambient (room) air. Therefore, the inspired oxygen concentration is dependent on the flow of oxygen through the unit, the patient's respiratory rate, and the patient's own tidal volume. Dyspneic patients with high respiratory rates and tidal volumes entrain a high volume of room air, which will result in a lower FiO_2 delivery. Oxygen via nasal cannula is prescribed in liters per minute. With each increase of 1 liter of oxygen, the inspired oxygen concentration increases by approximately 4%. The normal range of prescribed flow is 1 to 6 L per minute. This flow in a patient with a normal respiratory rate and tidal volume will deliver an FiO_2 of approximately 24% to 44%. Flows greater than 6 L per minute may result in irritation to the nasal and pharyngeal mucosa and possibly contribute to air swallowing. Humidification at a 1 to 6 L per minute flow rate is not required but is frequently utilized to prevent mucosal drying. Mouth breathing will not affect the concentration of delivered oxygen unless there is complete obstruction of the nares because oxygen will be inhaled from the anatomic reservoirs: the oropharynx and nasopharynx. There are multiple advantages of the nasal cannula system. Nasal cannulae are comfortable, well tolerated, and relatively inexpensive. They also allow the patient to communicate, eat, drink, and cough without disrupting oxygen flow. A disadvantage of the nasal cannula system is the variability of oxygen delivery with changing respiratory rates and tidal volumes. Nasal cannula systems may also cause pressure sores around the nose and ears. Care of the patient with this type of device would include close assessment of skin for signs of breakdown around the ears, cheeks, and nares and lubrication of the nares if the humidity is not being utilized and cleaning of the equipment as needed.

Oropharyngeal Catheter

The oro- or nasopharyngeal catheter is rarely utilized because of the need to move the catheter daily to minimize pharyngeal damage. A possible scenario in which it may be used is the short-term delivery of oxygen in low to moderate concentrations. As with the nasal cannula, oxygen delivery varies with respiratory rate and tidal volume.

Figure 4-11. Simple face mask.

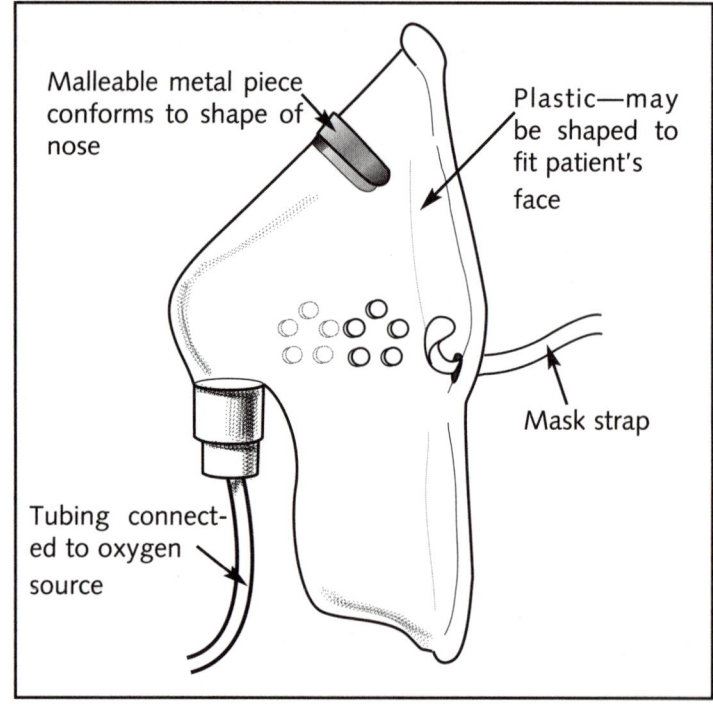

Malleable metal piece conforms to shape of nose

Plastic—may be shaped to fit patient's face

Mask strap

Tubing connected to oxygen source

Simple Face Mask

Face masks are generally well tolerated by adults (Figure 4-11). Openings cut into both sides of the mask stop a possible accumulation and rebreathing of expired air, which is high in CO_2. Oxygen flow rates in a simple mask should exceed 5 L per minute. This rate facilitates flushing out of expired air. The recommended flow rate through a simple mask is 5 to 8 L per minute. At this flow, the simple face mask can provide oxygen concentrations between 40% to 60%. However, as noted with the nasal cannula, the FiO_2 in a simple face mask is diluted by room air and can be affected by respiratory rate and tidal volume. Care of patients being treated with oxygen therapy via a simple mask includes recognition of the risk for aspiration of vomitus, assessment of facial skin and ears for irritation or breakdown, maintaining oxygen flow at greater than 5 L per minute, maintaining adequate water in the system for the provision of humidity, emptying connecting tubings of condensed water, and cleaning the masks when necessary.

Face Mask With an Oxygen Reservoir

Face masks with an oxygen reservoir bag are divided into two groups: partial rebreathing and nonrebreathing (Figure 4-12). These systems provide a constant flow of oxygen into an attached reservoir bag. The design of the partial rebreathing mask is similar to that of the simple face mask. The difference between the two is that the partial rebreathing mask has an oxygen reservoir bag attached. The purpose of the partial rebreathing mask is to increase FiO_2 by allowing it to be breathed from a reservoir. Exhaled air will also enter the reservoir bag, allowing some rebreathing of CO_2. In order to achieve an FiO_2 greater than 60%, a nonrebreathing mask must be used. A nonrebreathing mask consists of a face mask with an attached reservoir bag and a one-way valve between the reservoir bag and the mask. The one-way valve between the reservoir bag and the mask prevents exhaled air from reentering the reservoir bag and diluting the FiO_2. At a flow of 6 L per

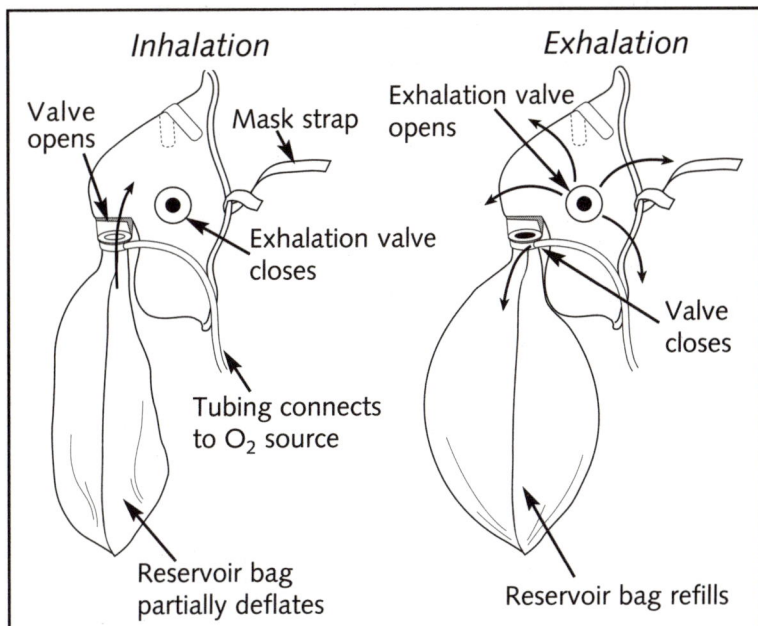

Inhalation

Valve opens

Mask strap

Exhalation valve closes

Tubing connects to O_2 source

Reservoir bag partially deflates

Exhalation

Exhalation valve opens

Valve closes

Reservoir bag refills

Figure 4-12. Rebreathing and nonrebreathing masks.

minute, an FiO_2 of approximately 60% can be achieved. Each additional liter per minute of oxygen flow will increase the FiO_2 by approximately 10%. This system can deliver the highest oxygen concentration in spontaneously breathing patients. At flows of 12 to 15 L per minute, a one-way valve between the reservoir and the mask and one-way valves covering both ports in the mask's sides preventing inhalation of room air, this system can deliver almost a 100% oxygen concentration. However, because a tight fit is seldom achieved with these masks, room air may be pulled in around the mask, diluting the FiO_2 to 80% to 90%. Care of patients being treated with oxygen therapy via a partial or non-rebreather mask mirrors that of a patient in a simple mask but also includes monitoring of the reservoir bag to assure continuous inflation and adjusting mask fit to minimize leaks.

Venturi Mask

In the Venturi (Venti) mask, oxygen under pressure is forced through various-sized orifices (Figure 4-13). As the oxygen exits the orifice, it creates a subatmospheric pressure, which entrains room air into the system. The size of the orifice and oxygen flow rate dictate the oxygen concentration. The Venturi mask can be adjusted to deliver the following fractions of inspired oxygen: 24, 28, 35, 40, and 60 (see Table 4-9). This system is used frequently in patients with chronic hypercarbia (COPD), who rely on an hypoxic drive for respiration and are at high risk of respiratory depression due to sudden increases in PaO_2 because it offers a more precise inspired oxygen fraction. Oxygen therapy via a Venturi mask at an FiO_2 of 24% is usually used initially. The patient's response to this dose of oxygen is then evaluated and the mask titrated to the desired level of SaO_2 or PaO_2. Care of patients treated with oxygen therapy via the Venturi mask is the same as patients being treated via a simple mask.

Transtracheal Catheter

This is a small catheter percutaneously inserted between the second and third tracheal cartilage. This option may be used for patients who require home oxygen therapy. The

Figure 4-13. Venturi mask.

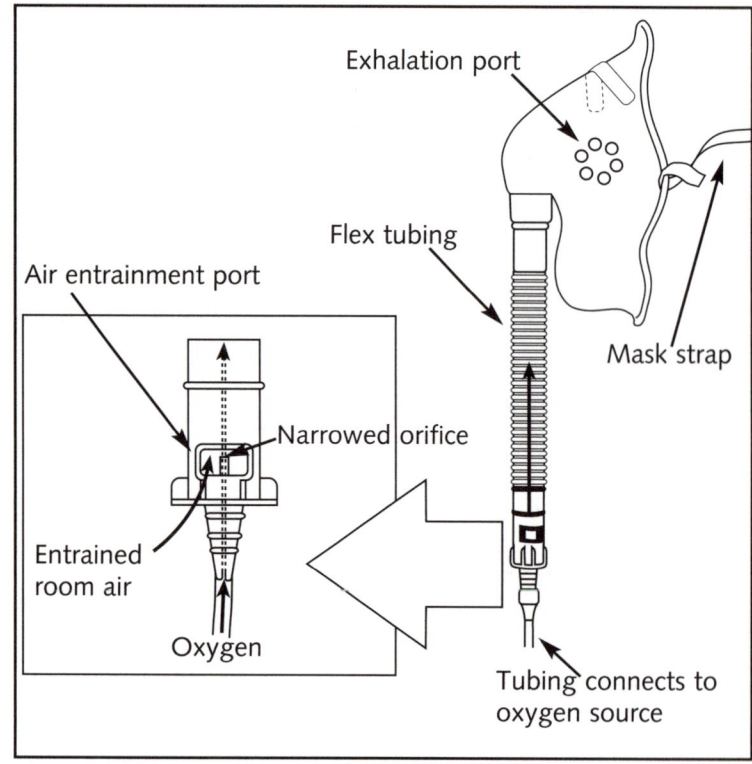

advantages of this oxygenation technique is that they are cosmetically more appealing, and the catheter may be concealed by clothing. These catheters do not interfere with eating, drinking, or talking. Patients with these catheters report an improved sense of taste and smell and an improved appetite. The disadvantages of transtracheal catheters include the risk of infection, the need for meticulous care, a possibly difficult insertion technique, and the possibility of subcutaneous emphysema should the catheter be dislodged before a mature tract is formed. Care of patients with these devices include teaching patients how to recognize and report evidence of infection: fever, warmth, erythema, edema at insertion site; a change in the color, consistency, and/or amount of secretions; and assessment of their catheters for patency.

Continuous Positive Airway Pressure and Bilevel Positive Airway Pressure Mask

CPAP is continuous positive airway pressure, pressure above atmosphere, at the airway opening throughout a spontaneous breathing cycle. CPAP systems deliver oxygen via a nasal or facial mask while applying CPAP. CPAP improves oxygenation by enhancing the transport of oxygen across the pulmonary capillary membrane and reducing the shunt created by collapsed alveoli. The positive pressure at the end of expiration (PEEP) helps to prevent alveolar collapse. A CPAP device is used to alert patients whose oxygen requirements cannot be met despite the delivery of maximum supplemental oxygen. CPAP systems consist of a face or nasal mask with an inflatable cushion and head strap to hold the mask tightly in place; a PEEP valve is incorporated into the exhalation port to maintain positive expiratory pressure and in the face mask version, a port through which nasogastric suction may be accomplished. BIPAP (bilevel positive airway pressure) provides pressure support ventilation by assisting inhalation, which increases tidal volume , PEEP, and minute ventilation (minute ventilation = tidal volume x respiratory rate). BIPAP is delivered via nasal or facial mask. Patients using CPAP or BIPAP must be able to protect their airway.

The advantage of utilizing a CPAP/BIPAP device is improved oxygenation with lower levels of inspired oxygen. Disadvantages include oral and nasal dryness, burning, bleeding, eye irritation, and interference with talking, eating, and expectorating sputum. These devices also put the patient at high risk for aerophagia, aspiration, the development of pressure sores, and decubitus ulcers under the perimeter of the mask. The care of patients being treated with these devices includes vigilant skin assessment, possible treatment with nasogastric tubes for decompression, antigas medications, and hydration measures for the oro- and nasopharynx.

Hazards of Oxygen Therapy

Obviously oxygen therapy is a highly beneficial treatment, however, it is not without risks. Most adverse effects of oxygen therapy occur when treatment has been prolonged and at an FiO_2 greater than 50%. Adverse effects include pulmonary oxygen toxicity and hypoventilation. Pulmonary oxygen toxicity is a result of higher than normal amounts of oxygen in the lower airways for a prolonged time period, $FiO_2 > 50\%$ to 70% for > 48 to 72 hours. This prolonged exposure may lead to ciliary dysfunction, impaired mucus removal, fibrosis of the alveolar capillary membrane, and respiratory distress syndrome. Early signs and symptoms of oxygen toxicity include increased respiratory rate, dyspnea, coughing, fatigue, lethargy, malaise, restlessness, paresthesias in the extremities, nausea, vomiting, and anorexia. Later symptoms include cyanosis, severe dyspnea, use of accessory muscles or respiration, and asphyxia. Hypoventilation may occur in patients who need a hypoxic drive to breathe. As the PaO_2 increases with supplemental oxygen, the stimulus for respiration can be blunted or removed. This could result in hypoventilation and possibly respiratory arrest. Signs and symptoms of hypoventilation include a decrease in the rate and depth of respiration and a decreasing level of consciousness.

MECHANICAL VENTILATION

Mrs. P., a 76-year-old white female with a history of COPD secondary to cigarette smoking (50 pack years) and hypertension (HTN), transient ischemia attack (TIA), and CAD presents to the ER with complaints of increasing shortness of breath (SOB) and chest pressure. She states this began approximately 5 hours ago when she returned from a shopping trip with her friend. She has taken three nitroglycerin tablets without relief of her chest pain and has used her Ventolin inhaler five to six times without any change in her SOB. Physical exam reveals an anxious, elderly, obese female who is pale, cool, diaphoretic, and using accessory muscles to breathe. Vital signs: temperature—96.5°F, AP—143 and irregular, BP—194/102 mmHg on the right and 198/104 mmHg on the left, RR—40 breaths per min and labored, SaO_2 is 84 on 100% oxygen via nonrebreathing mask. Lung sounds: inspiratory and expiratory crackles; posterior: T3 (thoracic vertebrae) down bilaterally; anteriorly: fourth intercostal space down bilaterally. The quality of the crackles does not change with deep breathing and coughing. Jugular venous distention is noted bilaterally with the patient sitting at a 75-degree angle. A systolic murmur and an S3 heart sound are auscultated. EKG reveals 4 mm ST segment elevation across the precordium (anterior septal leads). Arterial blood gas (ABG): pH—7.16, PCO_2—74, PO_2—47, SaO_2—84. A diagnosis of anterior septal myocardial infarction (MI) and pulmonary edema with resulting respiratory failure is made. The ER physician directs the RN to institute nitroglycerin IV and titrate up until relief of chest pain, maintaining a systolic blood pressure (SBP) of > 90 mmHg, give furosemide 60 mg IVP, give 2 mg MSO_4 IV every 3 minutes if SBP > 90 mmHg, until relief of chest pain, and directs the respiratory therapist to prepare for endotracheal intubation and mechanical ventilation.

Mechanical ventilation is indicated when a patient's lungs are incapable of delivering an adequate amount of oxygen to the tissues and/or removing a sufficient amount of carbon dioxide. This condition can be the result of a myriad of diseases or injury processes, such as drug overdose, COPD, asthma, pneumonia, inhalation injury, multiple trauma, neuromuscular disease, shock, multisystem failure, and postoperative states where anesthesia is not reversed or the integrity of the muscles of breathing are compromised.

Endotracheal Intubation

A patient who can no longer maintain adequate gas exchange or a patent airway and requires intervention with mechanical ventilation must have an artificial airway inserted. This artificial airway can be either an endotracheal tube (ETT) or a tracheostomy tube. The rationale for use of a tracheostomy tube as the initial artificial airway is described on page 141, in the tracheostomy section. The most common artificial airway utilized for short-term airway management and ventilatory support is the ETT. The ETT is a polyvinylchloride tube that is passed via either the nares or mouth through the vocal cords into the trachea with the tip positioned approximately 2 to 3 cm above the carina. Intubation is usually performed by an experienced professional, trained in the technique (ie, an anesthesiologist, pulmonologist, nurse anesthetist, or specially trained RN or RCP). The ETT design is standardized. The connector has a 15 mm standard outside diameter that facilitates connection to standard ventilatory equipment: ventilator circuitry, manual resuscitator bag (MRB), or anesthesia devices. The ETT body has a radiopaque stripe that runs the length of the tube to facilitate tube location on chest radiograph. The body also has centimeter markings that allow for the determination of depth of insertion. This distal tip of the ETT is beveled to allow easier passage. At the distal tip is a cuff that when inflated produces a seal in the trachea, allowing for the application of positive pressure ventilation and minimizing aspiration. When the cuff is inflated, no air can pass through the vocal cords to the nose and mouth, therefore the patient cannot speak. The inflating system for the cuff consists of a small bore tube that is fused to the body of the ETT with a pilot balloon at the proximal end. This pilot balloon has a spring-loaded, one-way valve that is activated by the insertion of a syringe. Air can be inserted or withdrawn from the cuff through this valve.

ETTs are available in a variety of sizes. Adult sizes range from 5 to 10 mm. The tube size is determined by its internal diameter and marked on the connector/adapter and/or tube body. Adult women are commonly intubated with a 7 to 8 mm tube; men with an 8 to 9 mm tube.

After the ETT is inserted, its position is assessed by auscultation with a stethoscope over the lung fields and abdomen. Many institutions now use a capnography device to aid in the assessment of proper positioning of the ETT. The gold standard of assessment for ETT position is the chest radiograph. Once the tube is determined to be in proper position, it is stabilized by either taping it to the face or with a variety of stabilizing devices. The depth of the tube at either the teeth, lip, or nares opening should be documented.

The goals of mechanical ventilation are:
1. Provide an adequate amount of oxygen delivery to the lung.
2. Maintain alveolar ventilation (the elimination of carbon dioxide).
3. Reduce the work of breathing.

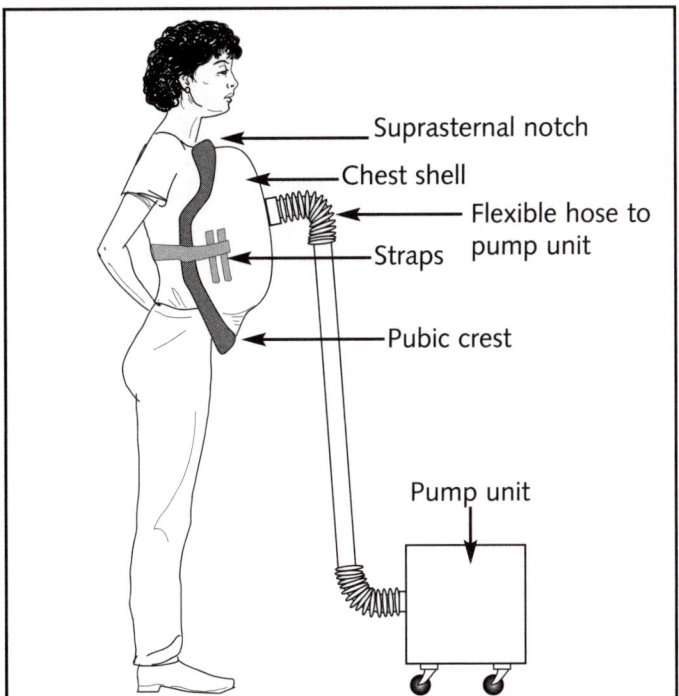

Figure 4-14. Negative pressure ventilator—chest shell.

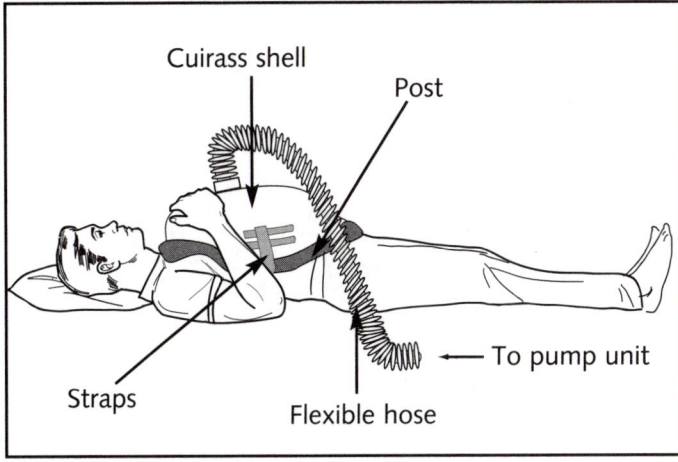

Figure 4-15. Negative pressure ventilator—cuirass shell.

Mechanical ventilation will not cure diseased lungs. It is used as adjunctive therapy to support the patient through a period where lung function is inadequate. Therapy during mechanical ventilation is aimed at correcting the underlying disease process and preventing the possible complications of mechanical ventilation. Once the patient is capable of maintaining adequate tissue oxygenation and alveolar ventilation (removal of CO_2), ventilatory support can be withdrawn.

Classification of Ventilators

Mechanical ventilators can be either negative pressure or positive pressure devices. Negative pressure ventilators—Drinker respirator tank (iron lung), chest cuirass (tortoise shell), and the body wrap (pneumowrap)—are rarely utilized in the treatment of acute respiratory failure (Figures 4-14 and 4-15). They are most commonly used as home night-

Figure 4-16. Negative pressure ventilator—inspiration.

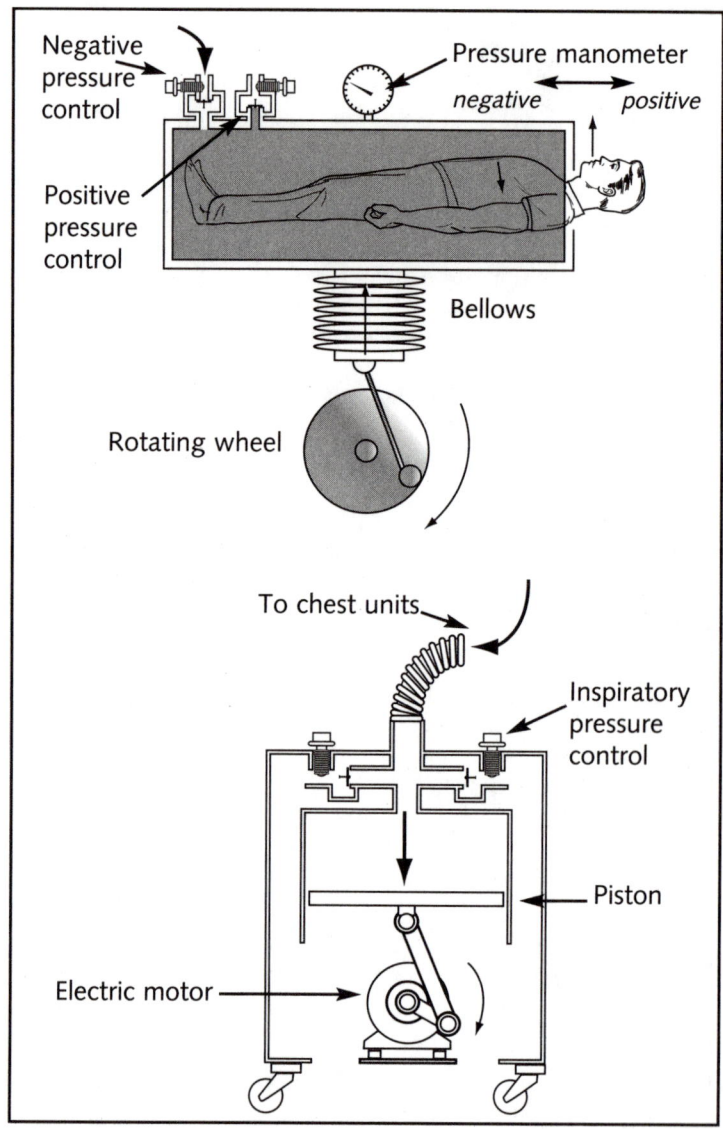

time ventilatory support by polio survivors and persons with neuromuscular disease, CNS disorders, COPD, or spinal cord injuries. Negative pressure ventilators do not require intubation. They are air tight devices that enclose either the chest wall cavity (tortoise shell, pneumowrap) or the entire body (iron lung), leaving the head exposed (Figures 4-16 and 4-17). They function by creating negative pressure around the thoracic cavity during inspiration, promoting air entry into the lungs, then negative pressure is stopped, allowing air to flow passively out of the lungs. Persons using these devices must have compliant lungs and be able to clear their own secretions. Positive pressure ventilators are the type most commonly used in the acute care setting. Positive pressure ventilators force gas into the lungs under positive pressure via an artificial airway (endotracheal tube or tracheostomy tube) during inspiration. Expiration occurs passively when the flow of gas from the mechanical ventilator ceases.

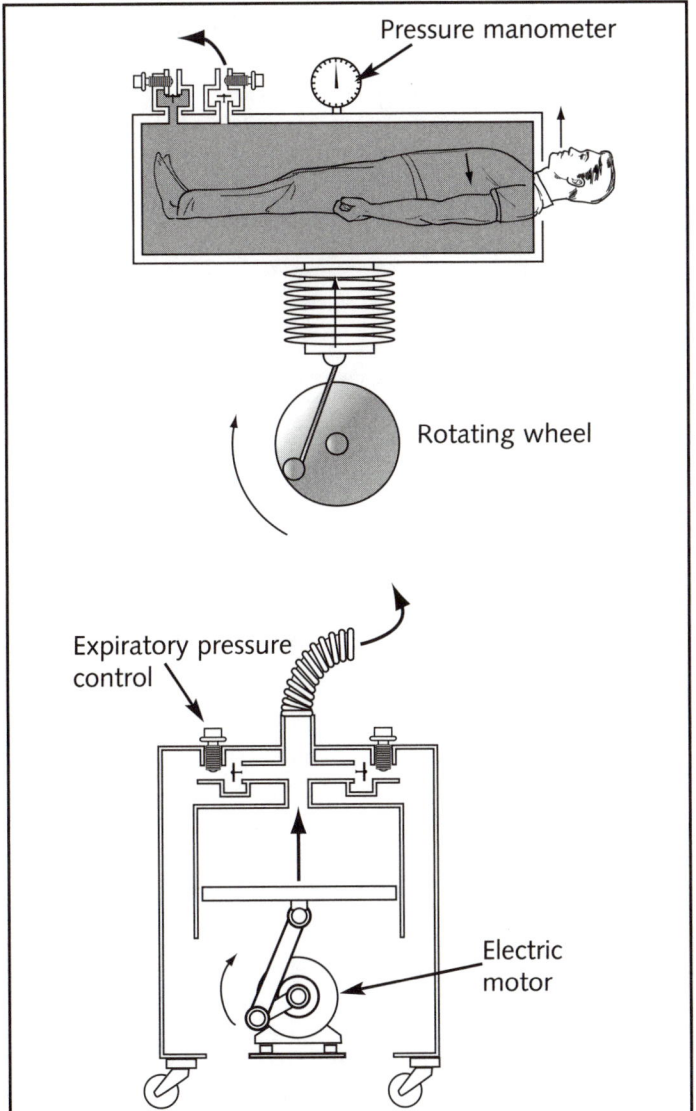

Figure 4-17. Negative pressure ventilator—exhalation.

Positive pressure ventilators are classified by the predetermined parameter, which terminates the aspiratory phase. Inspiration can be terminated or "cycled" by three parameters: volume, pressure, or time. Volume-cycled ventilators deliver gas to a preset volume. When the preset volume is reached, gas delivery is terminated, inspiration ends, and passive expiration begins. Puritan Bennett MA-1, MA-2, and 7200 A, and the Bourns Bear I-V are examples of volume ventilators. Pressure-cycled ventilators deliver gas until a preset pressure in the airway is attained. At this pressure gas, delivery is terminated and expiration begins. The volume of gas delivered will be affected by any variable that alters airway resistance or chest wall/lung compliance. If airway resistance increases or lung/chest wall compliance decreases, the volume of gas will decrease. If airway resistance decreases or lung/chest wall compliance increases, the volume of gas will increase. The Byrd Mark 6 is an example of a pressure-cycled ventilator. Time-cycled ventilators deliver gas for a preset amount of time. The volume of gas delivered is determined by the flow rate of the gas and the preset time internal. Changes in airway resistance or chest

Figure 4-18. Physiologic sequelae to positive pressure ventilation.

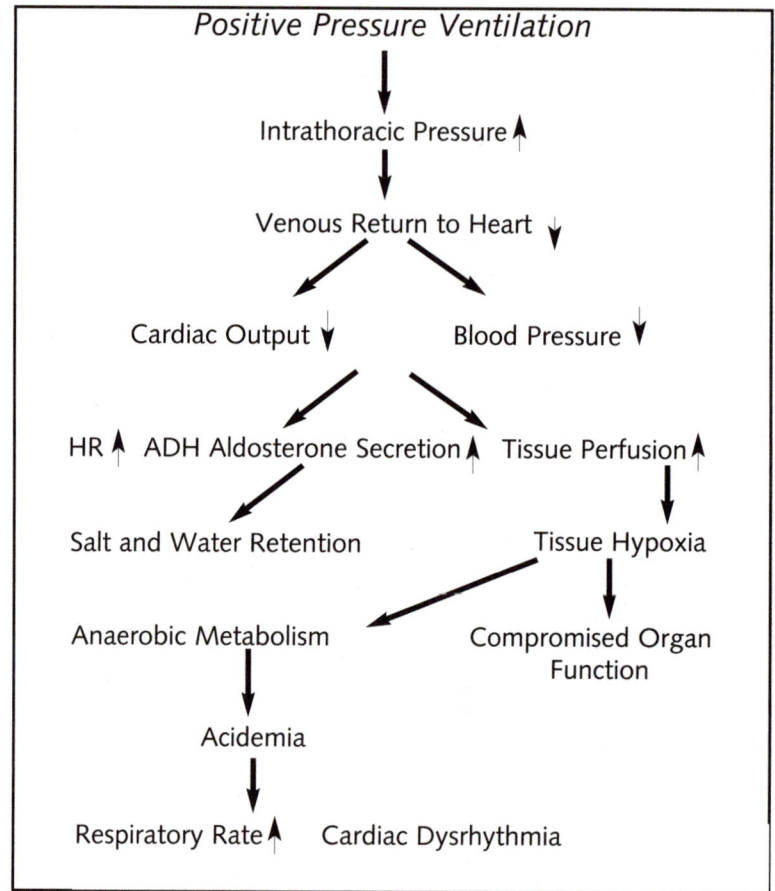

Positive Pressure Ventilation

Intrathoracic Pressure

Venous Return to Heart

Cardiac Output   Blood Pressure

HR ADH Aldosterone Secretion Tissue Perfusion

Salt and Water Retention   Tissue Hypoxia

Anaerobic Metabolism   Compromised Organ Function

Acidemia

Respiratory Rate   Cardiac Dysrhythmia

wall/lung compliance will also affect the volume of gas delivered by a time-cycled ventilator. This type of ventilation is used more commonly in neonatal and pediatric populations. The Siemens Seno 900 series is an example of a time-cycled ventilator. Many microprocessor-driven ventilators are capable of functioning in a variety of inspiratory flow patterns. The majority of positive pressure ventilators have built-in safety features with alarm functions to prevent the delivery of excessively high pressures, rates, or volumes to the patient being treated with mechanical ventilation (Figure 4-18).

Ventilator settings/controls—the volume-cycled ventilator is currently the most commonly used ventilator in acute care. Each of these ventilators has a number of parameters prescribed by the physician and set or adjusted by the nurse caring for the patient receiving mechanical ventilation. The parameters requiring physician prescription and universal to most ventilators include mode: SIMV, assist/control, PSV; respiratory rate (RR), breaths per minute (BPM), or frequency (f); tidal volume (Vt); fraction of inspired oxygen (FiO$_2$); positive end expiratory pressure (PEEP); continuous positive airway pressure (CPAP). Parameters such as inspiration to expiration ratio (I:E ratio); sensitivity; sighs; pressure limits; flow rate; flow wave patterns; pressure and/or flow triggers and alarms may be dictated by the type of ventilatory mode utilized or may be adjusted by the nurse responsible for ventilator management.

Respiratory rate, breaths per minute, frequency—these terms are the number of breaths the ventilator delivers every minute. The patient's respiratory rate equals the number delivered by the ventilator plus the patient's own spontaneous breaths.

Tidal volume—volume of gas delivered with each breath. This is usually set between 5 to 15 cc per kg.

FiO_2—the percent of oxygen being delivered with each breath. It is recommended that the lowest FiO_2 possible to meet the patient's needs be utilized.

PEEP—amount of pressure, measured in cm of H_2O, exerted by the ventilator during the expiratory phase of ventilation. PEEP improves oxygenation by enhancing gas exchange and preventing atelectasis. PEEP set at 3 to 5 cm H_2O is considered physiologic. Persistent hypoxemia despite high FiO_2s may be treated by increasing the amount of PEEP. PEEP, by increasing intrathoracic pressure, may decrease venous return to the heart, thereby possibly decreasing BP and cardiac output.

CPAP—application of positive airway pressure throughout the entire ventilatory cycle, inspiration and expiration, in spontaneously breathing patients. CPAP aids in alveolar recruitment during inspiration and prevents alveolar collapse during expiration. CPAP is indicated for the treatment of sleep apnea and is also used as a method to wean patients from ventilatory support.

I:E—determined by the preset volume being delivered and the rate of inspiratory flow. Normal I:E ratio is 1:2.

Sensitivity—the amount of negative pressure the patient must generate to trigger the ventilator to respond. Sensitivity is adjusted to require minimal patient effort, usually around 2 cm H_2O.

Sighs—volumes of air that are 1.5 to 2 times the preset Vt delivered 6 to 10 times an hour. Sighs are used to prevent atelectasis in certain circumstances.

Pressure Limits—settings utilized to limit the pressure the ventilator can use to deliver a specified volume. The pressure limit is usually set 10 to 15 cm H_2O greater than the pressure it takes to deliver a normal breath to a patient. Once a preset pressure limit is reached, the ventilator will stop delivering volume, even if the preset Vt is not obtained, to protect the patient against barotrauma. This is accompanied by an alarm system.

Alarm systems—visual and audible warning that alerts caretakers that certain conditions exist (eg, low or high pressures, low volumes, disconnection, inappropriate I:E ratio or FiO_2). Various tones are utilized for specific conditions, allowing the RN or RCP to expedite their trouble shooting when specific alarm conditions exist.

Modes of Ventilation

The mode of ventilation (Figures 4-19 and 4-20) describes the pattern by which the ventilator delivers breaths to the patient. There are five basic modes of ventilatory support: controlled mechanical ventilation (CMV), assist/control ventilation (A/C), synchronized intermittent mandatory ventilation (SIMV), pressure support ventilation (PSV), and pressure-controlled ventilation (PCV).

Controlled Mechanical Ventilation

CMV is the least frequently used mode of ventilation. During CMV, the patient receives a preset FiO_2, rate, and tidal volume. No spontaneous breaths are allowed. This mode is only utilized in patients who are not capable of spontaneous respiratory effort (ie, patients who are totally anesthetized or paralyzed).

Assist/Control Ventilation

In A/C ventilation, a preset Vt is delivered at a preset rate (control), but the patient may also initiate breaths (assist). The ventilator delivers the preset volume each time it "senses" the patient initiating a breath. Therefore, every breath the patient receives will be at the preset Vt. In this mode, the work of breathing may be significantly decreased. A/C

Figure 4-19. Modes of ventilation (I).

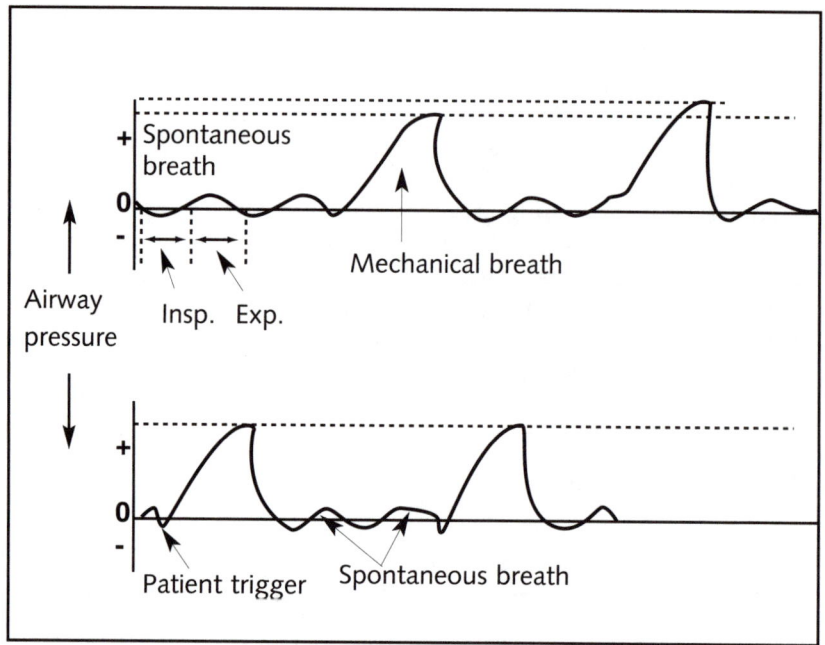

Figure 4-20. Modes of ventilation (II).

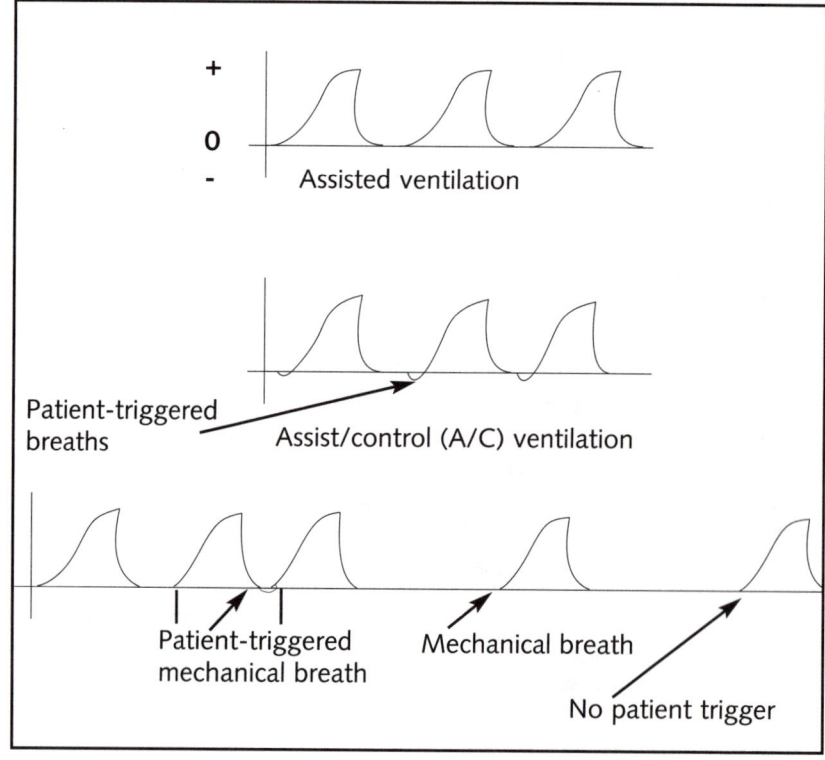

mode also allows for complete rest for the muscles of respiration. A/C is the most commonly used mode for the treatment of acute respiratory failure.

Synchronized Mandatory Ventilation

SIMV mode is similar to the A/C mode in that a preset rate, Vt, and FiO_2 are programmed into the ventilator. However, in the SIMV mode, the ventilator synchronizes its delivery of the preset volume breath to coincide with a patient's spontaneous effort within a specified time. It accomplishes this by having a control algorithm that has the ventilator wait a specified period of time to sense a spontaneous inspiratory effort. For example, if the preset rate is 6, the ventilator will wait for 10 seconds (if the rate were 4, the ventilator would wait for 15 seconds) to sense an inspiratory effort. If one is sensed, then the preset Vt is delivered with that effort. Any additional breaths initiated by the patient within that time frame will have a volume dependent on the patient's inspiratory effort. If no inspiratory effort is sensed in that time frame, the ventilator will deliver a breath at the end of the prescribed time period. This mode allows the patient to breathe spontaneously at variable volumes between ventilator breaths. It also assures that a minimum ventilatory pattern is maintained. The FiO_2 is constant for both ventilator and patient-initiated breaths.

Pressure Support Ventilation

In PSV, the patient's spontaneous inspiratory effort is augmented by the delivery of a preset level of positive inspiratory pressure. When the patient initiates inspiration, the preset amount of pressure support is delivered and held constant throughout inspiration, facilitating the flow of gas into the lung. In the PSV mode, Vt is variable, dependent on patient effort, and the amount of PS selected. The compliance and resistance of both the patient's lungs and the ventilator circuit PSV is utilized to assist the patient to overcome the increased resistance and work of breathing imposed by the disease process, as well as the implements of mechanical ventilation (ie, endotracheal tubes, inspiratory valves, and tubing).

Pressure Control Ventilation

In PCV, there is a preset number of breaths per minute with every breath being augmented by a preset amount of inspiratory pressure. When a preselected pressure is reached, the flow of gas is stopped and passive expiration begins. In PCV, there is no preset Vt. The Vt the patient receives is determined by the set inspiratory pressure, the inspiratory time, the patient's lung compliance, and the resistance of both the patient's airways and the ventilator circuit. The RN and RCP must carefully monitor Vt and minute ventilation because any factor which increases resistance or decreases compliance will negatively impact Vt and minute ventilation. Conversely, any situation which decreases resistance or improves compliance may result in an increase in Vt and subsequent overdistention and excessive ventilation.

Management of Patients Requiring Mechanical Ventilation

Patients requiring mechanical ventilation require a multidisciplinary approach to successfully manage their care. This team usually consists of a nurse, physician, respiratory therapist (RT), nutritionist, occupational and/or physical therapist, speech therapist (ST), social worker, pharmacist, and pastoral care provider. If possible, a team meeting involving the patient and family prior to the initiation of mechanical ventilation could help allay some fear and anxiety. The team should explain, in language the patient can comprehend, the reason(s) for mechanical ventilation, frequently reported sensations and experiences, possible duration of treatment, risks and benefits, strategies employed to facilitate weaning from mechanical ventilation, and what rights and responsibilities the patient and family have during this experience. Many times, however, patients are intubated and placed on mechanical ventilation as a result of an emergency situation. The nurse, in that scenario, plays the invaluable role of patient advocate and educator. The nurse is the patient's vital link to the health delivery system, acting as a direct caregiver and coordinator of essential services. It is imperative that the nurse understands the underlying pathology that resulted in the patient's need for mechanical ventilation. Understanding the disease process will guide the nurse in the provision and coordination of care. A patient who is ventilated for respiratory failure secondary to pneumonia will have different needs than a patient ventilated for respiratory failure secondary to cardiogenic shock. There are, however, many collaborative diagnoses common to patients requiring mechanical ventilation. By successfully managing these issues, the nurse has an enormous impact on the experience of the intubated, ventilated patient and his or her family. The nurse's primary goal is to monitor and evaluate the patient's response to mechanical ventilation. Parameters which must be closely monitored include vital signs, HR, BP, RR, SaO_2, breath sounds, breathing pattern, and arterial blood gases. The nurse will be the person at the bedside with the knowledge of the patient's response to mechanical ventilation, who will collaborate with the other disciplines to maximize this patient's care.

Potential Collaborative Diagnoses of Patients Requiring Mechanical Ventilation

High Risk for Inadequate Gas Exchange/Ineffective Breathing Pattern

Patients on ventilators may experience inadequate gas exchange and/or ineffective breathing patterns due to a variety of factors, such as occluded/partially occluded endotracheal tube or tracheostomy tube, dysynchrony due to "fighting/bucking" the ventilator, hemothorax, pneumothorax, pulmonary embolus, exhaustion, and any other condition that would increase airway resistance (asthma) or decrease lung compliance (ARDS). The nurse must carefully assess the patient for increased work of breathing, increased use of accessory muscles, fear, agitation, confusion, any factors that indicate fatigue and increased RR, and dysynchronous respiratory pattern. The nurse must also look for decreases in tidal volumes, increased HR and BP, decreased SaO_2, adventitious breath sounds, increased airway pressures, and decreased lung compliance. The ventilator function must also be carefully assessed to rule out any possible mechanical failures. Ventilator settings must be evaluated to ensure they are appropriate for the patient's current condition. The underlying problem must be discovered and appropriate interventions undertaken.

Ineffective Airway Clearance

The ability of the patient to expectorate his or her own secretions can be affected by multiple factors: length and diameter of the endotracheal tube, muscle strength, viscosity of the secretions, and level of sedation. If the patient cannot clear the airway, it is the responsibility of the RN or RT to suction the airway. Over the past 10 years, there has been excellent research done in the area of suctioning. Deep endotracheal or tracheostomy suctioning in the health care facility is a sterile procedure. The patient should be well oxygenated with 100% oxygen either through the ventilator circuit or via manual resuscitation bag prior to the initiation of the procedure. Suctioning should only be performed if indicated: coughing, visible secretions, increased work of breathing, decrease in SaO_2, high peak inspiratory pressures, and/or breath sounds revealing coarse wheezing or crackles. It has been well-supported that the ritual of instillation of normal saline prior to suctioning does not liquefy or break up secretions. It may stimulate the cough response. It also may introduce into the lower respiratory tract bacteria, which are present on the distal end of the ETT or TT, thereby putting patients at higher risk of nosocomial pneumonia. Instead of the instillation of NS, the cough response can be stimulated using the "sigh" setting on the ventilator or by using a manual resuscitation bag. Wall suction should be regulated not to exceed a maximum of 120 mmHg. The suctioning event should not exceed 10 to 15 seconds, and the patient should be allowed to return to baseline vital signs, HR, RR, SaO_2, and color between suctioning events. The nurse must be cognizant of the possible complications of suctioning: hypoxemia, hypoxia, tissue trauma to the tracheal and/or bronchial mucosa, cardiac dysrhythmias/arrest, bronchospasm, pulmonary bleeding, hemorrhage, infection, hyper/hypotension, and be prepared to intervene if they should occur.

Impaired Communication

Any patient being mechanically ventilated either via endotracheal (ET) or tracheostomy (T) tube will be unable to speak. Endotracheal tubes pass directly through the vocal cords. A tracheostomy tube is situated below the vocal cords but with the cuff inflated (required for positive pressure ventilation) precludes the passage of air through the vocal cords. Many of these patients have manual dexterity and/or visual impairment that limit their ability to communicate via the written word. Patients with ETTs have had dentures removed, altering the musculature in the face, and also the tube will be taped to their mouths or faces, making lip-reading difficult. The nurse working with the RCP and speech therapist must establish a form of communication to handle at the very least basic needs (ie, pain, toileting, and thirst). The inability to communicate engenders anxiety, and anxiety can play a major role in a patient's ability to tolerate mechanical ventilation. Inability to communicate also produces feelings of isolation. By establishing a communication system, the nurse will assist her patient to regain some control over the environment. There are valves on the market that can be utilized in mechanically ventilated patients to facilitate speaking. These valves require intense manipulation and monitoring of ventilatory parameters and are commonly only used for very short periods of time.

Fear/Anxiety

Many patients report fear as a dominant experience during mechanical ventilation. Ventilators have many alarms which when investigated may be benign (eg, high pressure secondary to a cough or hiccup), but the patient experiences the alarms as something seriously wrong with him or her or the life support machinery. They interpret these alarms as possibly life threatening. They may experience extreme dyspnea as a result of a disconnect from the ventilator and they are unable to call for help. It is of utmost importance for the nurse to provide support to these patients, assure them of their safety, and educate them as to the response time of the staff.

Powerlessness

All patients requiring mechanical ventilation are tethered to a machine. This condition limits their ability to communicate, toilet themselves, and even change position. Many mechanically ventilated patients are receiving drugs that alter their sensorium and judgment, which in turn may mandate measures to ensure their safety (eg, wrist restraints, side rails, bite blocks to prevent biting down on the ETT interrupting gas flow and possibly damaging the conduit to the cuff). This experience engenders powerlessness. The nurse can mitigate some of this by offering choices as to the routine of care: scheduling treatments, rest periods, and positioning. The nurse also needs to elicit the patient's desires/needs and incorporate these into the plan of care.

Isolation/Sensory Deprivation

Mechanically ventilated patients are unable to easily communicate, are often in a single room, and are limited in their physical activity. This can lead to sensory deprivation and loneliness. This is an area where nurses have an enormous impact. Interview the patient and family to discover this patient's interests and incorporate them into the plan of care. Watching baseball on TV, listening to show tunes, affixing a bird feeder to the window, or arranging for family, friends, and/or volunteers (or nurses if time permits) to read or play cards with the patient will go a long way toward lifting spirits. There are also many complementary therapies that could be employed to help allay fear and isolated feelings, such as massage, guided imagery, healing touch/therapeutic touch, and acupressure.

Alteration in Nutrition

All patients on mechanical ventilation will be unable to eat normally. The ETT bypasses the protective reflex of epiglottis closure, making normal eating impossible. The tracheostomy tube cuff impinges into the esophageal space, possibly compromising the ability to swallow. Malnutrition is a common problem in this population. Malnutrition leads to a loss of muscle mass and strength. The diaphragm, the major muscle of ventilation, is weakened early on by malnutrition. This weakening of the diaphragm can produce an ineffective breathing pattern. This will cause fatigue, further compromising the patient's ability to wean from the ventilator. The nurse needs to consult with the dietitian to formulate a plan for the institution and monitoring of nutritional support. Enteral feedings are the preferred method if the patient can tolerate this. Electrolytes must be monitored closely. Adequate amounts of calcium, magnesium, and phosphorous are essential for respiratory muscle contraction.

The inability to take anything by mouth intensifies the patient's need for excellent oral hygiene. Most intubated patients have their mouths partially kept open by the ETT, exposing the mucus membranes to dehydration. Also, many patients are being diuresed for their underlying medical problems. This combination makes thirst and oral discomfort difficult issues in this population. Many products exist to cleanse and hydrate the oral mucosa. Oral care is a task easily taught to family members. The provision of oral care by a family member provides the patient much comfort and relief and helps the family member feel more involved in the care.

Alteration in Bowel Function: Diarrhea

As a result of the necessity of enteral tube feeding, many ventilated patients suffer with diarrhea. Research at this time does not support the use of one feeding method, bolus or continuous, over another. The nurse must provide for adequate toileting, skin protection, and medication to alleviate diarrhea. Electrolyte levels, especially potassium, need to be closely monitored in patients experiencing diarrhea.

Alteration in Bowel Function: Ileus

Many patients who require mechanical ventilation are receiving high doses of analgesic and anxiolytic medications. These medications, especially when coupled with inactivity and low fiber enteral feedings, decrease bowel motility and can lead to an ileus. Patients receiving enteral feedings must have comprehensive abdominal assessments, which include observation of the size of the abdomen, auscultation of bowel sounds, palpation to detect firmness or pain, and careful monitoring for the frequency and quality of bowel movements, and quantity of residual tube feedings in the stomach after a predetermined time. The nurse should collaborate with the physician around the use of a pro-

Table 4-9

Complications of Mechanical Ventilation

Mechanical

1. Failure in ventilator function/alarm system.
2. Loss of electrical power.
3. Inadequate humidification.
4. Overheating of inspired air leading to mild hyperthermia.
5. Volume overload due to humidification of inspired air.

Physiologic

1. Barotrauma: pneumothorax, pneumomediastinum, subcutaneous emphysema.
2. Cardiac dysrhythmias.
3. Decreased cardiac output: tachycardia, hypotension, tissue hypoxia, water and salt retention.
4. Oxygen toxicity.
5. Tracheal/laryngeal damage.
6. Stress ulcer/gastritis.
7. Aspiration of gastric contents.
8. Nosocomial pulmonary infection.

motility agent to possibly prevent the development of an ileus. The use of stool softeners and laxatives to maintain adequate bowel function, is frequently necessary due to inadequate fiber in commercially prepared enteral feeding formulas, medications which slow bowel function and relative lack of physical activity.

Disuse Syndrome

Many ventilated patients are initially confined to bed by their underlying medical problem and confined to a limited geographic area as a result of being tethered to a ventilator. As soon as the patient is stable, the nurse, OT/PT, and the patient should formulate a conditioning program. Physical exercise improves overall muscle tone and strength, facilitates gas exchange, promoting oxygen delivery to the tissues, and improves mood. Improved muscle strength enhances a patient's ability to wean from ventilatory support. Family members can also be encouraged to participate in training by being taught the regime and acting as coaches for their loved one.

Complications of Mechanical Ventilation

Intubation and mechanical ventilation may produce many adverse sequelae (Table 4-9). A manual resuscitation bag with an oxygen source must be readily available in case of equipment failure/malfunction or loss of electrical power. Many ventilators do not have back-up battery systems.

Positive pressure ventilation can cause serious physiologic complications. Pulmonary barotrauma related to overdistention of the alveolar units may result in pneumothorax, pneumomediastinum, and subcutaneous emphysema. Positive pressure ventilation increases intrathoracic pressure, thereby decreasing venous return to the heart. This can result in decreased cardiac output that may cause a compensatory increase in HR. Decreased cardiac output also may decrease blood pressure, thereby decreasing blood and oxygen delivery to the tissues. Decreased oxygen to the tissues can result in tissue hypoxia and possible anaerobic metabolism, leading to acidemia. Decreased cardiac output may also trigger a compensatory increase in the secretion of ADH and aldosterone that will lead to salt and water retention. The nurse must be cognizant of these possible sequelae—recognize, report, and intervene when appropriate. For example, the prescribing physician may decide it is appropriate to treat cardiac dysrhythnias by increasing the FiO_2. Signs and symptoms of decreased cardiac output may be treated by decreasing the amount of PEEP or Vt. Careful assessment of the patient's volume status is an integral part of managing patients requiring mechanical ventilation.

To utilize positive pressure ventilation, the endotracheal tubes must have a cuff that seals the trachea during ventilation. This cuff exerts pressure. If the pressure exceeds capillary arterial perfusion pressure, approximately 30 to 32 cm H_2O in a patient with normal hemodynamics, then blood flow to the tracheal tissues will be compromised. Because venous and lymphatic flow occurs at even lower pressures, ideally the cuff pressure should be maintained at 25 cm H_2O. Higher pressures will result in a decrease in bloodflow and subsequently oxygen delivery to the tracheal tissue. This in turn may cause tissue erosion and ischemic damage leading to the development of tracheomylasia and possible tracheoesophageal fistula. To prevent this, cuff pressure should be measured at least every 24 hours. Pressures may be measured with a standard sphygmomanometer or aneroid cuff pressure manometer, such as the cufflator. If pressure exceeds 25 cm H_2O, the physician should be notified and steps taken to remedy the situation. These steps may include administering sedative agents to reduce tracheal muscle tone or possibly changing the endotracheal tube to one with a smaller diameter.

Also, because the ETT can move due to a variety of circumstances, there are incidences in which the cuff does not totally occlude the trachea. If the cuff is not occluding the trachea, the patient may aspirate oral or gastric content into the lung. Endotracheal and tracheostomy tubes bypass the normal lines of defense for the lung. This compromise of normal defenses puts patients at higher risk for acquiring a nosocomial and aspiration pneumonia.

Research has demonstrated that patients being treated with mechanical ventilation are at very high risk of developing stress ulcers/gastritis. Nurses must be cognizant of this risk and monitor the patient for complaints of gastric discomfort or the presence of blood in the gastric aspirate or stool. Most physicians prescribe stress ulcer prophylaxis (ie, a hydrogen ion blocker or proton pump inhibitor) for mechanically ventilated patients.

The use of mechanical ventilation places enormous responsibility on all the disciplines caring for the patient. We must be hypervigilant to ensure safe and effective treatment.

Weaning/Liberation From Mechanical Ventilation

No simple parameters exist that indicate when weaning/liberation from mechanical ventilation should be attempted. The underlying condition which precipitated the institution of mechanical ventilation should be resolved or at least improving. Weaning is usually not attempted until the FiO_2 is < 50%, PEEP is < 10 cm H_2O, the patient is hemodynamically stable and possesses intact protective (cough, gag) reflexes. Research demonstrates that if a patient cannot generate a negative aspiratory force (NIF: the amount of negative pressure the patient can generate when inhaling against a closed valve) of < -20 cm H_2O and a vital capacity (quantity of gas exhaled after the deepest possible inhalation) of > 10 to 15 cc/kg, then the probability of a successful wean is very low. Research has been unable to identify any parameters that can predict weaning success. A variety of methodology and ventilatory modes are employed to wean patients from ventilatory support. These techniques include T-piece, CPAP, IMV, and PSV. One has not been proven to be more efficacious than another.

The collaborative team should begin to prepare the patient and family for the experience of weaning as soon as it is appropriate to do so. The process of weaning and the patient's and staff's role in weaning must be carefully and repetitively explained in order to avoid fear and undue anxiety. The patient must be reassured that he or she will not be alone and struggling for breath, and that a team member will be closely monitoring the condition/progress. Team members/family can act as emotional support and/or as coaches and cheerleaders. The patient should be placed in a position which will facilitate diaphragmatic movement. Sitting or semirecumbent positions are usually the best tolerated. The airway should be cleared of any secretions. The use of complementary therapies, such as music therapy, guided imagery, bio-feedback, and other energy-based therapies should be explored with the patient. As stated above, there are no indicators supported by research to predict who will be able to sustain spontaneous ventilation after the withdrawal of mechanical support. Common practice is to attempt extubation, removal of the ETT, if the patient has intact protective reflexes (cough and gag), is capable of generating a Vt of 5 cc/kg, a VC of 10 cc/kg, a NIF more negative than -20 cm H_2O, a minute volume of 6 to 10 L/minute, SaO_2 > 92%, and RR, HR, and BP within 10% to 20% of baseline. If these criteria are met, then extubation will occur. If these criteria are unable to be met, then depending on the patient, family, and durable power of attorney's wishes, the option of either a tracheostomy (see Tracheostomy section) or terminal wean will be pursued.

Extubation

If a patient has been successfully weaned, either the MD, RN, or RCP will remove the ETT. The procedure is explained to the patient. Usually patients who have been intubated require supplemental oxygen after extubation, therefore this should be set up and ready for use prior to extubation. Then, with the patient in an upright or semirecumbent position, the ETT and mouth are suctioned. The tape is removed, the patient is instructed to take a deep breath, and the cuff is deflated via aspiration of the pilot balloon. The patient is told to cough while the tube is swiftly removed. The rationale for the cough during extubation is to force any secretions remaining above the cuff into the oropharynx, thereby reducing the risk of aspiration. Supplemental oxygen, if prescribed, should be administered at this point and titrated to maintain prescribed SaO_2. The patient should be asked to speak and cough. Patients need to be closely monitored post extubation for the development of upper airway obstruction due to vocal cord or laryngeal edema. In this case, the patient will become stridorous and dyspneic. This is an emergency and the physician should be contacted immediately. Cool mist and/or nebulized racemic epinephrine may be utilized to reduce edema. If these treatments are unsuccessful and the patient's airway is compromised, immediate intubation or tracheostomy is indicated. Many patients post extubation experience hoarseness and difficulty swallowing. Food and fluids are usually withheld for a period of hours post extubation. Ice chips are normally allowed. When fluids are begun, water is first given so that the nurse can assess the patient's ability to swallow.

Tracheostomy

A tracheotomy is a surgical incision into the trachea in the area of the second, third, and fourth tracheal rings (see Figure 4-7). A tracheostomy is the resulting opening, or stoma, that is made during a tracheotomy procedure. A tracheostomy tube is inserted into the stoma. A tracheostomy is utilized for a variety of reasons; however use of a tracheostomy tube implies that an artificial airway will be necessary for a prolonged period of time. A tracheostomy is performed when a patient has been unsuccessful in his or her attempts to wean from ventilatory support. This usually occurs between 2 weeks and 4 weeks after intubation.

Indications for tracheostomy:

1. Long-term secretion management.
2. Airway protection from aspiration.
3. Acute upper airway obstruction: trauma, burns.
4. Prophylaxis against airway obstruction: radical neck, neurological surgeries, laryngectomy.
5. Prolonged intubation, mechanical ventilation.

Tracheostomy is generally better tolerated than endotracheal intubation. Tracheostomy tubes create less airflow resistance, allow for improved oral care and intake, and may, dependent on patient condition and tube design, allow for talking. Tracheostomy tubes are available in a number of materials, sizes, and designs: cuffed or uncurbed, plastic, nylon or metal, single or double lumen, and fenestrated or nonfenestrated. Generally tracheostomy tubes consist of a neck flange, which rests flush against the neck. The flange has openings at both sides through which cloth or Velcro ties are inserted for securing the airway. The flange should be secured against the skin of the patient's neck to prevent movement of the tube in the stoma, minimizing airway trauma. The tube itself usually has a 15 mm adaptor on the proximal end, allowing easy interface with ventilatory devices. Most plastic tracheostomy tubes have a radiopaque stripe for radiologic position identification. On the proximal end of cuffed tubes is a cuff, whose design and function mirror that of an ETT (see Endotracheal Intubation). An obturator is included with the tracheostomy tube. When inserted into the tube, its smooth, rounded tip slightly protrudes from the body of the tube. The function of the obturator is to prevent injury to the tracheal wall during insertion. It must be removed to allow air to pass through the tube. It is usually kept at the bedside should emergency reinsertion of the tube be necessary.

Tracheostomy care (Table 4-10) is necessary to keep the tracheostomy tube and stoma clean, dry, and free from secretions and mucus, thereby preventing infection and maintaining a patent airway. In acute care, the tracheostomy tube is suctioned prior to the onset of tracheostomy care to remove any excess secretions. The nurse must assure the tracheostomy tube is secure at all times to prevent accidental dislodgment. Prior to tracheostomy care, what type of care is necessary? Is the tube single or double lumen? If single lumen, only stoma care is required. If double lumen, the inner cannula may need to be changed or cleaned. If the inner cannula is disposable, current recommendations allow for its replacement every 24 hours. If the inner cannula is nondisposable, recommendations are for cleansing every 8 hours and when necessary with half-strength hydrogen peroxide. Tracheostomy ties are usually changed every 24 hours and when necessary. Velcro or other manufactured devices are changed as needed. A properly applied tracheostomy-securing device allows space for one finger to be placed between the tie and the neck. Tracheostomy dressings should be changed whenever they are wet. Wetness irritates the skin and coupled with bacteria provide an excellent medium for the growth of bacteria. Some tracheostomies are sutured into place to prevent dislodgment. The sutures are normally left in place for 7 to 14 days, allowing for a tracheostomy tract to form. Care must be taken to assess the effect the sutures have on the peristomal skin and report any breakdown.

Table 4-10

Tracheostomy Care (in the Acute Setting)

1. Assemble the following equipment
   - Goggles
   - Sterile gloves
   - Scissors (if tracheostomy ties are in place)
   - Sterile normal saline
   - Suctioning equipment
   - Tracheostomy care components or kit is available
     - H_2O_2
     - Sterile, precut tracheostomy dressing (precut, sewn-edge dressings necessary to prevent threads from falling into the stoma and possibly lung)
     - Tracheostomy securing devices: ties, Velcro holder
     - Pipe cleaners; brush cleaner; cotton-tipped swabs
     - Forceps
     - 4x4 sterile gauze pads; two sterile bowls
     - Sterile inner cannula (if indicated)
2. Wash hands
3. Explain procedure to patient
4. Place patient in position of comfort (this allows RN easier access to tracheostomy
5. Suction the tracheostomy tube
6. Remove soiled dressing and discard in appropriate receptacle
7. Pour half-strength H_2O_2 into one bowl and plain Normal Saline into other
8. Wear sterile gloves
9. Remove inner cannula and either discard or cleanse it (according to institutional policy)
   - Immerse inner cannula in half-strength H_2O_2
   - Use brush and pipe cleaners to remove secretions
   - Immerse cannula in N/S and remove excess solution with sterile gauze
   - Reinsert cannula, assuring it is locked in place. If patient is ventilator dependent or outer cannula diameter is not correct size, attach an adapter or spare inner cannula to ventilator to assure uninterrupted ventilation
   - Wet sterile gauze or cotton-tipped swabs with sterile N/S and clean peristomal skin
   - Change tracheostomy ties

Decannulation

If the indications for tracheostomy have been resolved and the patient is stable, then the physician will make the decision to proceed with either immediate decannulation or gradual decannulation. In immediate decannulation, the tracheostomy tube is removed and the stoma covered by a sterile, nonocclusive dressing. If air loss is a problem, then the stoma may be covered with a petroleum-impregnated gauze and covered by a dry gauze.

The patient will immediately need to use their natural airway for ventilation and secretion removal. There are multiple techniques for gradual decannulation. The tracheostomy tube is replaced at prescribed intervals by a tube of a smaller size—downsizing. Downsizing allows for gradual closing of the stoma. The tracheostomy tube may also be plugged for a prescribed period of time and the patient assessed for the tolerance of this procedure. If it is well-tolerated, immediate decannulation may ensue. A tracheostomy button may be placed in the tracheal stoma after decannulation. The button prevents the stoma from closing, thereby allowing for immediate access should that be necessary. With the button in place, the patient must use his or her natural airway for ventilation and secretion removal.

Tracheostomy care may be done with two people; one person securing the tube while the other removes the ties and performs the care. If the nurse performs tracheostomy care alone, the old ties must remain intact until the new ties are secured.

Changing tracheostomy ties:
1. Manufacturer's devices should be used according to their instruction.
2. If using cloth ties:
   - Assure skin on the neck is clean, dry, and without breakdown. If breakdown is present, treat according to institutional guidelines.
   - Cut hole 3/4 of an inch from end of tape.
   - Pass cut end through the hole in flange of tracheostomy tube.
   - Thread noncut end through hole and pull tightly. Do this on both sides.
   - Bring ties to side of neck and tie with a square knot. Knot must be secured so only one finger can be placed between tie and neck.
3. Place new tracheostomy dressing.

BIBLIOGRAPHY

Black JM, Matassarin-Jacobs E. *Medical-Surgical Nursing: Clinical Management for Continuity of Care*. Philadelphia, Pa: W.B. Saunders Company; 1997.

Burrell L, Gerlach M, Pless B. *Nursing Management of Adults with Respiratory Problems*. Stamford, Conn: Appleton & Lange; 1997.

Dossey BM, Guzzetta C, Kenner CV. Critical Care Nursing 3rd ed. New York, NY: JB Lippincott Co; 1992:219-229.

Ignatavius DD, Bayne M. *Medical Surgical Nursing: A Nursing Process Approach*. Philadelphia, Pa: W.B. Saunders Co; 1991:2013-2030.

Ignatavius DD, Workman ML, Mishler MA. *Medical-Surgical Nursing: A Nursing Process Approach*. Philadelphia, Pa: W.B. Saunders Co; 1995.

McGowan C. Noninvasive ventilatory support: use of bi-level positive airway pressure in respiratory failure. *Critical Care Nurse*. 1998;18(6):47-53.

Norris J, ed. Critical Care Skills: A Nurse's PhotoGuide. Philadelphia, Pa: Springhouse Corporation; 1996:317-336.

Roberts N. Selective approach to successful stoma management. *ORL Head and Neck Nursing*. 1995;13(4):12-16.

Ruppert S, Kernicki J, Dolan J. *Dolan's Critical Care Practice Survey*. 2nd ed. Philadelphia, Pa: FA Davis Co; 1991.

Ulrich SP, Canale SW, Wendell SA. *Medical-Surgical Nursing Care Planning Guides*. Philadelphia, Pa: W.B. Saunders Co; 1998.

Weilitz P, Dettenmeien P. Test your knowledge of tracheostomy tubes. *Am J Nurs*. February 1994:46-50.

Wilkinson M, Muzzarelli K. *Tracheostomy Care Practice Survey*. Society of Otorhinolaryngology, Head and Neck Nurses, and AACN; 1996.

MULTIPLE-CHOICE QUESTIONS

1. When Mr. J. is receiving oxygen via nasal prongs, the nurse understands that this method does all of the following except:

   A. Delivers a precise concentration of oxygen

   B. Does not require humidification

   C. Is traumatic to the respiratory tract

   D. Does not require a written order

2. If Mr. J.'s O_2 saturation does not respond to oxygen delivered by nasal prongs, then a facial mask with a reservoir bag may be needed. The risks of higher inspired oxygen (FiO_2) include all of the following except:

   A. Dryness of the mucus membranes

   B. Risk of hypoventilation

   C. Potential for oxygen toxicity

   D. Excessive, watery pulmonary secretions

3. After a chest x-ray, a diagnosis of left lower lobe pneumonia is made. Chest physical therapy and an incentive spirometer are ordered. All the following actions show that the patient understands how to use the spirometer except:

   A. The patient holds the spirometer in the upright position

   B. The patient places the spirometer in his mouth and completely exhales

   C. The patient places the spirometer in his mouth, takes a deep breath, and holds it for 2 to 5 seconds before removing the mouthpiece and exhaling

   D. The patient tries to cough after using the spirometer

4. Mr. J.'s fever has resolved and he is being discharged with theophylline, as well as with clarithromycin, an antibiotic. Your teaching about theophylline would include all of the following except:

   A. Take theophylline on an empty stomach

   B. Report signs of theophylline toxicity such as nausea, dizziness, rapid heart rate, or muscle twitching to the health care provider

   C. Decrease caffeine and chocolate intake as theophylline has similar effects

   D. Take theophylline at regular intervals

CHAPTER 4 ANSWERS

1.   D
2.   D
3.   B
4.   A

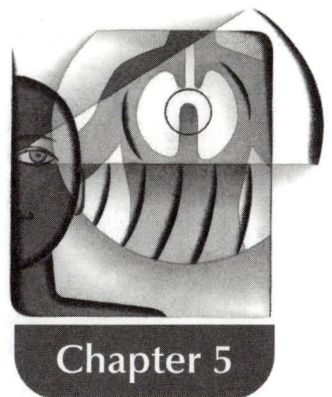

Chapter 5

Anatomy and Physiology of the Cardiovascular System

Mr. M. is a 76-year-old man with newly diagnosed coronary artery disease. Sometimes he has chest pain when exerting himself. When this happens, he stops what he is doing, sits down, and the pain usually subsides in a few minutes. Today, he wants to know why he has chest pain.

While the respiratory system provides oxygen to the body, it is the cardiovascular system that moves the oxygen to the cells. The heart works as a pump to move oxygenated blood throughout the arterial system and returns deoxygenated blood to the heart and lungs via the venous system. This process of pumping and circulating is called *perfusion*, and without it the other processes—ventilation and diffusion—would not provide oxygen to the cells.

The cardiovascular system is comprised of two parts: the heart that pumps the blood and the vascular network through which blood is channeled. The vascular network consists of arteries and veins: the arteries carry blood away from the heart, and the veins return blood to the heart. In this chapter, the heart and the components of the vascular network will be discussed. Each part of the cardiovascular system will be reviewed as it pertains to the process of oxygenation.

THE HEART

The heart is an amazing organ and the cardiovascular system could not function without it. It is small, about the size of a clenched fist in an adult, but it can pump 100,000 times a day. The heart rate can be alternated, depending on the needs of the body. It is finely regulated by neural and hormonal mechanisms to ensure the oxygenation of the tissues.

The heart is a muscular organ that lies near the center of the thoracic cavity (Figure 5-1). It is somewhat anterior in the chest and is situated directly behind the sternum. The heart lies within a pericardial cavity, which is lined by a thin, serous membrane called the

Figure 5-1. Position of the heart in the thoracic cavity.

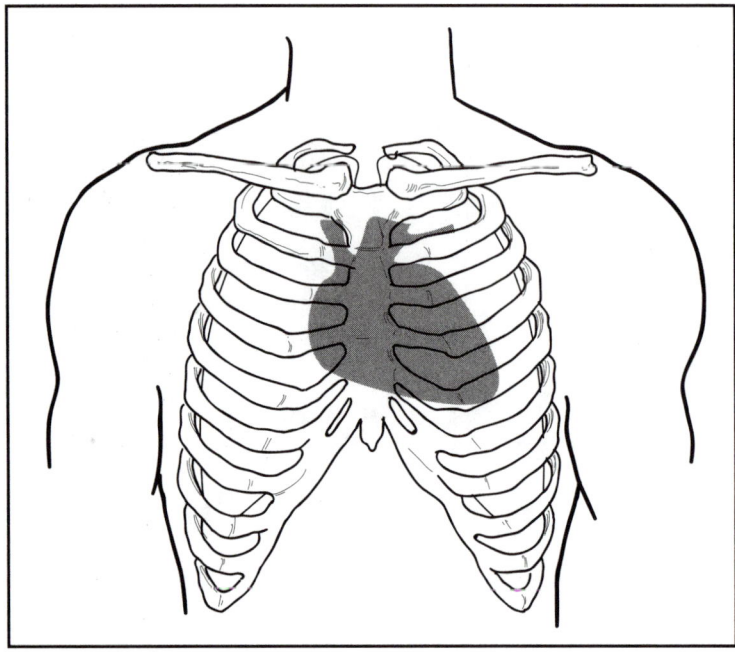

Figure 5-2. The chambers and the layers of the heart.

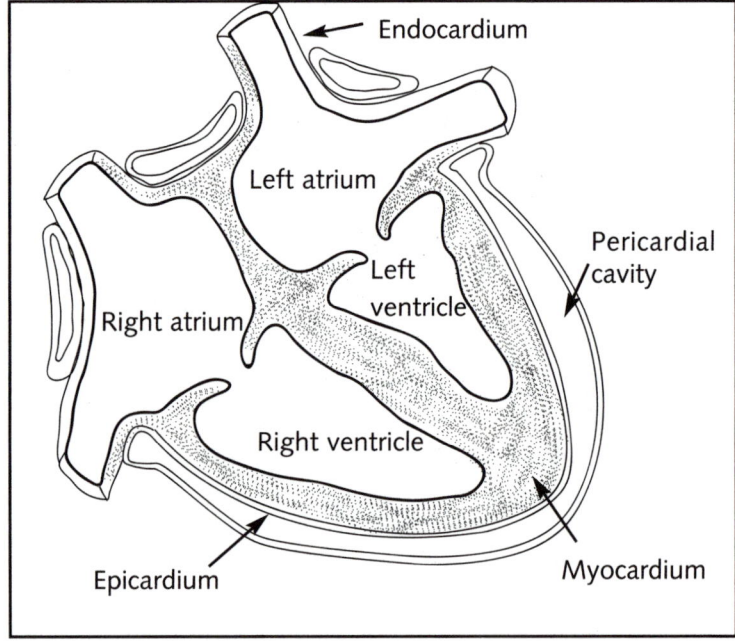

pericardium. A membrane called the *epicardium* surrounds the heart itself. Pericardial fluid is the lubricant between the pericardium and the epicardium. There is only about 10 cc of pericardial fluid, but it reduces friction between the surfaces of the two membranes.

The heart is composed of three layers: the *epicardium,* the *myocardium* or cardiac muscle, and the *endocardium* that lines the inner surfaces of the heart's chambers. The heart is divided into four chambers: the *right atrium,* the *right ventricle,* the *left atrium,* and the *left ventricle* (Figure 5-2). The myocardium contracts rhythmically to move blood through the

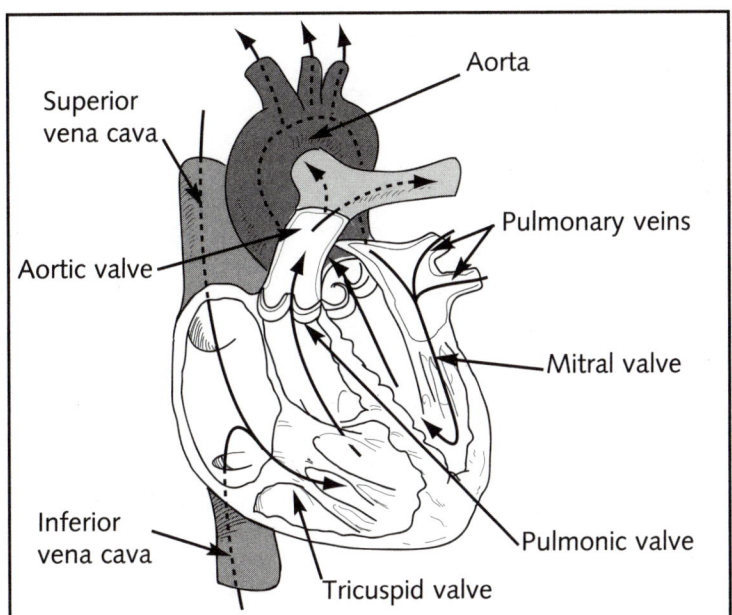

Superior
vena cava

Aortic valve

Inferior
vena cava

Aorta

Pulmonary veins

Mitral valve

Pulmonic valve

Tricuspid valve

Figure 5-3. The heart valves.

heart, into the pulmonary vasculature, and out again into the systemic vasculature. The atria serve to collect blood as it returns to the heart, draining it into the ventricles to be pumped into the circulation. The atria contract at the end of diastole, providing the "atrial kick"—a 30% increase in blood return to the ventricles, which is particularly useful during times when increased cardiac output is needed.

The two cycles of the heart are referred to as *diastole* and *systole*. Diastole is when the chambers of the heart are filling with blood. Systole is the contraction of the heart muscle, expelling blood from the heart. Venous blood enters the right atrium from the superior and inferior vena cavae. It flows into the right ventricle and then leaves the right side of the heart via the pulmonary artery. Blood passes through the pulmonary vasculature in the lungs, where gas exchange takes place at the alveoli. Reoxygenated blood returns to the left side of the heart at the left atrium via the pulmonary vein. It moves into the left ventricle and is pushed into the aorta by the contraction of the myocardium, where it begins its journey to the systemic tissues.

Valves control the flow of blood between the atria and ventricles of the heart and some of the blood vessels that are connected to the heart (Figure 5-3). They alternately open and close to ensure one-way blood flow through the heart. There are four valves in the heart: the *tricuspid, pulmonic, mitral,* and *aortic* valves. There are no valves where the large vessels drain into the atria.

Circulation through the heart valves flows in an orderly sequence when the valves are working properly. Blood drains from the superior and inferior vena cavae into the right atrium. It passes the tricuspid valve lying between the right atrium and right ventricle. During systole, the pulmonic valve opens and blood flows from the right ventricle into the pulmonary artery. After a trip through the pulmonary vasculature, reoxygenated blood flows through the pulmonary vein and into the left atrium. It passes the mitral valve between the left atrium and left ventricle. The final valve that blood passes through is the aortic valve, which lies where the left ventricle connects to the aorta. The closing of the heart valves can be heard as heart sounds (the assessment of heart sounds will be reviewed in Chapter 6).

Figure 5-4. Cross section of arteriosclerotic plaque in an arterial wall.

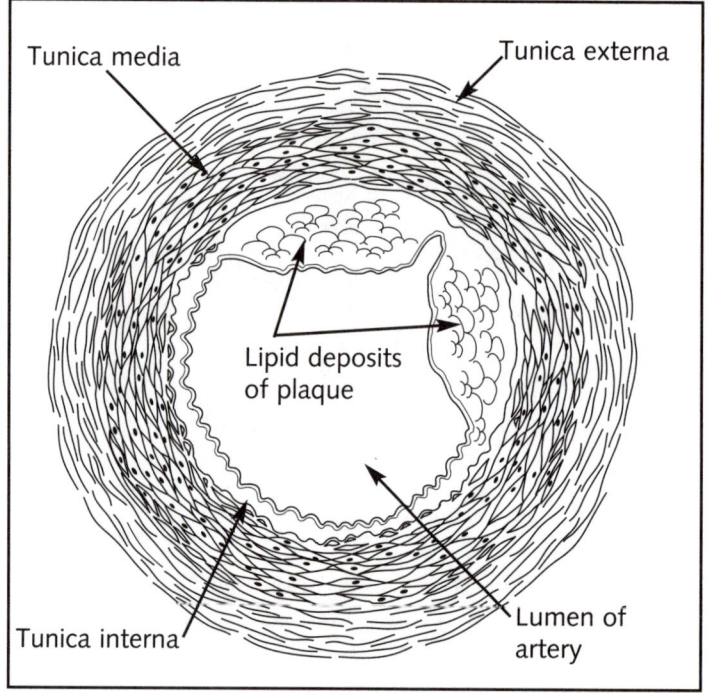

Blood flows from an area of higher pressure to an area of lower pressure. As blood moves from the heart through the circulatory system, it slowly loses pressure. The blood pressure in the aorta is approximately 120/80 mmHg. The mean arterial pressure is 70 to 100 mmHg. Mean capillary pressure is 40 mmHg. As blood travels in the venous circulation, the mean pressure is 10 mmHg, and when it reaches the right atrium the pressure is only 2 to 5 mmHg.

The heart muscles work continuously, requiring oxygen and nutrients just like other tissues. The muscles of the heart are supplied with oxygen by the coronary circulation. The coronary arteries begin at the ascending aorta just past the aortic valve where blood pressure is the highest in the systemic circulation. They branch into smaller arteries to supply different parts of the heart muscle. When coro-

> Atherosclerosis is the process in which fatty substances, lipids, accumulate in the endothelial lining of the arteries. The result is a layer of fatty tissue or plaque that protrudes into the lumen of the artery. Plaques can encourage clot formation or break loose and occlude blood vessels.

nary arteries are blocked by atherosclerosis or clots, hypoxia occurs in the heart muscle distal to the blockage (Figure 5-4). Patients with hypoxic cardiac tissues may experience chest pain or angina. If hypoxia continues and the heart muscle does not receive enough oxygen, the muscle dies. This is called a "heart attack" or myocardial infarction. This part of the heart muscle no longer functions. Depending on the location and extent of the tissue death, the myocardial infarction may make the heart incapable of maintaining adequate blood flow and the patient can die.

The myocardium contracts due to an electrical conduction system contained within the muscle walls (Figure 5-5). The electrical system stimulates the muscle fibers to contract.

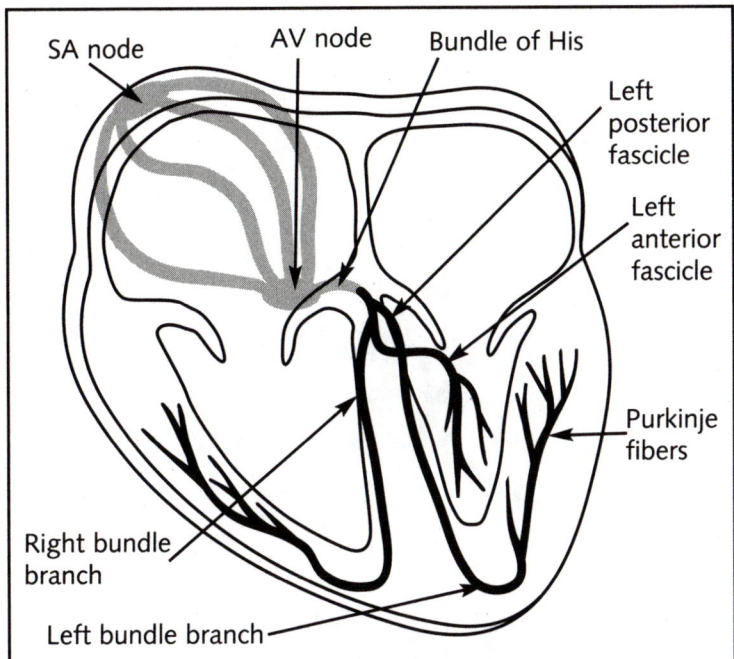

Figure 5-5. The conduction system of the heart.

The atria fill and contract first and then the ventricles fill and contract. In this rhythmic pattern the heart fills and then pushes blood out into the pulmonic and systemic circulation. The conduction system originates in the sinoatrial node (SA node) in the right atrium. The SA node is considered the pacemaker of the heart. The electrical impulse or depolarization then travels down the fibers to the atrioventricular node (AV node) at the base of the right atrium. At least four smaller branches, including Bachmann's bundle, travel from the right atrium to the left atrium, allowing for synchronized contraction of both atria. At the AV node, the conduction pathway branches into the right and left bundle branches, which innervate the ventricles of the heart. Special cells called Purkinje fibers carry the impulses to the myocardial cells of the ventricles. The electrical activity in the heart can be recorded on an electrocardiogram (EKG). The EKG is used to represent the mechanical activity of the heart during the cardiac cycle (the use of the EKG in the assessment of the heart will be reviewed in Chapter 6).

THE VASCULAR NETWORK

The miles and miles of blood vessels that distribute oxygen and nutrients to the cells and remove waste products make up the vascular network. This network can be further divided into two main circuits: the *systemic* circuit and the *pulmonic* circuit (Figure 5-6). The systemic circuit supplies all the body's tissues with blood except the lungs. The lungs are provided with blood via the pulmonic circuit. Both circuits are made up of a pump (the heart and the vessels), arteries, veins, and capillaries. The pump for the pulmonic system is the right ventricle of the heart, and the pump for the systemic circuit is the left ventricle. Both circuits are connected and depend on the adequate and equal functioning of the other. The circulatory system is a closed, pressurized system; if one side of the heart fails, then the other side is affected. For example, if a patient is in a right-sided heart failure, then blood backs up in the venous vasculature. Or, if the left side of the heart

Figure 5-6. The vascular circuits: pulmonic and systemic.

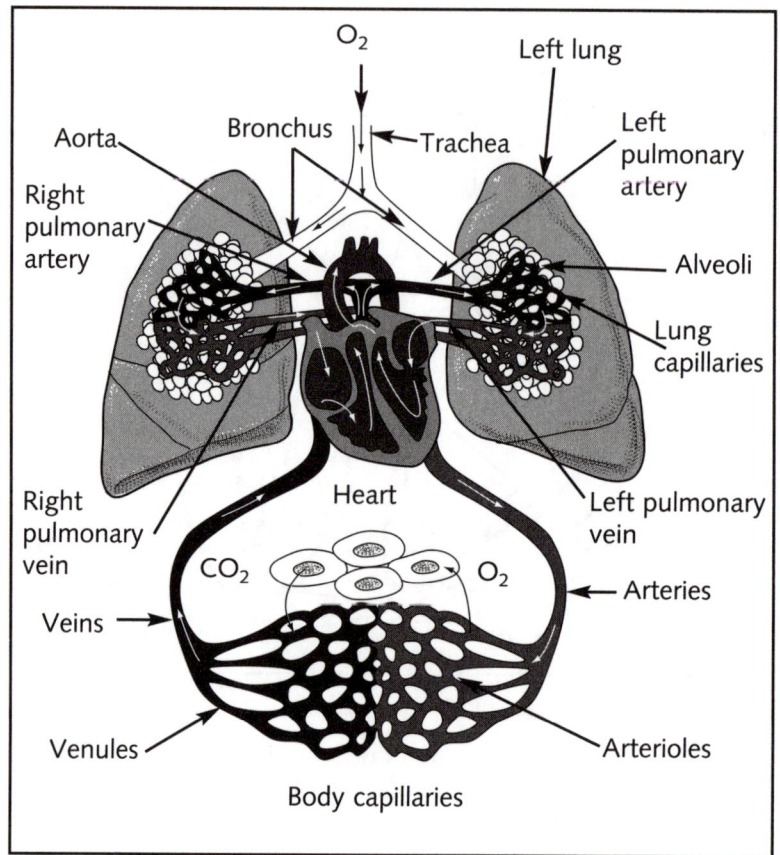

could not keep up with the right side, then blood would accumulate in the pulmonary vasculature.

The Arterial System

The arterial system begins at the heart as the aorta leaves the left ventricle. The aorta is a large vessel, about 2.5 cm in diameter. The aorta begins to branch into smaller and smaller arteries and then into arterioles. Arteries and arterioles have a large number of elastic fibers that allow them to stretch and recoil with changing blood pressures of the cardiac cycle. Blood then moves from the arterioles into the capillaries, the tiny, thin-walled vessels that supply the tissues with oxygenated blood.

The arterial system is a high-pressure system and the vessels are constructed to withstand changes in pressure. Different types of arteries have different proportions of elastic fibers and smooth muscle depending on their function. Elastic arteries are large vessels that have a high proportion of elastic fibers and less smooth muscle. The pulmonary artery and the aorta are examples of elastic arteries. They are very resilient and stretch during changes in blood pressure. Muscular arteries are medium-sized arteries that distribute blood to the organs. These arteries have proportionately more smooth muscle, which allows the vessels to change diameter and blood flow to distal tissues. The carotid arteries are an example of muscular arteries.

The Capillaries

Capillaries are the tiniest vessels in the circulatory system and the only ones that permit the exchange of gases and nutrients between the tissues and the circulating blood. Their thin walls are comprised of a single layer of endothelial cells. Gaps between the endothelial cells and the specialized basement membrane allow diffusion of oxygen and carbon dioxide, as well as nutrients and cellular waste products. The average diameter of a capillary is only 8 μm. Blood flow also slows in the capillaries, allowing adequate time for diffusion. The capillaries form a network of communicating vessels called a capillary bed or *plexus*. The entrance to each capillary is guarded by a band of smooth muscle called a *precapillary sphincter* (Figure 5-7). This sphincter controls the flow of blood into the capillary and is influenced by neural and hormonal impulses. Capillary walls are also involved in the secretion and removal of vasoactive substances in the circulation.

The Venous System

The venous system begins when capillaries in the tissues drain deoxygenated blood back into small vessels called *venules*. The return trip to the heart and lungs is the reverse of the arterial system, with small venules merging with others to create larger and larger veins. Veins continually join together on the return path to the heart until they reach the right side of the heart as the two largest veins: the inferior and superior vena cavae.

Veins are structured differently from arteries because the venous system is a low-pressure system. The blood pressure in the veins is only 10% of that in the ascending aorta, the beginning of the arterial system. The walls of veins are thinner and more elastic because they have less smooth muscle (Figure 5-8). Veins do not have to withstand wide pressure changes like arteries, but they do have to compete with the force of gravity. A system of valves is needed to prevent backflow of blood in the smaller veins (Figure 5-9). Large veins like the vena cavae do not have valves.

In addition to valves, the muscles of the extremities and the thoracoabdominal pump assist in returning venous blood to the heart. The skeletal muscles in the extremities push blood through the venous system as they contract and relax during activity. The thoracoabdominal pump refers to the pressure changes in the chest during breathing. On inhalation, the negative pressure in the chest pulls venous blood into the thoracic cavity and back to the right side of the heart.

The Pulmonary Circuit

The pulmonary circuit, as previously discussed in this chapter, is separate from the systemic vasculature. It delivers the blood from the right side of the heart to the lungs for removal of carbon dioxide and reoxygenation, and returning blood to the left side of the heart for delivery into the systemic circuit (see Figure 5-6). Blood leaves the right side of the heart for delivery to the lungs via the pulmonary artery. It is the only artery in the body that carries deoxygenated blood. This artery branches into smaller arteries in the lungs and then into capillaries surrounding the alveoli. The walls of the alveoli are very thin, allowing for diffusion of gases. Carbon dioxide diffuses across the capillary membrane and alveolar wall into the alveoli to be exhaled. Oxygen in the alveolar air crosses over the alveolar wall into the blood. The reoxygenated blood begins its return trip to the heart via the pulmonary venules and then the larger veins. The blood returns from the lungs to the left atrium via the pulmonary vein. It is the only vein in the body that carries oxygenated blood.

The pulmonary circuit is shorter than the systemic circuit, and the vessels are much shorter. The heart and lungs are only centimeters apart. The pressure required to pump

Figure 5-7. Structure of capillary bed with precapillary sphincters.

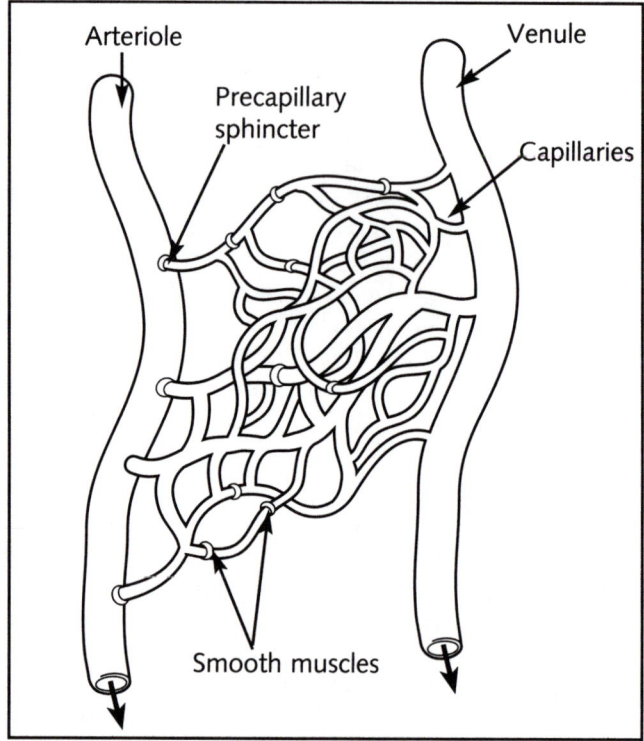

Figure 5-8. Structure of arteries versus veins.

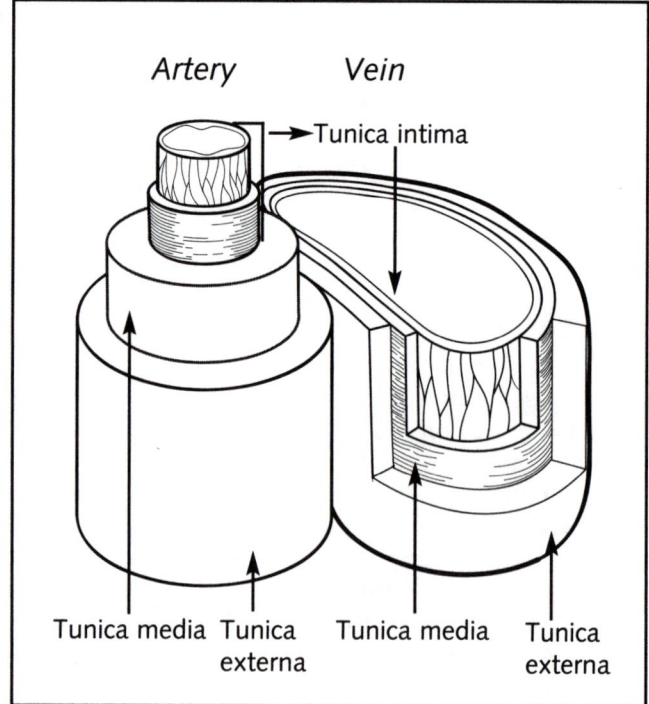

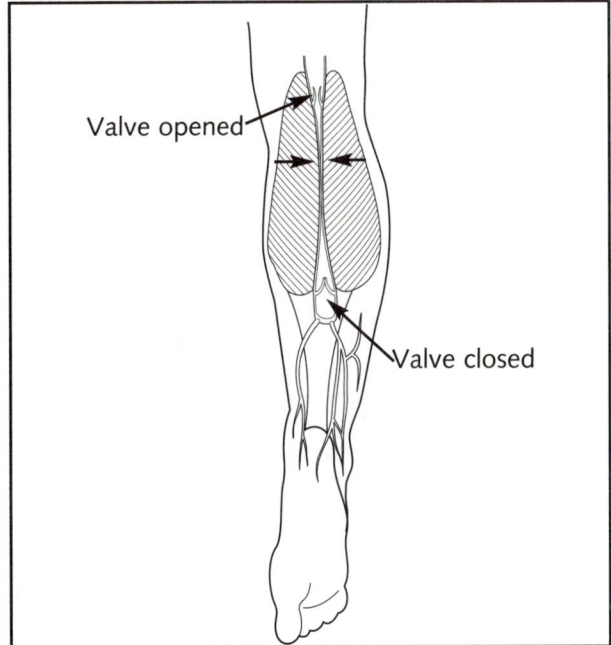

Figure 5-9. Valves of the venous system preventing backflow of blood.

blood from the right side of the heart through the pulmonary circuit and back to the left side of the heart is only about 15 mmHg. This is much less than the pressure that must be generated by the left side of the heart for the systemic circuit (about 120 mmHg.)

The Structure of Arteries and Veins

Arteries and veins are hollow pipes comprised of three cellular layers (Figure 5-10). The exterior of the vessels is called the *tunica externa*. It is a connective tissue sheath that protects and supports the vessel. The middle layer of a blood vessel, the *tunica media*, is made of concentric layers of smooth muscle within a matrix of collagen and elastic fibers. The smooth muscle constricts to control the diameter of the blood vessel and regulate blood flow. The *tunica intima* is the innermost layer that lines the inside of the vessel. It has a smooth layer of endothelial cells that promotes blood flow and prevents platelet adherence and clotting.

Distribution of Blood in the Vasculature

The total blood volume is not divided evenly between the arterial and venous vasculature (Figure 5-11). The arterial system (ie, the heart, arteries, and capillaries) holds only 30% to 35% (about 1.5 L) of the total volume. The remaining 65% to 70% is in the venous system (about 3.5 L). The veins are thinner-walled and more elastic than the arteries and can stretch eight times more than an artery. The venous system can act as a reservoir of blood for the body. This reservoir or venous reserve can be called upon to increase arterial blood flow if needed. For example, if severe hemorrhaging occurs, the medulla activates the smooth muscles around the veins. The veins contract and blood leaves the venous system and contributes to the general circulation to increase the blood pressure in the arterial system.

Figure 5-10. Layers of blood vessels.

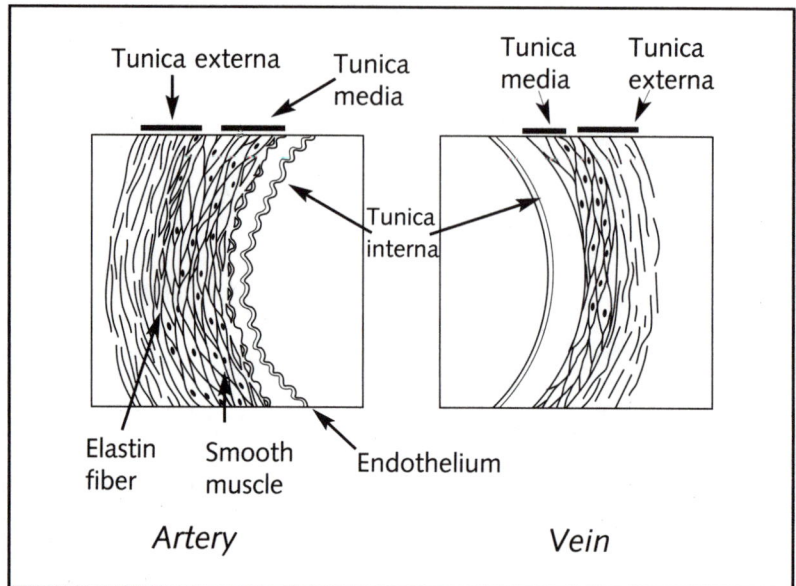

Figure 5-11. Distribution of blood in the circulatory system.

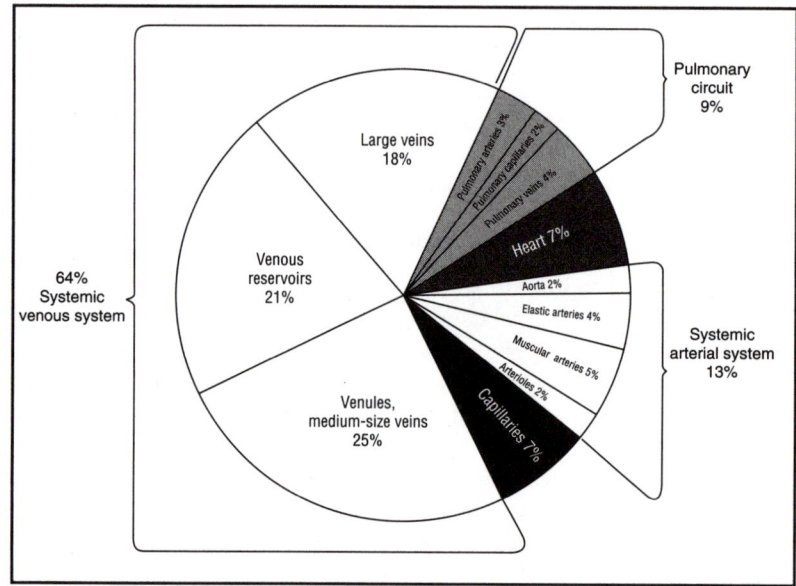

THE PHYSIOLOGY OF THE CIRCULATORY SYSTEM

The main function of the cardiovascular system is to maintain an adequate blood flow. As simple as this may sound, it takes a complex system of checks and balances to keep pace with the changing needs of the different tissues in the body. Normally, blood flow is equal to the cardiac output. But there are two factors that affect the flow of blood: pressure and resistance.

Pressure

Fluids flow from areas of high pressure to areas of lower pressure. Flow is proportional to the difference in pressure. Blood pressure is the force needed to move blood through the arterial system into the relatively lower pressures of the venous system and back to the heart. The pressure difference between the aorta, where the arterial system begins, and the right atrium, where the venous system ends, is called the pressure gradient. Blood flow through the capillaries at the cellular level is directly proportional to the arterial blood pressure. Blood pressure must be kept relatively high because of the force working against it: namely resistance.

Resistance

Resistance is the force that opposes movement. The relationship between blood flow and resistance is inversely proportional: the greater the resistance, the lower the blood flow. *Total peripheral resistance* (TPR) or *systemic vascular resistance* (SVR) is the resistance of the entire circulatory system to blood flow. Since the greatest pressures are in the arterial system, the term *peripheral resistance* refers to the resistance of the arterial system. For perfusion to occur, the circulatory pressure must be greater than the peripheral resistance. The diameter of the arterioles is the most important factor in determining peripheral resistance—the larger the diameter, the lower the resistance.

Sources of resistance include vascular resistance, blood viscosity, and turbulence. Vascular resistance is the friction caused by blood moving along the vessel wall. Any decrease in the diameter of the blood vessel, particularly of the arterioles, will decrease the blood flow. The wider the diameter of the blood vessel, the more quickly the blood flows through it.

Viscosity refers to the resistance to flow caused by the friction of molecules in a liquid. The number of molecules or particles suspended in the liquid interacts to make fluids more or less viscous. A thin liquid, like water, has a low viscosity and can be moved at low pressures. A thicker liquid such as corn syrup flows at relatively higher pressures. Whole blood is about five times more viscous than water. Blood viscosity remains relatively stable except in pathological states such as dehydration or polycythemia (a high percentage of red blood cells in whole blood), which can change the viscosity of blood and the peripheral resistance.

Turbulence occurs in areas of high flow, in areas of changing surfaces, and in areas of changing diameters. Normally, blood flow is relatively smooth, but it becomes more turbulent when it flows through the chambers of the heart and the large vessels. An example found in nature would be the water flow over rocks in a river, causing rapids. Turbulence slows the blood flow. It also creates sounds that can be heard with a stethoscope. Turbulence through incompetent valves in the heart may be heard as murmurs. Arteriosclerotic plaques can cause turbulence in larger vessels like the carotid arteries, producing sounds called bruits.

Blood Pressure

Blood pressure is actually three different pressures: arterial, venous, and capillary. As was previously reviewed, the rate of blood flow is dependent on the pressure and the diameter of the blood vessel through which it is flowing. The pressure is highest at the beginning of the arterial system where the aorta leaves the left ventricle (about 120 mmHg). As blood travels away from the heart, the blood vessels become narrower and resistance increases. Blood pressure decreases continually until it reaches the capillaries where the pressure is very low and the blood moves very slowly. This slowed flowing allows diffusion to take place. The lower pressure in the capillaries also protects the thin walls from damage. As the blood leaves the capillary beds and enters the venous system, the vessel diameters begin to increase, thus decreasing resistance. Flow increases even

Figure 5-12. Arterial pulses.

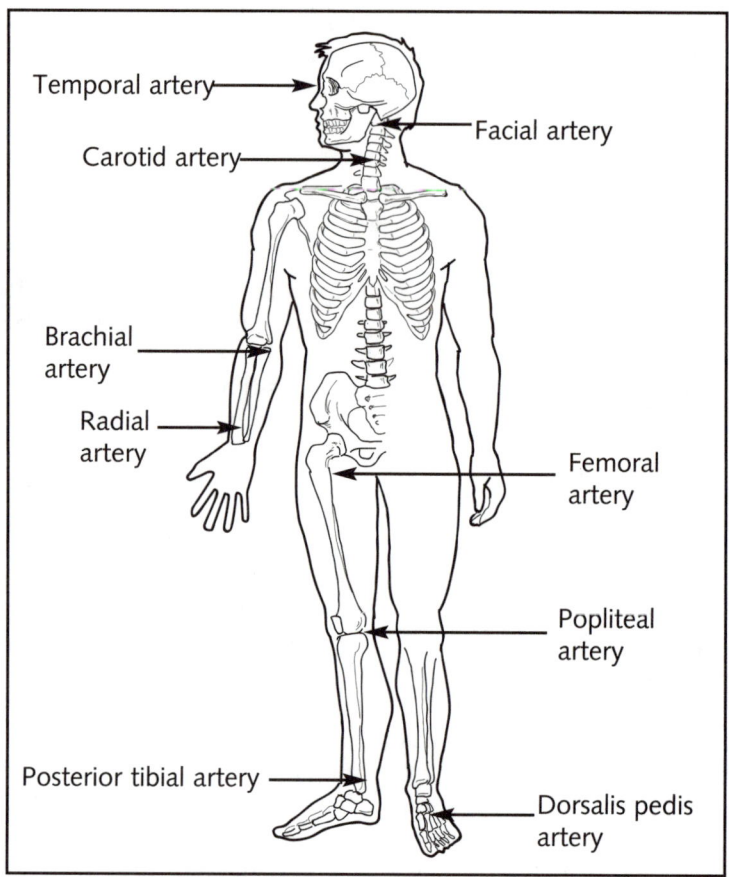

though the pressures are low. The venous blood pressure is one-tenth of the arterial system, but the system of valves, the muscular pump, and the thoracoabdominal pump all assist in returning venous blood to the heart. The blood pressure is lowest as blood enters the right atrium at the end of the venous system. In the pulmonary circuit, pressures are quite low when compared to the systemic circuit because the system is much shorter and the vessels are more elastic, providing less resistance.

Blood pressure fluctuates depending on the cardiac cycle. It is highest when both ventricles are contracting (systolic pressure) and lowest when the ventricles are filling (diastolic pressure). Blood pressure can be measured because it not only pushes blood through the circulatory system; it also pushes outward against the vessel walls. It can be measured using a *sphygmomanometer*. This is an inflatable cuff used to exert pressure over a muscular artery to the point that blood flow can be obstructed and then the pressure lowered so that the pressure at which blood flow returns can be heard by a stethoscope and measured. (Chapter 6, page 172 will review how to take a blood pressure). Different arterial pulse points in the body can be palpated and used to measure the blood pressure against the vessel walls (Figure 5-12).

Blood pressure is measured in millimeters of mercury (mmHg) with systolic pressure listed over the diastolic pressure. The difference between the systolic and diastolic pressures is referred to as the *pulse pressure:*

- Systolic pressure/diastolic pressure: 120/80 mmHg.
- Systolic pressure – diastolic pressure = pulse pressure.

- If BP is 120/80, then 120 − 80 = 40 mmHg (pulse pressure).

If only a single value is used to record the blood pressure, it is referred to as the *mean arterial pressure* (MAP). A mean arterial pressure (MAP) is about 90 to 100 mmHg. The formula for the MAP is:

- 1/3 pulse pressure + diastolic pressure = mean arterial pressure.
- If BP = 120/90 then PP = 30, so 1/3 (30) + 90 = 100.

Blood pressure varies depending on the cardiac output, the peripheral resistance, and the blood volume. Cardiac output and blood pressure can increase or decrease depending on the heart rate, stroke volume, and venous return to the heart. Peripheral resistance can be increased by vasoconstriction and decreased by vasodilation. Changes in resistance change the blood flow and pressure. Changes in blood volume will affect the venous return to the heart. For example, if a patient is hemorrhaging, less blood will return to the heart, and the cardiac output and blood pressure will drop. How the body alters blood pressure and blood flow to compensate for the changing needs of the tissues will be reviewed in the next section.

REGULATION OF THE CARDIOVASCULAR SYSTEM

Many mechanisms are involved in maintaining adequate perfusion of the tissues. All cells require oxygen and nutrients to function and need to have waste products removed. Whether blood reaches the cellular level depends on the cardiac output, the blood pressure, and the peripheral resistance (Figure 5-13).

Cardiac output (CO) is the volume of blood pumped every minute into the systemic circulation by the heart. It is normally equal to peripheral blood flow. Cardiac output is affected by the heart rate, the stroke volume, and the peripheral resistance (Figure 5-14). The formula for calculating the cardiac output is:

$$\text{cardiac output (CO)} = \text{stroke volume (SV)} \times \text{heart rate (HR)}$$

For example: SV is 80 mL x HR of 60 beats per minute = 4800 mL/minute or cardiac output = 4.8 L/min. A discussion of each factor influencing the cardiac output, heart rate, stroke volume, and peripheral resistance will clarify how important the heart's pumping action is to the oxygenation of the tissues.

Heart Rate

The heart rate is influenced by local, neural, and hormonal factors. The SA node of the heart is the pacemaker of the heart and sets the heart rate, which is normally 60 to 100 beats per minute. This intrinsic rate can be altered by the autonomic nervous system (ANS). The cardiac centers for the ANS are located in the medulla and receive input from the hypothalamus and the peripheral chemoreceptors and baroreceptors. The chemoreceptors in the aortic arch and carotid bodies provide information about the oxygen and carbon dioxide levels in the blood. The baroreceptors provide information about the blood pressure. All this information is coordinated to adjust the functioning of the cardiovascular system. For example, if the oxygen levels or the blood pressure fall or the carbon dioxide levels rise, then the heart rate (and cardiac output) can be increased to ensure that the vital organs and tissues receive adequate circulation.

The ANS provides sympathetic and parasympathetic innervation of the heart (Figure 5-15). The sympathetic division increases the heart rate and cardiac contractility. The

Figure 5-13. Factors influencing blood pressure.

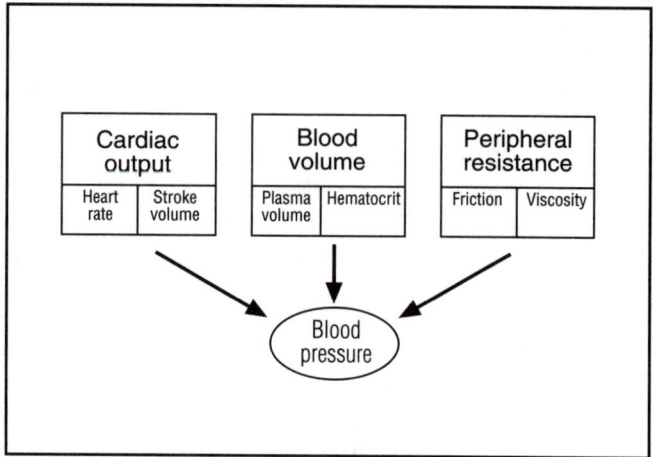

Figure 5-14. Pressure wave.

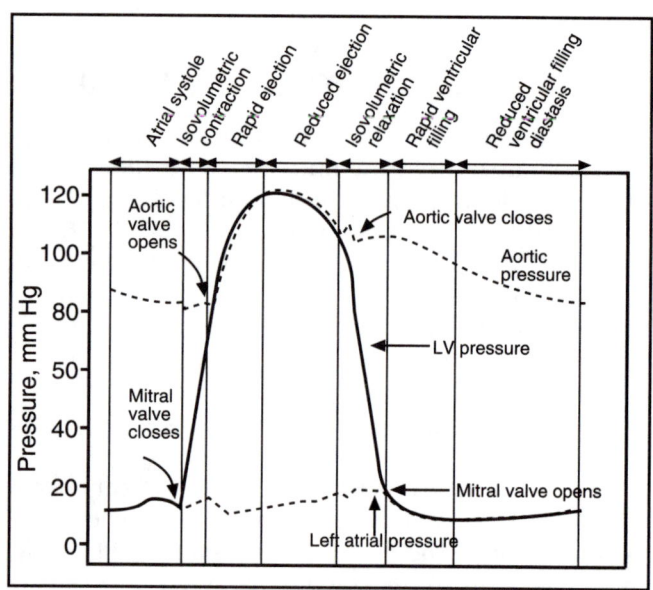

parasympathetic division decreases the heart rate via the vagus nerve. The heart can vary its rate by 2.5 times. As the heart rate increases, the cardiac output increases. However, at higher heart rates, less time of the cardiac cycle is spent in filling the ventricles (diastole), and the cardiac output can actually decrease.

The hormones epinephrine and norepinephrine are produced by the sympathetic neurons in the heart and by the adrenal glands. They can also increase the heart rate, cardiac contractility, and cardiac output. The so-called "fight or flight" mechanism can be triggered in times of stress or physical exertion, increasing the heart rate and cardiac output to allow increased circulation and performance.

The autonomic nervous system allows the circulatory system to respond to a variety of stresses of everyday life. When a patient moves from the lying to the standing position, 20% of the blood in the heart and lungs is redistributed to the legs. The venous return to the heart drops and the blood pressure falls. The baroreceptors are stimulated and the sympathetic nervous system increases the heart rate and the peripheral vascular resistance. These mechanisms increase the blood pressure and compensate for the postural

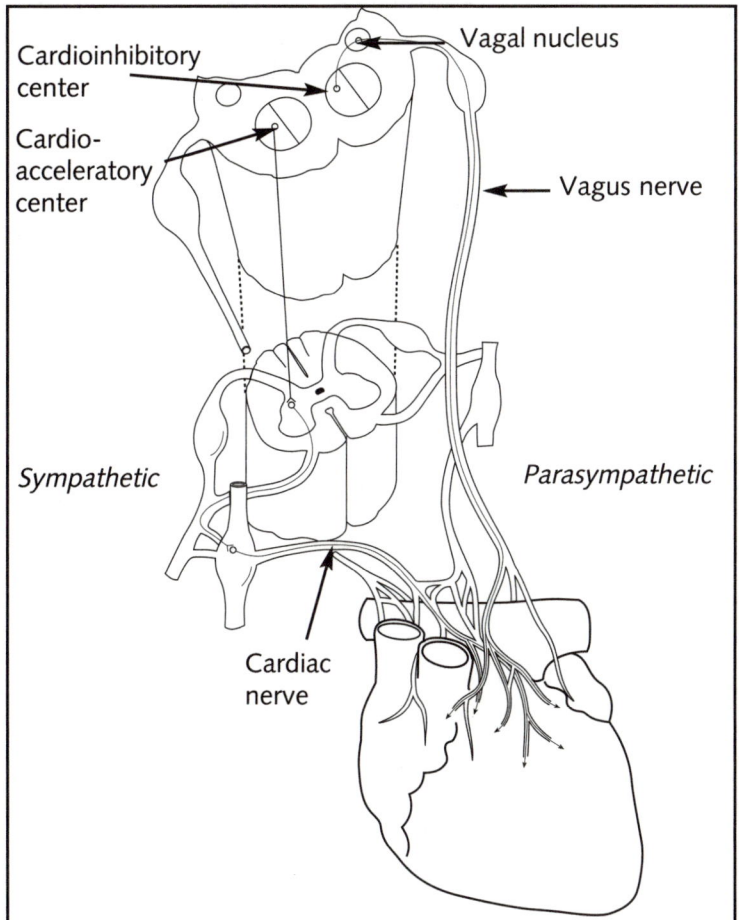

Figure 5-15. Regulation of heart rate by the autonomic nervous system.

Cardioinhibitory center

Cardio-acceleratory center

Vagal nucleus

Vagus nerve

Sympathetic

Parasympathetic

Cardiac nerve

redistribution of the blood volume. During exercise, the skeletal muscle pump also contributes to the venous return to the heart. Decreased responsiveness to postural stimulation of the sympathetic nervous system can cause postural hypotension, a significant drop in blood pressure when changing position.

Stroke Volume

The stroke volume is the amount of blood ejected from the ventricle during systole. It is normally 55 to 100 mL per beat. Since both sides of the heart must function equally, if the left ventricle pumps out 80 mL, then the right atrium must also receive 80 mL. When the ventricles contract, they do not eject every millimeter of blood. This residual volume, the end-systolic volume, is the amount of blood remaining in the ventricles after systole.

The specialized muscle cells of the myocardium contract more forcefully when they are stretched. The greater the venous return to the heart, the more the myocardium is stretched and the more strongly it will contract. This general rule of "more in = more out" is named Starling's law of the heart after the physiologist who discovered it. The filling of the ventricles at the end of diastole just prior to contraction produces a pressure in the wall called *preload*. Starling's mechanism works best if the cardiac muscle fibers are stretched to 2.5 times their resting length. If the stretch is excessive, then the strength of the contraction can decrease.

Figure 5-16. Regulation of blood flow.

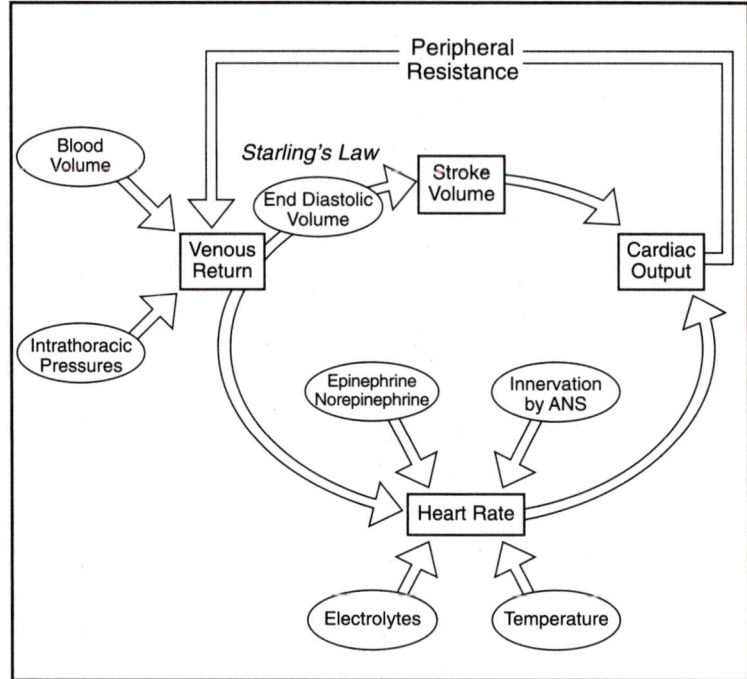

Resistance

When the preload pressure has been reached, the ventricle begins to contract. On the left side of the heart, the aortic valve opens when the left ventricle overcomes diastolic pressure (Figure 5-16). As it continues to contract, systolic pressure is achieved as it pushes against resistance in the arterial system. Afterload is the pressure created in the ventricular wall to achieve systolic pressure. Systemic vascular resistance (SVR) is the clinical measure of the left ventricular afterload. Preload and afterload also apply to the right side of the heart. Pulmonic vascular resistance (PVR) is the clinical measure of the right ventricular afterload.

Systemic vascular resistance can be increased and decreased by the arterioles and the capillaries. The capillaries can regulate their blood flow through the precapillary sphincters. Local, hormonal, and neural impulses can dilate or contract the sphincters, altering the blood flow in the capillary beds. Local tissue factors are released that dilate the sphincters and increase circulation to the tissues. For example, during exercise, the precapillary muscles respond to the needs of the tissues and dilate to allow greater blood flow to the muscles. Conversely, if the patient is hemorrhaging, then the sphincters can contract in response to sympathetic hormones like epinephrine. This shunts more blood into the systemic circulation to maintain blood pressure and blood flow to vital organs like the heart and brain.

In summary, the cardiovascular system is a well-tuned machine, consisting of a pump and blood vessels. The pump (the heart) is well suited for pushing blood throughout the systemic and pulmonary circulation. The arteries, veins, and capillaries are each constructed to serve their individual functions. Many neural and hormonal mechanisms allow regulation of the system to provide oxygen and nutrients to the tissues. Every cell in the body must be provided with oxygen and nutrients, and the cellular waste products and carbon dioxide need to be removed. The cardiovascular system ensures the perfusion of the tissues with oxygen.

BIBLIOGRAPHY

Bates B. *A Guide to Physical Examination and History Taking*. 6th ed. Philadelphia, Pa: J.B. Lippincott Co; 1995.

Goldman L, Braunwald E. *Primary Cardiology*. Philadelphia, Pa: W.B. Saunders Co; 1998.

Martini F. *Fundamentals of Anatomy and Physiology*. 2nd ed. Englewood Cliffs, NJ: Prentice Hall Inc; 1992.

Porth CM. *Pathophysiology: Concepts of Altered Health States*. 4th ed. Philadelphia, Pa: J.B. Lippincott Co; 1994.

MULTIPLE-CHOICE QUESTIONS

1. The main function of the atria of the heart is to:
    A. Contract and push blood into the systemic circulation
    B. Collect blood from the pulmonary and systemic circuits
    C. Be the pacemaker of the heart
    D. Sense changes in the carbon dioxide and oxygen levels

2. Arteries and veins are structured differently because:
    A. The veins need to withstand higher pressures
    B. The arterial system is a low pressure system
    C. Arteries need valves to help push the blood to the tissues
    D. Veins operate in a tenth of the pressure of the arteries

3. The heart rate is regulated by the "pacemaker of the heart":
    A. The sinoatrial node in the left ventricle
    B. The Purkinje fibers in the ventricles
    C. The SA node in the right atrium
    D. Bachmann's Bundle

4. The relationship between resistance and blood flow could be summarized as:
    A. The lower the resistance, the more pressure is needed to make blood flow
    B. The higher the resistance, the faster the flow
    C. The lower the resistance, the faster the flow
    D. The higher the resistance, the less pressure is needed to make blood flow

5. Both diastole and systole are important in the cardiac cycle because:
    A. The chambers of the heart fill with blood during diastole
    B. The ventricles contract during diastole to move blood throughout the circulation
    C. The atria and ventricles fill during systole
    D. When ventricles stretch less during diastole, they expel more blood during systole

CHAPTER 5 ANSWERS

1. B
2. D
3. C
4. C
5. A

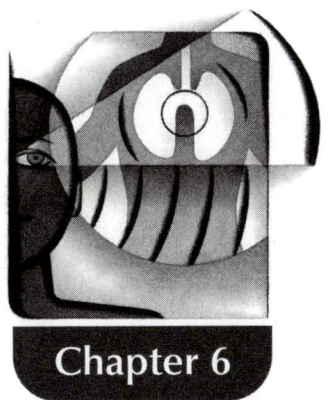

Chapter 6

Assessment of the Cardiovascular System

Al has a long-standing history of chronic obstructive lung disease, high blood pressure, and is 60 pounds overweight. He continues to smoke despite urgings from his physician to quit. He called this morning because his chest felt tight and he could not catch his breath. When the nurse asked him what he did to help the pain, he said that he laid down an hour ago but the pain did not go away. Suspecting that his pain could be cardiac in origin, the nurse asks if his son is available to take him to the hospital or can he call an ambulance. This scares Al but the nurse reassures him that this is the best place for him because they can get to the root of his pain and make him feel better. The nurse reminds him not to smoke any more cigarettes. Vital signs, an EKG, blood work, and pulse oximetry are done on Al's arrival in the emergency department. His vital signs are as follows: HR—108 beats per min, RR—32 breaths per min, and BP—176/94 mmHg. The SaO_2 is 86%. The nurse starts oxygen via nasal cannula at 4 L per min. His EKG shows ST segment elevations and his chest pain is not fully relieved by sublingual nitroglycerine, so a cardiac catheterization is ordered.

- How would you explain the purpose of the cardiac catheterization to Al?
- What allergies would you ask Al about prior to the procedure?
- What feelings should Al report to the nurses in the Cath Lab during the procedure?
- Why is bedrest important after the catheterization?

Assessment of the cardiovascular system involves evaluating the adequacy of tissue perfusion. The perfusion process is similar to plumbing: the heart acts as the pump to deliver oxygenated blood to the cells and the vascular network functions as the pipes. Perfusion through the cardiovascular network is a closed system that responds to changes in pressure. Unlike plumbing, the cardiovascular system is also responsive to changes in the tissue demands and can alter flow to meet the demands of the body. This chapter will review the assessment of the cardiovascular system as it pertains to tissue perfusion and cell oxygenation.

GENERAL ASSESSMENT

A general overview of the patient's functioning provides clues to the overall health and the efficiency of the cardiovascular system. Examine the patient and estimate his apparent age. A comparison of his apparent and stated age may reveal that the patient looks older because of smoking, sun exposure, or poor health. Notice any cyanosis around the mouth and nose or in the extremities. Central cyanosis could indicate poor oxygenation or circulation. Assess the patient's facial expression, posture, and body language. These may allude to problems with breathing, pain, or anxiety. Pallor may indicate anemia or low cardiac output. Diaphoresis may suggest hypotension or myocardial infarction. Note the patient's respiratory patterns during activity. Increased breathlessness during a mild activity like disrobing may indicate problems with the respiratory or cardiovascular systems. While these are only general clues, they can direct a more detailed assessment of the heart and circulatory system.

ASSESSMENT OF THE CARDIOVASCULAR SYSTEM

An assessment of the cardiovascular system begins with questions about the patient's family health history. Any history of heart disease in the patient's family is important in understanding the patient's health risks. Family history would include congenital heart disease, angina, myocardial infarction, elevated cholesterol levels (hyperlipidemia), high blood pressure, and strokes. Other diseases associated with heart problems include a family history of diabetes and thyroid disease.

The nurse asks about the patient's own health history including:

1. Heart disease (acute, chronic, or congenital), hypertension, diabetes, hyperlipidemia, heart murmurs, rheumatic fever, or varicose veins.

2. Lifestyle, including occupation, hobbies, sleep habits, stressors, exercise, smoking, and alcohol intake.

3. Medications, including cardiac medications, antihypertensive, over-the-counter medications, oral contraceptives, herbal remedies, and nutritional supplements.

4. Nutritional habits, including caloric, fat, salt, and caffeine intake.

The patient's health history should include questions about the presenting problem plus nonspecific symptoms. Ask the patient about what brought him to seek a health care provider and use follow-up questions to determine the timing of the symptom(s), alleviating

> Chest pain—It is important to note the quality, character, location, radiation, frequency, and any precipitating factors when assessing chest pain.

factors, and how they impact on the patient's functioning. Nonspecific symptoms might include fatigue, cough (refer to Chapter 2), dizziness, palpitations, or problems with sleep. Some common signs and symptoms of patients with cardiovascular disorders include:

- **Chest pain**—including arm, shoulder, and neck pain, as well as timing of the pain to activities.

- **Pain in the extremities on exertion**—relieved by rest (intermittent claudication) or heaviness in the extremities (varicose veins).

- **Dyspnea on exertion or with ordinary activities**—note the timing, the precipitating activity, and the alleviating factors.

- **Orthopnea or difficulty breathing when recumbent**—note the timing of the orthopnea (paroxysmal nocturnal dyspnea, or PND, occurs shortly after falling asleep and is relieved by sitting up). Ask about the number of pillows that the patient uses to sleep.

- **Palpitations** (awareness of heart beating)—note any precipitating factors like caffeine, nicotine, alcohol, sugar, or stress. Also ask about awareness of skipped beats.
- **Edema of the extremities**—note location, unilateral or bilateral swelling, any discoloration of the extremities, presence of ulcerations, and time during the day when the edema is noticeable.
- **Episodes of dizziness or fainting**—these may indicate cardiac arrhythmias, postural hypotension, or a vasovagal response.

Physical Assessment of the Cardiovascular System

To begin a more specific examination of the cardiovascular system, the patient needs to be disrobed and well draped. The room should be warm, well lighted, and quiet. The nurse needs only her eyes, ears, hands, and a stethoscope to examine the patient. Start by assessing the skin and mucus membranes, looking at the color, pigmentation changes, temperature, and hair distribution on the extremities, lesions, or ulcers. Patients with venous insufficiency may have brownish pigmentation on the lower extremities. Those with arterial insufficiency may present with reddened and swollen extremities that are hairless. Check the nail beds for clubbing (see page 26).

Pulses

Assess the adequacy of the arterial perfusion by palpating the peripheral pulses (Figure 6-1). The pulses which are palpable include the temporal, carotid, brachial, radial, femoral, popliteal, dorsalis pedis, and posterior tibial pulses. Using the pads of the index and middle fingers, gently palpate over the pulse and grade it on a scale of 0 to 4. Too much pressure can obliterate the pulse. Assessing and grading the pulses allows the nurse to evaluate perfusion by documenting the patient's baseline status, monitoring changes in circulation, and comparing the corresponding pulses on the opposite side of the body. The nurse documents the findings in the patient's chart.

Sometimes the pulses are difficult to palpate, especially when there is arterial insufficiency of the extremities. A Doppler ultrasound (DUS) may be used to listen for the presence of a pulse. The DUS apparatus has a special stethoscope with a transducer and an audio unit. The transducer is applied to the skin, and ultrasound waves detect the movement of red blood cells in the blood vessels. The pressure wave of increased blood flow after the heart contracts is detectable by the transducer as a pulse. A water-soluble gel is used on the skin to enhance the transmission of the sounds. The pulse sites may be marked with a waterproof marker so that they are easier to locate during subsequent assessments.

> The stethoscope was invented by Rene Laennec in 1816. He is known as the "father of auscultation." The word *stethoscope* comes from a Greek word meaning the "spy of the chest." The diaphragm is used to hear high-frequency sounds and is held firmly on the skin. The bell is used to hear low-frequency sounds and is held lightly on the skin.

The pulses may be weak or absent in the extremities if there is arterial insufficiency. Capillary filling may be slowing (greater than 1 second), and the affected extremity starts to blanch when elevated above the heart for 1 to 2 minutes. When patients have venous insufficiency of the extremities, the pulses are present but may be difficult to palpate due to edema.

Figure 6-1. Sites for palpating arterial pulses.

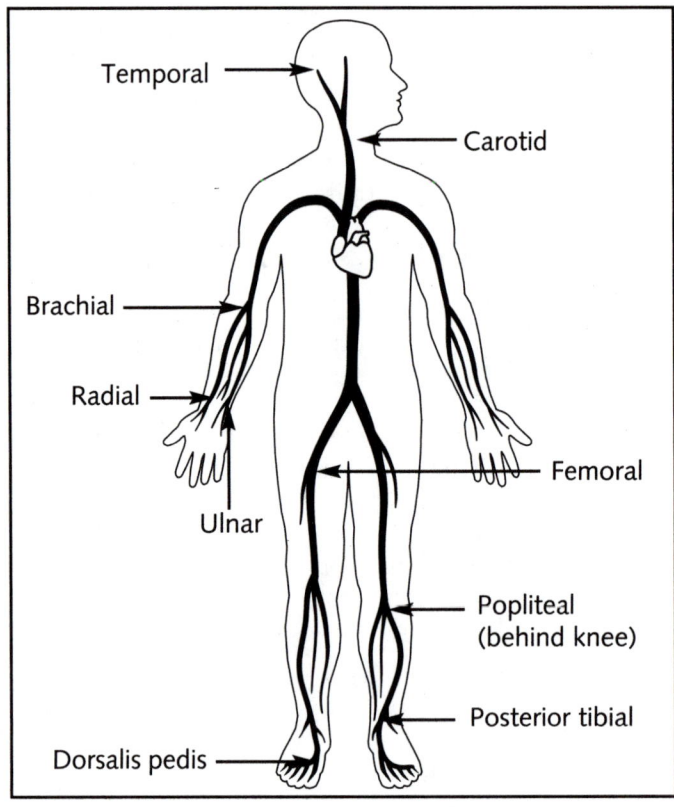

Pulse Rate

Using the patient's radial pulse on the wrist, count the pulsation for a full minute to get a sense of the heart rate and regularity. Use the finger pads of the middle fingers pressed lightly over the pulse. If the pulse is regular, count the pulsation for 30 seconds and multiply by 2 to get the 1-minute pulse rate. If the pulse is irregular, count the pulsation for a full minute.

The most accurate method for obtaining the heart rate, especially when the pulse is irregular, is by listening to the apical pulse for a full minute. (See Cardiac Assessment on page 173 for how to obtain the apical heart rate.) An irregular pulse may represent premature beats that may not be palpable peripherally at the radial pulse because left ventricular filling was incomplete prior to systole. When a pulse is irregular, note the type of irregularity: regularly irregular (ie, beat, beat, pause, beat, beat, pause), irregular with respiration (ie, an increasing rate with inspiration and decreasing rate with expiration), or totally irregular. Alternately, take a radial and apical pulse rate and note any discrepancies. Normally, these are identical but may not be in cases of varying cardiac output.

Grading Pulses

0 = Absent
1 = Weak and thready
2 = Normal
3 = Strong
4 = Bounding

Blood Pressure

The blood pressure is an important determinant of cardiovascular functioning. As the heart relaxes and contracts, it sends a pressure wave of blood through the circulatory system. The pressure wave is what produces the impulse detected as an arterial pulse and the Korotkoff sounds that are heard when auscultating a blood pressure. Normally, the blood pressure is finely controlled by neural and hormonal influences that maintain adequate tissue perfusion. Measuring the blood pressure can assess the adequacy of the circulation and the regulatory mechanisms.

Blood pressure can be measured either directly or indirectly. Direct measurement requires the insertion of a catheter into an artery. Indirect blood pressure readings are done with a blood pressure cuff and auscultation of Korotkoff sounds or Doppler reading of the pressure wave. Using a sphygmomanometer (a blood pressure cuff attached to a manometer) and a stethoscope, the blood pressure is usually taken on the upper arm. A mercury sphygmomanometer aneroid instrument may be used to take a blood pressure (Table 6-1).

Ranges for Heart Rates	
Normal	60 to 100 beats per minute
Bradycardia	less than 60 beats per minute
Tachycardia	more than 100 beats per minute

Blood pressure should be taken on both arms. When hypertension is suspected, the blood pressure should be repeated on three separate occasions, and the patient should refrain from smoking cigarettes or drinking caffeine for 30 minutes before the reading. In patients with symptoms of dizziness and syncope, the blood pressure should be taken in the reclined, sitting, and standing positions. Changing from the reclined to the standing position does not normally change the systolic pressure and may only slightly increase the diastolic pressure. But a decrease in the systolic blood pressure of more than 20 mmHg constitutes postural or orthostatic hypotension. Dehydration (hypovolemia) and certain antihypertensive medications are common causes of postural hypotension.

Paradoxical blood pressure is a decrease of greater than 10 mmHg in the systolic pressure during inspiration. This change is sometimes called *pulsus paradoxus*. It can be assessed by taking the blood pressure twice during inspiration and during rest. First, palpate the systolic pressure while the patient stops breathing for a moment. Then, auscultate the blood pressure during inspiration and note when the sounds are first heard. Subtract the second number from the first and note any discrepancy between the two systolic pressures. Causes of pulsus paradoxus include pericardial tamponade, pulmonary hypertension, and restrictive pericarditis.

Blood pressure ranges for normal and high blood pressure have been labeled by the Joint National Committee on Detection, Evaluation and Treatment of High Blood Pressure in the United States. Values for normal and abnormal blood pressures are seen in Table 6-2.

High blood pressure can be categorized in different ways. If both pressures are elevated, the highest pressure determines the category of hypertension. When only the systolic or diastolic pressure is elevated, it is called *isolated systolic* or *diastolic* hypertension.

Examination of the Chest

The examination of the chest allows assessment of the structure and functioning of the cardiovascular system. To review, the landmarks are established by the anatomy of the thorax: the midsternal line, the midclavicular line, the sternal notch, the intercostal spaces between the ribs, the midscapular line, and the midaxillary line (Figure 6-3). Several key

Table 6-1

Measuring Blood Pressure

1. Choose a cuff of the appropriate size: width should be 40% of the upper arm circumference (about 12 to 14 cm) (Figure 6-2). The bladder should be 80% of the circumference. A cuff that is too small may give an abnormally high reading.

2. Palpate the brachial pulse and position the arm at the level of the patient's heart with the palm facing up.

3. Wrap the cuff around the upper arm and brachial artery so that the bottom of the cuff is about 2.5 cm above the brachial pulse. It is best to have no clothing on the arm when taking a blood pressure.

4. To know how high to inflate the cuff, first take a palpable systolic reading. Palpate the radial pulse and rapidly inflate the cuff until the radial pulse disappears. Then, while deflating the cuff, palpate the return of the radial pulse. This is the palpable systolic pressure. Add 30 to this number and use this as the highest pressure to which the cuff is to be inflated.

5. Place the stethoscope over the brachial pulse. The bell of the stethoscope picks up the low-pitched sounds (Korotkoff sounds) better than the diaphragm.

6. Inflate the cuff to the predetermined number (30 above the palpable systolic pressure) and slowly deflate the cuff (2 to 3 mmHg per second), listening for two consecutive sounds. Note this number as the systolic pressure. Continue deflating the cuff until the sounds become muffled and disappear. This is the diastolic pressure. The point of disappearance gives the best measure of diastolic pressure.

Figure 6-2. Blood pressure cuff—appropriate size for accurate measurement.

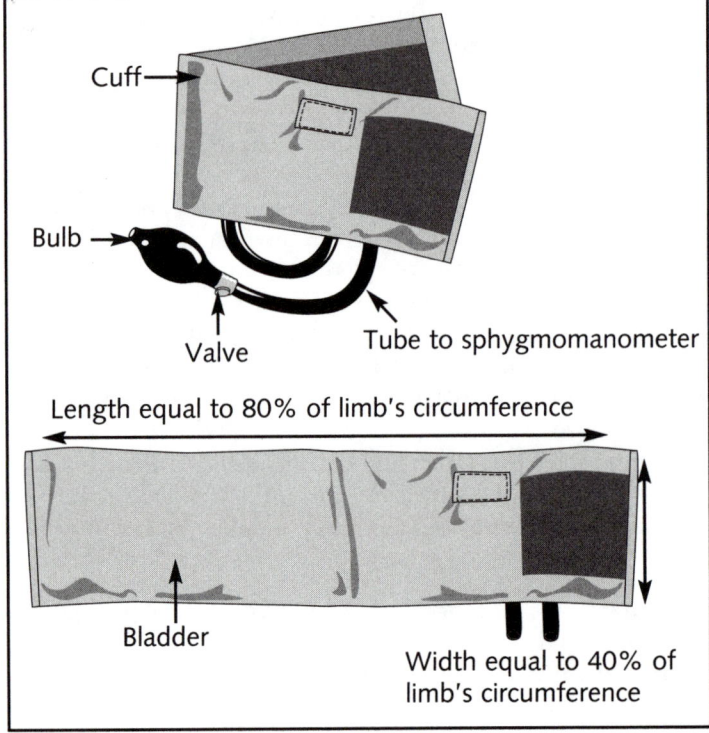

Table 6-2

Normal and Abnormal Blood Pressures

Category	Systolic	Diastolic
Normal	<130	<85
High normal	130-139	85-89
Mild hypertension	140-159	90-99
Moderate hypertension	160-179	100-109
Severe hypertension	180-209	110-119

landmarks are used in cardiac assessment as they approximate the location of cardiac structures within the bony thorax (Figure 6-4). These cardiac landmarks are used during palpation and auscultation of the chest wall and heart.

The examination of the chest follows three steps: inspection, palpation, and auscultation. Start examining the patient by looking at the anterior chest while the patient is sitting. Take care to drape female patients as much as possible while allowing for adequate visualization. Notice any pulsation, retractions, or movements of the chest wall. Inspect the large vessels of the neck: the carotid arteries and the jugular veins. Note their location and how high up the neck the pulsations are visible.

The jugular veins can be used to estimate the venous pressure and the pressure in the right atrium of the heart. A noninvasive method of estimating venous pressure is to observe the jugular vein in the neck. Assess the jugular venous distention using the following steps:

1. Position the patient in a supine position with the head of the bed at a 30-degree angle and turn his head slightly away from the side being inspected.
2. Use oblique lighting and observe the neck for the pulsation of the jugular vein on either side of the neck. It is usually above the sternal notch or just posterior to the sternocleidomastoid muscle.
3. Find the highest point up the neck where the jugular venous pulsation is visible.
4. Measure from the sternal angle (the connection of the second ribs to the sternum and manubrium) to this level using a vertical ruler and a horizontal reference point to the highest point of jugular venous pulsation (Figure 6-5).
5. Measurements greater than 3 to 4 cm above the sternal angle may indicate elevated venous pressure. Central venous pressure can also be measured using central lines and electronic equipment.

Cardiac Assessment

After inspecting the thorax and the neck veins, the nurse can begin palpating the chest wall. The patient can remain in the supine position with the head of the bed at a 30-degree angle. The nurse should be on the patient's right side. Using the cardiac landmarks in Figure 6-4 (aortic, pulmonic, Erb's point, tricuspid, and mitral areas), palpate with the finger pads along the chest wall, noting any thrills or vibrations. Thrills are vibrations that may accompany loud, rumbling heart murmurs. (Heart murmurs are addressed more specifically on page 177). Vibrations may accompany murmurs or extra heart sounds.

Figure 6-3. Thoracic landmarks.

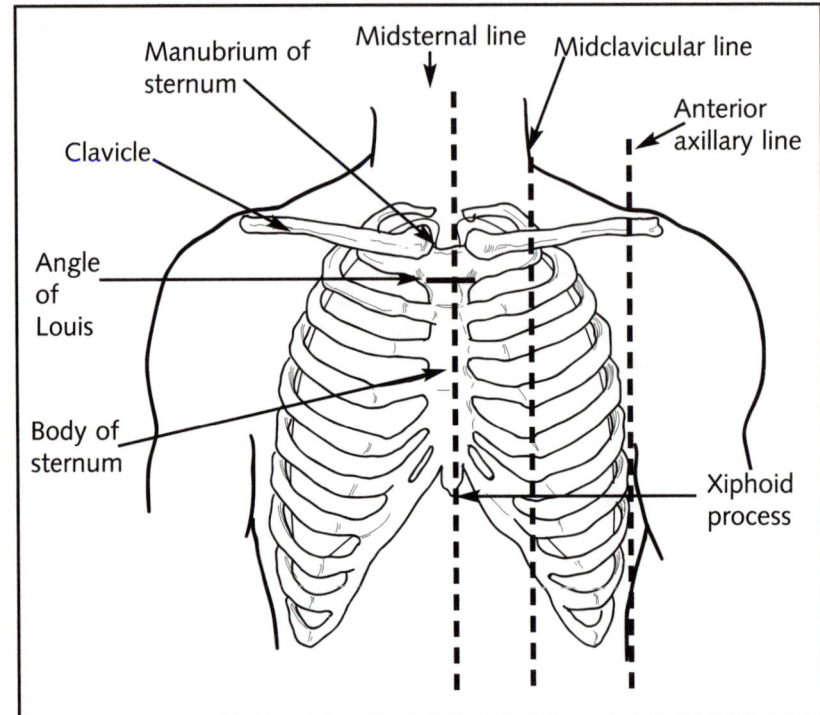

Figure 6-4. Cardiac landmarks.

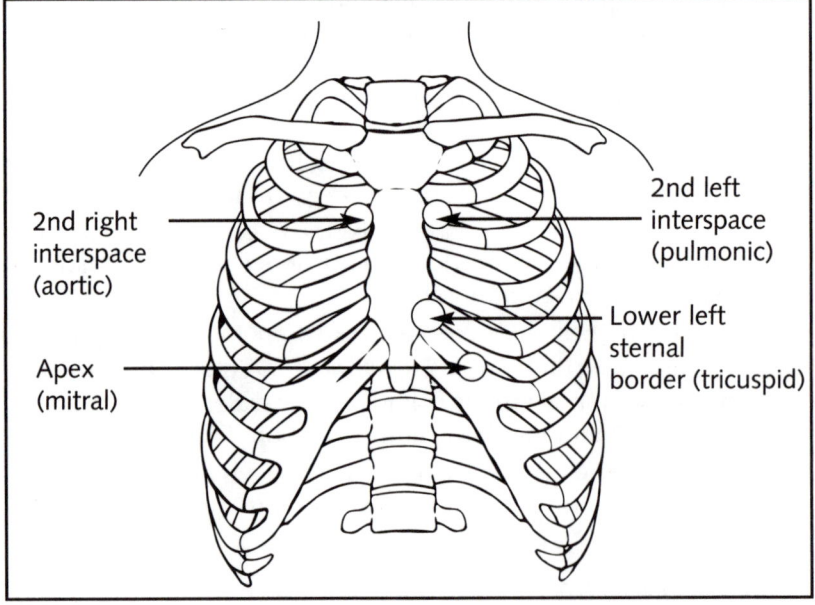

Locate the apical pulse by palpating along the fourth and fifth intercostal spaces and slightly medial to the midclavicular line. Remember that the intercostal spaces are labeled by the rib above them (eg, the second intercostal space is just below the second rib). In female patients with large breasts, move the breast gently upward or ask the patient to do this. This will allow better palpation of the chest wall. Note the location, amplitude, and regularity of the apical pulse.

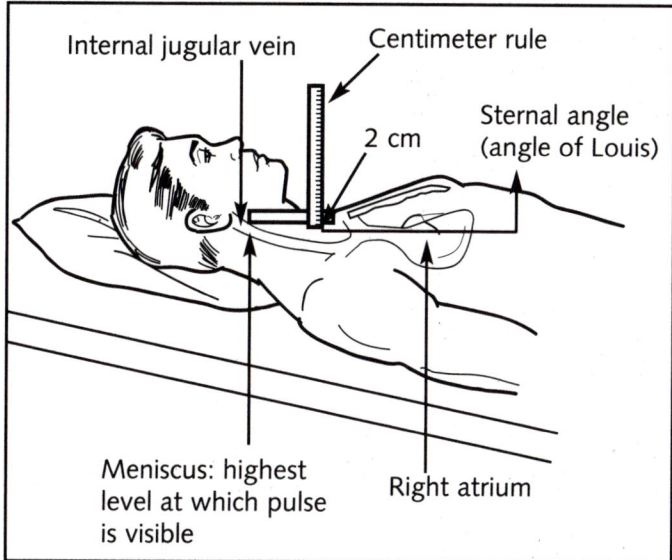

Figure 6-5. Measuring jugular vein distention.

Auscultation is one of the most frequently used techniques for assessing cardiac functioning and one which requires much practice in order to become proficient. Clean and warm the stethoscope prior to applying it to the patient. With the patient in the supine position with the head of the bed at a 30-degree angle, begin listening to the heart using the bell of the stethoscope and then repeat the same steps using the diaphragm. Begin listening at the same cardiac landmarks that were used for palpation of the chest wall. Start at the base of the heart (the aortic and pulmonic sites) and progress to the apex of the heart (the tricuspid and mitral sites). Do not forget to listen at Erb's point (the third intercostal space at the left sternal border), as extra heart sounds and murmurs are often heard here.

The first heart sounds the nurse should listen for are the "lub" and "dup" sounds of the heartbeat, or S1 and S2. Each "lub-dup" or S1 and S2 equals one heartbeat. Identifying the two sounds takes some practice and knowledge about the physiologic basis for the sounds. Heart sounds are caused by the closing of valves and the rapid distending of the chambers of the heart with blood. It is easiest to think about heart sounds as the valves closing during the cardiac cycle. "Lub" or S1 is the sound that accompanies the

> Auscultation of the chest is an important part of assessing the cardiovascular system. Lung sounds provide clues to cardiac as well as pulmonary disorders. Crackles are often a sign of congestive heart failure and may be more pronounced on the dependent side. Wheezes and rhonchi may indicate left-sided heart failure.

closing of the atrioventricular valves (tricuspid and mitral valves) just before contraction of the ventricles (systole). "Dup" or S2 is the sound that accompanies the closing of the aortic and pulmonic valves after the ventricles have emptied and the heart enters the filling phase of the cardiac cycle (diastole). Using the first letter of each valve to represent each valve closing, think about the heart sounds and the cardiac cycle using Table 6-3.

The opposite pair of valves is open during each heart sound, allowing blood to fill the chambers. For example, when S1 is heard, the tricuspid and mitral valves are closing to allow blood to fill the atria. At the same time, the aortic and pulmonic valves are

Table 6-3

Cardiac Cycle

	——One heartbeat——		——One heartbeat———	
	Lub	Dup	Lub	Dup
Heart sound	S1	S2	S1	S2
Valves closing	T-M	A-P	T-M	A-P
	Systole	Diastole	Systole	Diastole

T = Tricuspid valve	Diastole = ventricular filling
M = Mitral valve	Systole = ventricular contraction
P = Pulmonic valve	A = Aortic valve

opening as the ventricles contract and are pushing blood into the systemic and pulmonic circulation.

Using the cardiac landmarks, listen for S1 and S2 at each site. S2 will be loudest at the base of the heart at the aortic and pulmonic sites. S1 will be loudest at the apex of the heart, the tricuspid, and mitral sites. To identify S1, gently feel the carotid pulse while listening to the heart sounds. The carotid pulse will immediately follow S1. Sometimes it is easier to identify each heart sound by tapping the first and second fingers of the head with the "lub" and "dup" sounds to get the rhythm of the heart beat.

Occasionally in healthy, young adults, the second heart sound, S2, will be split into two parts. Each part represents a valve closing—first the aortic and then the pulmonic valve because they are not closing simultaneously. When the second heart sound is split on inspiration but the split disappears on expiration, this is called *normal* or *physiologic splitting*.

While listening to the heart sounds, assess the rate, rhythm, and quality of the heartbeat. Like assessing the pulse, label the rate as normal, bradycardic, or tachycardic. Note whether the rate is regular or irregular. While auscultating, listen for the intensity of the heart sounds during each beat and note whether they sound of the same strength or varying strengths with each beat. Take an apical pulse by listening to the apex of the heart for a full minute. Remember that the apical pulse is usually at the left fourth or fifth intercostal space at the midclavicular line. If the apical pulse has been located on palpation first, it is much easier to locate it when auscultating the apical pulse. Always compare the findings to the patient's baseline data by reviewing the chart.

Extra heart sounds are heard when the heart is not functioning properly. Extra sounds include S3, S4, heart murmurs, opening snaps, and friction rubs. Both S3 and S4 are diastolic sounds. S3, or a *ventricular gallop*, signals decreased ventricular compliance (stiffness). It may be one of the first signs of congestive heart failure. It is best heard with the bell of the stethoscope because it is a low-frequency sound. Listening at the tricuspid area at the left lower sternal border, S3 is heard immediately after S2 and the heart beat sounds like *Tennessee:*

S1		S2	S3	S1		S2	S3

The fourth heart sound, S4, is sometimes called a *presystolic* or *atrial gallop* and is heard with decreased ventricular compliance. It is also heard with the bell of the stethoscope at the apex of the heart. The heart beat sounds like *Kentucky:*

S4 S1	S2	S4 S1	S2

Opening snaps are made when a stenotic mitral valve opens. It is an early, diastolic sound and heard best with the diaphragm of the stethoscope.

Heart Murmurs

Heart murmurs are extra heart sounds that signal valvular dysfunction. Valves can become incompetent because they do not open and close properly. Stenotic valves may not close completely, allowing blood to flow backward (regurgitant flow). They also may not open fully, causing turbulent forward flow. The abnormal blood flow produces sounds that can be heard with a stethoscope and sometimes palpated as thrills.

Heart murmurs are described by their timing during the cardiac cycle, their location, the presence of radiation, the intensity, the pitch, and quality of the sound. Murmurs are first differentiated by whether they are systolic (occurring between S1 and S2) or diastolic (occurring between S2 and S1). The timing of the murmur during the cardiac cycle is important because it can help identify which valve is incompetent. Murmurs occur only during a particular point during the cardiac cycle (ie, pansystolic), during the whole systolic component of the cycle, or across the whole cycle (ie, continuous murmur).

> Other positions for a more specific evaluation of heart sounds include the left lateral recumbent position, leaning forward while sitting, squatting, and standing. The left lateral recumbent position may bring out S3, S4, and mitral murmurs. Leaning forward while sitting accentuates aortic valve murmurs.

The location of the maximal intensity and the presence of radiation of the sound to other locations like the neck or axilla should also be noted (Table 6-4).

The intensity of the murmur may vary during the cycle. The varying intensity or configuration may be described as increasing during the cycle (crescendo) or decreasing in intensity (decrescendo).

Pitch refers to whether the murmur is of high, medium, or low pitch. The stethoscope will help differentiate the pitch. The bell picks up low-pitched sounds and the diaphragm picks up the higher-pitched sounds. Quality is a more vague descriptor, comparing the murmur to other sounds that are generally recognizable. For example, a murmur may be described as blowing or harsh in quality.

Friction rubs are sounds made by inflamed pericardial tissue. The rubbing of the inflamed tissues as the heart rocks in the pericardial cavity causes harsh sounds that are somewhat "scratchy" in nature. The sound of a pericardial friction rub is similar to a pleural rub. To differentiate between a pericardial and a pleural rub, the nurse asks the patient to hold his breath for a couple of seconds. If the rub disappears during breath-holding, then it is a pleural friction rub. Causes of pericardial friction rubs include pericarditis.

Laboratory and Diagnostic Tests

A variety of tests are used to assess the functioning of the cardiovascular system. Some tests are more invasive and require more recovery time than others. The nurse's role is to understand the implications for the test and the patient's experience. She teaches the

Table 6-4
Murmur Intensity Scale

Grade 1—very faint
Grade 2—quiet but immediately heard with a stethoscope
Grade 3—moderately loud
Grade 4—loud
Grade 5—very loud, may be heard with stethoscope partly off the chest wall
Grade 6—can be heard with a stethoscope off the chest wall

patient about the test, the preparation that is needed, what to expect during the test, and what is involved in recovery. Patients also want to know what the test will reveal and how soon they will have information about their health. The nurse addresses these issues prior to the test to alleviate some anxiety. Some tests of cardiovascular functioning include:

- Blood tests
- Chest radiology
- Electrocardiograms
- Stress tests
- Echocardiograms, ultrasound, and Doppler studies
- Arteriograms
- Cardiac catheterization
- Radionuclide scans
- Hemodynamic monitoring

Blood Tests

Laboratory blood work is done by simple venipuncture in the outpatient setting or in the acute care setting if the patient is hospitalized. Preparation depends on the type of blood test. For example, a serum cholesterol is best obtained in the morning after fasting during the previous night. Refer to the guidelines of the facility or contact the laboratory for test-specific preparation. Some blood tests that are taken are:

- Electrolytes—sodium, potassium, magnesium, calcium, and phosphorus. These are involved in the maintenance of fluid balance, blood vessel tone, and cardiac muscle contractility. Blood glucose may be drawn if there is a question about diabetes.
- Cholesterol and triglycerides—to assess changes that could signal hyperlipidemia and risk factors for arteriosclerosis.
- Cardiac enzymes—troponin T, creatine phosphokinase (CPK), and CPK-MB fraction to assess cardiac muscle damage, lactic acid dehydrogenase (LDH), serum glutamic oxoloacetic transaminase (SGOT), and aspartate amino transferase (AST).
- Hematologic tests—including a complete blood count (CBC), coagulation times (activated partial thromboplastin time—APTT, and prothrombin time—PT), and erythrocyte sedimentation rate (ESR).
- Arterial blood gases—used to determine oxygenation of tissues, carbon dioxide levels, and acid-base balance (see Chapter 2 for more information an acid-base balance).

Chest Radiology

Chest x-rays are routinely taken to assess the shape, size, and location of the heart. Anterior-posterior films can be taken in a radiology department or at the bedside. Left lateral views may also be taken in radiology to provide more information about the heart. The x-rays provide information about cardiac and left-ventricular enlargement, pulmonary edema, and placement of catheters and endotracheal tubes.

Electrocardiograms

Electrocardiograms (EKG or ECG) are noninvasive tests that produce a graphic record of the electrical activity in the heart. The cardiac muscle contracts because of an electrical signal which travels along the conduction pathways of the heart. The electrical impulses stimulate the heart to contract. The electrical activity changes the polarity (negativity and positivity) of the cardiac muscle cells. The depolarization of the cells (ie, a wave of positive charge) occurs just prior to and during contraction. Then the cells repolarize (ie, cardiac cells return to their negative charge) to prepare for the next contraction. This change in polarity caused by the electrical stimulation can be captured and traced onto timed graph paper to provide a visual record of the heart's function and structure. Electrodes are skin sensors that are placed on the chest and extremities to capture electrical changes in the heart. They are connected to an EKG machine or telemetry unit where the graphic record is recorded. EKG can also be monitored by ambulatory units (Holter monitor) to assess patients with suspected cardiac dysrhythmias.

The cardiac rate, rhythm, and variations in the pattern can be read to reveal changes such as angina or myocardial infarction. A normal EKG (Figure 6-6) means that the heart has intact conduction pathways. A standard 12-lead EKG evaluates anterior, inferior, and lateral walls of the heart. Additional leads (eg, 15 or 18 lead EKG) may be necessary to evaluate the right ventricle and posterior wall. EKGs can also detect premature beats, blockages in the conduction system, myocardial ischemia, or electrolyte imbalances. Characteristic changes to the EKG occur during chest pain from angina and disappear when the pain subsides. Specific EKG changes in certain leads can identify the area and evolution of a myocardial infarction.

An EKG can be continuously displayed on a cardiac monitor so that the heart rate and rhythm can be continuously monitored and dysrhythmias can be quickly detected and treated. A printout of the EKG on special paper allows for more careful analysis of the heart's electrical activity. The paper is marked with squares allowing for rapid calculation of the heart rate and measuring the distances between landmarks on the waveform. Each tiny box on the EKG paper represents 0.04 seconds, and each large square represents 0.2 seconds. At the top of the EKG are vertical marks at every 3 seconds.

The tracings of an EKG indicate electrical changes within the myocardial cells. Electrical depolarization of the myocardial cells occurs immediately before contraction (systole). Repolarization of the myocardium occurs after contraction (diastole) as the intracellular environment regains its normal electrical charge. Myocardial cells must repolarize before they can effectively depolarize and contract again. The basic landmarks of an EKG are:

- P wave—indicates SA node function and atrial depolarization.
- P-R interval—indicates AV node conduction time (normal time 0.12 to 0.2 seconds).
- QRS complex—indicates ventricular depolarization (normal time 0.06 to 0.10 seconds).
- ST segment—indicates time between complete depolarization of the ventricles and complete repolarization.
- T wave—represents ventricular repolarization.

Figure 6-6. Normal EKG with labels (P, Q, R, S, T) for common features.

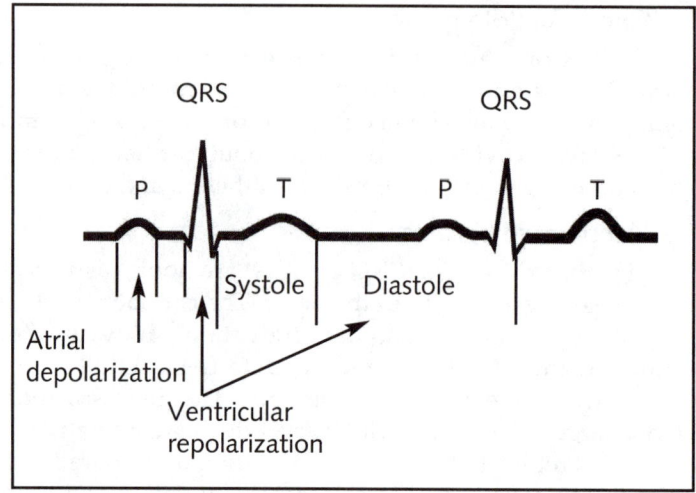

Figure 6-6. Normal EKG with labels (P, Q, R, S, T) for common features.

The Bibliography at the end of the chapter lists books on reading EKGs. Although it is beyond the scope of this book to describe all the different types of cardiac rhythms, all nurses should take a course on reading EKGs so they can better care for their patients.

Stress Tests

Stress tests or exercise EKGs are noninvasive tests used to evaluate cardiac function and perfusion with increasing levels of activity. They are useful in diagnosing ischemic heart disease. Electrodes are placed on the chest to monitor the heart rate and rhythm, and the blood pressure is monitored while the patient exercises on a treadmill or stationary cycle. If the patient develops chest pain, hypotension, or EKG changes, he or she may have coronary artery disease. A positive stress test indicates that more invasive tests may be needed. Stress tests also provide guidelines to safe activity levels for patients with known coronary artery disease.

Echocardiograms, Ultrasound, and Doppler Studies

Echocardiograms are used to assess left ventricular and valvular function. They can also visualize all four chambers of the heart, evaluate the motion of the left ventricular wall, and calculate the ejection fraction and left ventricular end diastolic pressures (LVEDP). An ultrasound transducer is moved along the skin of the thorax over the thoracic structures. A water-soluble gel is used to enhance transmission of the ultrasound waves. Transesophageal echocardiography involves placing a transducer into the esophagus to evaluate the wall motion of the cardiac chambers. It provides clearer images of the heart.

As previously described in the section on assessment of pulses, Doppler ultrasound can aid in diagnosing problems with blood flow in the heart and the extremities. Color Doppler studies are useful in evaluating blood flow in the heart, especially in cases of congenital anomalies or valvular regurgitation (backward flow). In the extremities, the test involves using a pressure cuff and ultrasound to detect the blood flow rates at different pressures.

Arteriograms

Arteriograms can be done with any of the arteries of the body, but they are commonly used in studying the aorta, cardiac valves, femoral arteries, and carotid arteries. (Coronary artery studies, a type of arteriogram, will be described in the next section on

Cardiac Catheterization.) An intravenous catheter is inserted into a large artery, a radiopaque dye is injected into the artery, and then x-ray pictures are taken. The blood vessel anatomy and valvular function are captured on film and help in diagnosing aortic aneurysm, valvular defects, and arterial blockages. Nursing care of patients undergoing arteriography includes:

1. Obtaining informed consent.

2. Assessing the patient's vital signs during the procedure and watching for reactions to the dye (dyspnea, numbness, or tingling).

3. Assessing the puncture site after the procedure for signs of bleeding and using sandbags for pressure as ordered.

4. Evaluating peripheral pulses distal to the perforation site to assess adequacy of circulation.

5. Ensuring adequate hydration to facilitate elimination of the dye and prevention of kidney damage from the dye.

Cardiac Catheterization

Cardiac catheterization is performed to evaluate the coronary arteries and valves. It is an invasive procedure, requiring admission to an outpatient or short-stay unit in an acute care setting. Admission to an acute care facility is necessary because emergent surgery may be required. The nursing care prior to cardiac catheterization includes:

1. Informed consent.

2. NPO (no oral intake of food) for 8 to 12 hours pretest.

3. Assess patient for allergies to dyes or iodine that may be used during the test.

4. Evaluate peripheral pulses prior to catheterization.

5. Record vital signs, height, and weight pretest.

6. Inform patient about fluttering feeling as catheter is inserted and to report dyspnea, itching, or numbness, which could signal an allergic reaction to the radiopaque dye.

A catheter is inserted and threaded up to the left or right side of the heart. If a right heart catheterization is being performed, the catheter is inserted into the antecubital vein and threaded into the superior vena cava and into the right heart. Right heart catheterization allows monitoring of pressures in the right atria, ventricles, and pulmonary arteries, and calculation of cardiac output. Continuous monitoring of circulatory pressures is useful in critically ill patients. Special hemodynamic catheters can be left in place after the catheterization to measure pressures and cardiac output in the intensive care setting.

If a left heart catheterization is being performed, a radiopaque catheter is inserted into the femoral or brachial artery and threaded into the aorta and left heart. The most common application of left heart catheterization is selective arteriography of the coronary arteries. This allows the evaluation of the patency of the coronary arteries and visualization of stenosis or blockage of the arteries. Other measurements that can be taken include the ejection fraction and pressures in the chambers and great vessels. Cardiac catheterization can be combined with interventions, such as balloon angioplasty or direct injection of thrombolytics (eg, streptokinase, t-PA) to reopen blocked coronary arteries.

Nursing care of patients after cardiac catheterization includes:

1. Maintaining bedrest (including straight leg for 8 hours) and activity levels per cardiologist; patients are at risk for bleeding at the arterial puncture site, and bedrest allows adequate clot formation at the puncture site.

2. Assessing site for bleeding and using sand bags for pressure on site as ordered (sandbags are used to prevent bleeding at the site).

3. Evaluating peripheral pulses (every 15 minutes for 1 hour, every 30 minutes for 1 hour, and every hour for 2 hours) distal to the puncture site to ensure adequate perfusion; patients are at risk for arterial occlusion at the puncture site, which could severely diminish blood flow to the periphery. Decreased blood flow would be demonstrated by decreased or absent peripheral pulses, cyanosis, or coolness of the extremities.

4. Continuing intravenous fluids (to aid in elimination of dye) and increasing diet per orders.

5. Evaluating adequacy of urinary output after the procedure.

Radionuclide Scans

Nuclear medicine studies can be performed to assess the perfusion of the heart muscle. Special dyes, such as Technetium 99m (^{99m}T) or Thallium-201 (^{201}Tl) are used to detect perfusion defects in the heart muscle and localize the area of infarction. Thallium may also be injected into the bloodstream prior to exercise (treadmill) to evaluate the effect of exercise on coronary perfusion. Cameras in the nuclear medicine department are designed to measure the radioactivity given off by the dye in the tissues. Defects are seen as areas with little or no uptake of the dye because the area is poorly perfused by the coronary arteries.

Radionuclide scans can be combined with other diagnostic tests to evaluate the perfusion of the heart by the coronary arteries, ventricular wall motion, and ejection fraction. They can be combined with arteriography to measure right- or left-sided ejection fractions. Multigated acquisition scanning (MUGA) combines the injection of technetium pertechnetate with scans to detect ventricular function, detect aneurysms, and evaluate coronary perfusion before and after exercise. Ejection fractions (EF) compares the amount of blood that fills a ventricle with the amount of blood ejected from the ventricle during systole. A normal ejection fraction for the left ventricle is 75% to 80%, meaning that when the ventricle fills with blood, it ejects 75% to 80% of that blood with each contraction. Radionuclide scans can also be combined with stress tests to evaluate blood flow in the coronary arteries during increasing levels of activity.

Hemodynamic Monitoring

Hemodynamic monitoring is useful in seriously ill patients when information is needed about central pressures. It provides direct measurement of pressures in the great vessels and the heart. This information can assess cardiac functioning and volume status.

A hemodynamic monitoring system requires a catheter, an infusion system, a transducer, and a monitor (Figure 6-7). To directly monitor central pressures, invasive lines must be inserted into the blood vessels and threaded toward the heart. A chest x-ray is needed to confirm the placement. The catheter is connected to a heparinized infusion system. The infusion system is delivered under pressure with a pressure bag to prevent back flow of blood into the catheter and possible occlusion of the catheter by thrombosis. The pressure in the catheter is relayed to a transducer that converts the mechanical pressure into electrical energy. The electrical energy is displayed as waveforms on a monitor. The transducer is calibrated according to the manufacturer's instructions and leveled to the patient's phlebostatic axis (Figure 6-8).

Hemodynamic monitoring provides information about the pressures of the heart and the systemic circulation. Different catheters are used to obtain specific information. Because of the risks involved, informed consent must be obtained from the patient or his family prior to the insertion of these catheters.

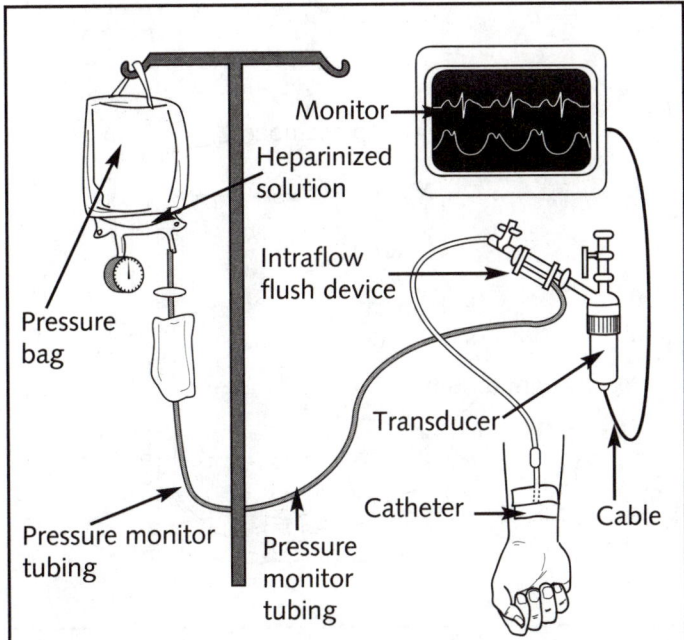

Figure 6-7. Components of hemodynamic monitoring system.

Figure 6-8. Phlebostatic axis.

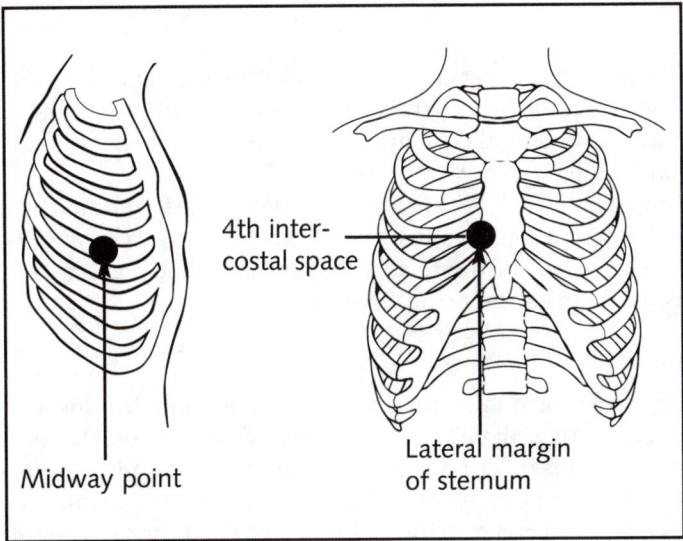

Arterial Lines

Intra-arterial monitoring directly measures arterial blood pressure. The physician inserts a catheter into the radial artery (see Figure 6-7) and connects it to a transducer that constantly reads the blood pressure onto the monitor. Directly measured blood pressures by intra-arterial monitoring are usually 10 to 15 mmHg higher than indirect measurements taken with a stethoscope and a sphygmomanometer. Intra-arterial catheters can also be used to obtain arterial blood gas samples and other blood tests. Assessment of the intravenous dressing over the puncture site in the radial artery must be done frequently because of the risk of bleeding.

Figure 6-9. CVP monitoring.

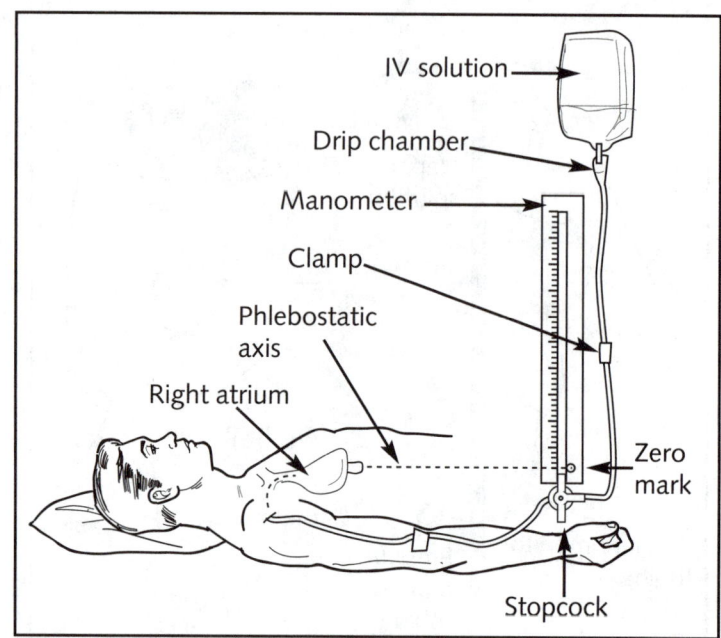

Central Venous Pressure

A pulmonary artery catheter or a central venous catheter monitors the central venous pressure (CVP). The physician inserts a catheter into the venous system and threads it into the right atrium. A chest x-ray checks placement. The intravenous infusion system is connected to a transducer and a monitor (Figures 6-9 and 6-10).

A normal CVP is 2 to 6 mmHg. A high CVP indicates right ventricular failure. Low CVPs may indicate hypovolemia. The intravenous site must be carefully observed and the dressing changed according to the protocol of the facility. Since the catheter is centrally placed, it can be a source of infection, thrombosis, and hemorrhage.

Pulmonary Artery Catheters

Pulmonary artery catheters are triple or quadruple lumen catheters that are inserted into a large vein, such as the internal jugular vein, by a physician (Figure 6-11). These catheters can read the right atrial pressures (CVP) directly and can indirectly measure the left atrial pressures. The catheter has three ports—one at the tip to measure pulmonary artery wedge pressure (PAWP), one in the right atrium to measure right atrial pressure, and one that can be used for cardiac output injectate. The right atrial pressure may be constantly observable on the monitor. Other calculations are done intermittently. The PAWP or "wedge" pressure approximates the left ventricular end diastolic pressure (LVEDP). It is measured by inflating a balloon at the end of the catheter and allowing it to float through the heart and into the pulmonary circulation until it occludes a branch of the pulmonary artery. The sensor then reads pressures in the left side of the heart.

Cardiac output (C/O) can also be obtained with the pulmonary artery catheter using the thermodilution technique. A known amount of D_5W at either cooled or room temperature is injected into the port. The thermistor on the catheter measures the mixing of D5W into the circulation. Cardiac output is calculated by machine and is useful in determining the functioning of the left ventricle. A normal C/O is 4 to 7 L per min. The normal homeostatic mechanisms adjust the cardiac output to respond to increased tissue demands for

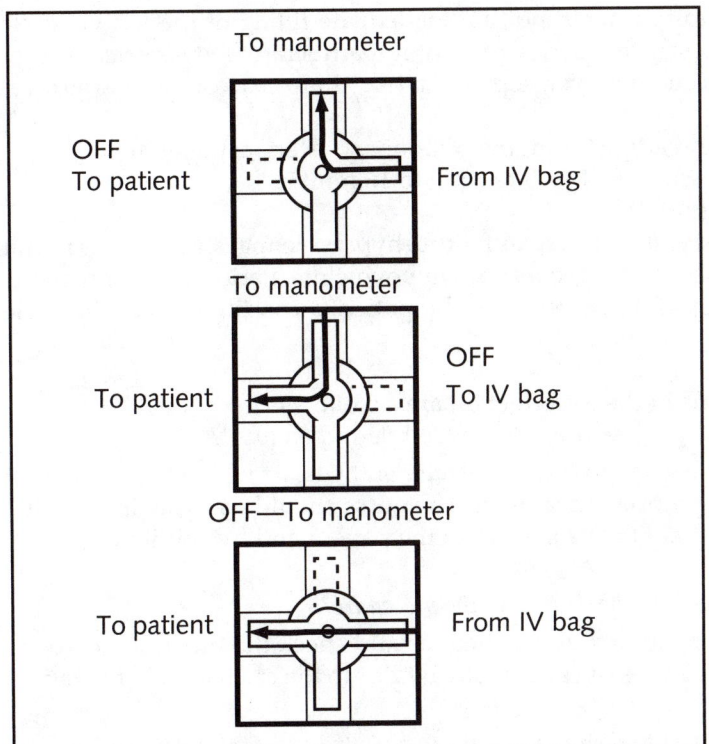

Figure 6-10. Stopcock to a water manometer for reading CVP.

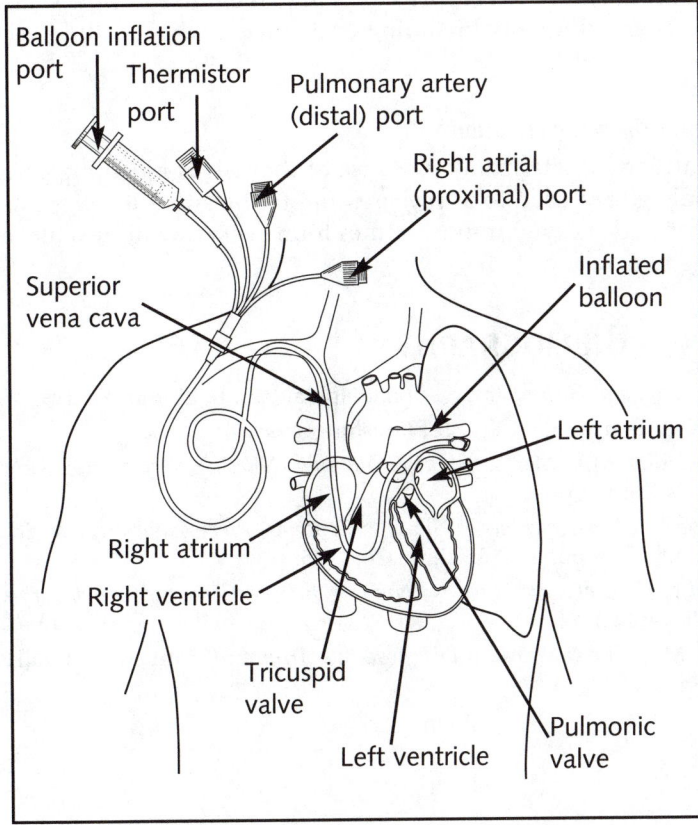

Figure 6-11. Pulmonary artery catheter for hemodynamic monitoring. The inflated balloon in a pulmonary artery indirectly reads pressure on the left side of the heart.

oxygen. Low resting cardiac output may indicate inadequate filling of the left ventricle because of valvular stenosis, restrictive pericarditis, or impairment of left ventricular contractility. High resting C/O occurs in fever, sepsis, anxiety, thyrotoxicosis, and arteriovenous fistula.

Normal values for different readings from the pulmonary artery catheter are:
- Pulmonary artery pressure (PAP): 20 to 30/5 to 16 mmHg
- PAWP: 6 to 12 mmHg

Elevated PAWP may indicate left ventricular failure, hypervolemia, shunting, or mitral valve regurgitation. A decreased PAWP occurs with hypovolemia. Periodic measurements of the PAWP allow the team to follow trends in the patient's condition and adjust the interventions appropriately.

The answers to the questions in the introduction are as follows:
- *How would you explain the purpose of the cardiac catheterization to Al?*

The cardiac catheterization is used to locate the area of the heart where the circulation is blocked and to direct the appropriate treatment. The nurse should use drawings or diagrams as necessary to help explain the procedure to the patient and his family.

- *What allergies would you ask Al about prior to the procedure?*

The nurse should ask the patient about his allergies and check the medical record for evidence of sensitivity to intravenous dyes or shellfish prior to the cardiac catheterization.

- *What feelings should Al report to the nurses in the Cath Lab during the procedure?*

During the cardiac catheterization, Al should report any pain to the nurse or physician. He should also tell them if he has any difficulty breathing or itchiness, which could indicate a sensitivity to the dye.

- *Why is bedrest important after the catheterization?*

Bedrest is important after cardiac catheterization because of the risk of bleeding from the catheter insertion site. Sandbags are used to apply pressure to the site. Vital signs as well as site assessment are performed every 15 minutes times four, every 30 minutes times two, and then every hour times two.

BIBLIOGRAPHY

Bates B. *A Guide to Physical Examination and History Taking.* Philadelphia, Pa: J.B. Lippincott; 1995.

Dubin D. *Rapid Interpretation of EKGs.* Tampa, Fla: COVER Publishing; 1994.

Ignatavius DD, Workman ML, Mishler MA. *Medical-Surgical Nursing: Nursing Process Approach.* Philadelphia, Pa: W.B. Saunders Co; 1995.

Kozier B, Erb G, Blais K, Wilkinson JM. *Fundamentals of Nursing: Concepts, Process and Practice.* 5th ed. Reading, Mass: The Benjamin/Cummings Publishing Co; 1995.

Swearingen PL, Keen JH. *Manual of Critical Care Nursing: Nursing Interventions and Collaborative Management.* St. Louis, Mo: Mosby Inc; 2001.

Tierney LM, McPhee SJ, Papadkis MA. *Current Medical Diagnosis and Treatment.* 34th ed. Norwalk, Conn: Appleton & Lange; 1995.

Multiple-Choice Questions

1. During the first heart sound, S1 or "Lub," what valves are closing?
   A. Aortic and pulmonic
   B. Tricuspid and mitral
   C. Aortic and mitral
   D. Mitral and pulmonic

2. All of the following are true about S3 except:
   A. It sounds like "Kentucky" with the other heart sounds
   B. It falls after S2
   C. It is called a ventricular gallop
   D. S3 may indicate congestive heart failure

3. Nursing care prior to cardiac catheterization includes all of the following except:
   A. Assess for allergies to dyes or iodine
   B. Evaluation of peripheral pulses
   C. Informed consent
   D. Clear liquids prior to the test

4. A normal central venous pressure (CVP) is:
   A. 15 to 26 mmHg
   B. 6 to 10 cmHg
   C. 2 to 6 mmHg
   D. 25 to 35 mmHg

5. Pulmonary artery wedge pressures (PAWP) are used to measure:
   A. Right ventricular pressures
   B. Central venous pressure
   C. Left ventricular end diastolic pressure
   D. Systemic blood pressure

CHAPTER 6 ANSWERS

1. B
2. A
3. D
4. C
5. C

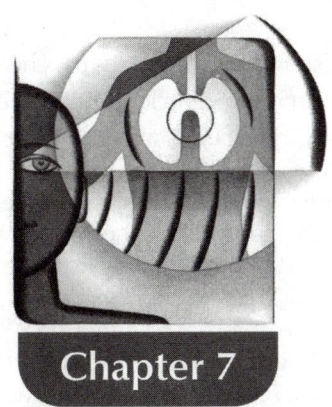

Chapter 7

Disorders of the Cardiovascular System

At the hospital, Al's chest pain (from Chapter 6) is somewhat relieved by nitroglycerine, but his EKG continues to show ST elevations. An emergent cardiac catheterization shows an 80% stenosis of the left anterior descending artery, and angioplasty is performed with stent placement. Al's pain subsides quickly after reperfusion, and he returns home 2 days later after his isoenzymes and EKGs continue to be negative. His discharge medications include propanolol and sublingual nitroglycerine. Al returns to the office for a follow-up 1 week later.

Mrs. B comes to the emergency room complaining of nausea and burning in her chest. She woke up this morning and "didn't feel well." She tried an antacid, but it did not provide any relief from the burning. Mrs. B's husband drove her here this morning because she looked "bad." Mrs. B is 68-years-old and has a history of obesity, hypertension, and diabetes. Today her blood pressure is 168/94 and her apical pulse is 120 beats per minute. Her respiratory rate is 30 breaths per minute with an O_2 Sat of 93%. She appears pale and diaphoretic. Per hospital protocol, you administer oxygen via nasal cannula at 4 L per minute. You connect her to the cardiac monitor and assess the cardiac rhythm. Her heart rhythm is sinus tachycardia with 6 to 8 premature ventricular contractions (PVCs) per minute.

- What are the risk factors for coronary artery disease?
- Why does Al's pain subside after stent placement?
- How does propanolol help patients with coronary artery disease?
- What teaching will you do regarding the use of sublingual nitroglycerine?
- Which risk factors are modifiable, and how will you incorporate teaching about these to Al now that he has been diagnosed with coronary artery disease?
- What risk factors does Mrs. B have for coronary artery disease?
- What medications may be used immediately when Mrs. B arrives in the emergency department?

- Why is oxygen administered to patients with chest pain?
- What is causing the premature ventricular contractions?

The functioning of the cardiovascular system is important to the process of oxygenation because this system allows perfusion of the tissues. Without the delivery system of blood vessels and a pumping heart, the process of breathing would be useless. Inhaled oxygen would never reach the cells. The respiratory and cardiovascular systems work together to bring oxygen into the body, deliver it to the cells, and remove carbon dioxide and metabolic waste products. This chapter will discuss disorders of the cardiovascular system as they pertain to the process of oxygenation.

There are many different diagnoses for disorders of the cardiovascular system, but not all of them are appropriately covered in a book that focuses on oxygenation. This chapter will focus on selected cardiovascular disorders that impact the delivery of oxygen to the cells. Atherosclerosis, coronary artery disease, heart failure, peripheral arterial disease, and cardiogenic shock will be covered in this chapter. The nursing diagnoses that focus on maintaining oxygenation will be discussed as they pertain to the particular disorders. Cardiovascular disorders require collaborative interventions by different members of the health care team to facilitate recovery from acute conditions, to minimize complications for patients with chronic conditions, and to maximize the patient's functional abilities.

ATHEROSCLEROSIS

Any discussion of diseases that affect the perfusion of the tissues must start with a discussion of *atherosclerosis*. It is the most common cause of arterial obstruction and can lead to peripheral arterial disease, coronary artery disease, and cerebrovascular accidents (CVA). *Arteriosclerosis* is a general term to describe a number of disorders in which the arterial walls thicken and lose elasticity. Where arteriosclerosis is a generalized disorder, atherosclerosis refers to the thickening of large and medium-size arteries with the deposition of fatty streaks or plaques that decrease the lumen of the artery (Figure 7-1). Atherosclerosis occurs because of:

- Accumulation of lipids in the connective tissue.
- Overgrowth of smooth muscle and accumulation of macrophages and T-cells.
- Formation of a matrix of connective tissue within the intima of the vessel.

Atherosclerosis is usually a silent disorder until the blood flow is so diminished that it cannot keep pace with the tissue's oxygen needs. When the lumen of an artery is obstructed to the point where blood flow is inadequate to meet the tissue demands, tissue hypoxia and ischemia develop distal to the blockage. Without sufficient oxygen, the tissue switches from aerobic to anaerobic metabolism. Lactic acid and other caustic waste products result from anaerobic metabolism, causing tissue irritation and pain. Tissue death or necrosis occurs when an artery becomes so blocked by plaques, thrombosis, or embolism that the cells can no longer survive even with anaerobic metabolism.

The etiology of atherosclerotic changes is unknown but many theories exist. One theory is that the intimal (inner) wall of an artery is damaged and platelets cluster or aggregate over the injury (the so-called platelet aggregation theory). The platelets stimulate proliferation of smooth muscle in the vessel wall, blocking the lumen of the artery. Another theory hypothesizes that lipids deposit over the injury on the intimal wall of the arteries and a fibrous plaque forms over this fatty core (the chronic endothelial injury theory.) The process of fatty deposition and plaque formation seems to be enhanced by other factors, such as genetic predetermination, diseases like diabetes and hypertension, and lifestyle habits like high fat intake and smoking. Over years, the disease progresses, block-

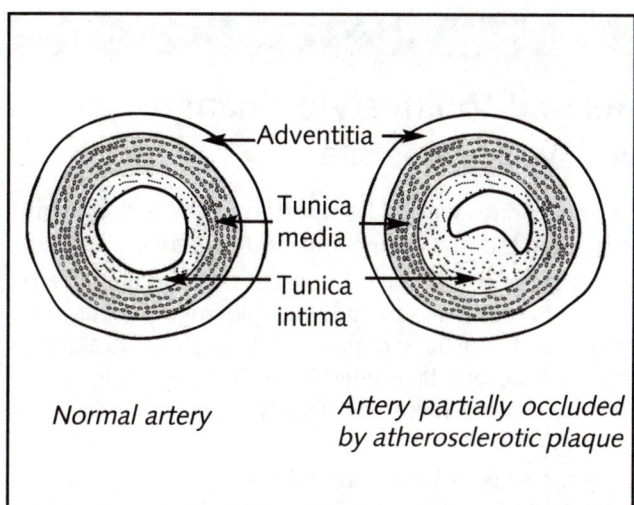

Figure 7-1. Atherosclerotic plaque narrowing the artery.

Adventitia

Tunica media

Tunica intima

Normal artery

Artery partially occluded by atherosclerotic plaque

ing the arteries and depriving distal tissues of oxygenated blood. Arteries to the heart may become blocked, causing angina and myocardial infarction. Arteries in the legs may become narrowed, and nonhealing ulcers or gangrene may develop on the feet and toes. Infection in the gangrenous tissue may become life-threatening, requiring amputation of the limb. Plaque in the carotid arteries can break off and block cerebral arteries, causing transient ischemic attacks or cerebrovascular accidents (CVAs or strokes.) The ramifications of atherosclerosis are astounding in terms of loss of productivity and quality of life.

Some factors which contribute to the atherosclerotic process are modifiable and can alter the disease course. Atherosclerosis is a silent disease until years of damage to the vessels have been done. There appears to be a genetic component to dyslipidemia. Two genetic predispositions to hyperlipidemia are e-4 allele and the pattern B form of high low-density lipoprotein (LDL) levels.

To screen for congenital dyslipidemia, total serum cholesterol should be performed on all people over the age of 20. The total serum cholesterol should be less than 200 mg/dL (milligrams per deciliter). Total cholesterol above 200 mg/dL is referred to as hyperlipidemia. If the total cholesterol is elevated, two components of the total cholesterol, high-density lipoproteins (HDL) and LDL components, are measured. HDLs are often referred to as the "good cholesterol" because elevations of this component are associated with lower risk for atherosclerosis. LDLs are sometimes referred to as the "bad cholesterol" because elevations have been linked to a higher risk for atherosclerosis and cardiovascular disorders. Detection of hyperlipidemia in early adulthood can allow time for lifestyle changes, dietary modifications, and sometimes medication before damage is done.

Triglycerides, other fatty substances in the blood, are measured separately from cholesterol levels. Hypertriglyceridemia is an elevation of the triglycerides level above 150 mg/dL and is also a risk factor for developing atherosclerosis. Hypertriglyceridemia is thought to be a congenital disorder, and its impact on the development of atherosclerosis is being studied. Triglycerides may also be elevated with excessive alcohol consumption.

One of the most common nursing diagnoses in patients with or at risk for atherosclerosis is Knowledge Deficit related to lifestyle changes to improve hyperlipidemia (Table 7-1).

Atherosclerosis and arteriosclerosis can lead to high blood pressure or hypertension. The diminished elasticity of the arteries and the thickening caused by plaque formation

Table 7-1

Knowledge Deficit Related to Lifestyle Changes to Improve Hyperlipidemia

- **Reduce weight.** Maintaining the appropriate weight is important for reducing lipids. Being overweight is a risk factor for high blood pressure and cardiovascular disorders.

- **Modify diet.** Decreasing total fat intake and especially saturated fats and cholesterol can lower LDLs, particularly in patients with congenital hyperlipidemia. If LDLs are between 130 to 159, a fat-modified diet is usually prescribed. If LDLs are greater than 160, both saturated fat and cholesterol intake need to be reduced. The American Heart Association recommends the following dietary proportions to decrease fat intake and serum cholesterol.

  Step 1: Diet—reduce total daily fat intake to less than 30% of total daily caloric intake, saturated fat intake to less than 10%, and total cholesterol to less than 300 mg/day.

  Step 2: Diet (if LDLs remain elevated after Step 1 diet)—reduce saturated fat intake to less than 7% and total cholesterol to less than 200 mg/day.

- **Exercise.** Moderate exercise (30 minutes a day, three to five times a week) appears to promote optimal lipid levels and decrease the risk of cardiovascular disease. Exercise may also promote collateral circulation and plaque regression. A stress test may be prescribed before starting an exercise program.

- **Stop smoking.** Smoking increases the risks for peripheral arterial disease, hypertension, low HDL levels (the "good cholesterol"), and cardiovascular disease. Even a half a pack of cigarettes a day can significantly increase the chances of a person dying from heart disease. Encourage all patients to quit smoking and especially those with hyperlipidemia (see page 72 for strategies for smoking cessation).

- **Control hypertension.** Take blood pressure medication regularly, get follow-up blood pressure measurements as prescribed.

- **Take cholesterol-lowering medications regularly** (if prescribed after dietary interventions alone are not working) to decrease total lipids. Types of medications include:
  - Bile-acid sequestrants (cholestyramine)
  - Nicotinic acid (niacin)
  - Fibric acid (gemfibrozil)
  - HMG-CoA reductase inhibitors (Lovastatin)

- **Control diabetes.** Follow prescribed dietary and medical treatment for diabetes if this is also a problem. Consultation with a dietician or diabetic teaching nurse may help the patient understand the disease and facilitate better control of blood sugar.

and smooth muscle proliferation can make the vessels less responsive to changes in blood pressure. Conversely, hypertension can cause arteriosclerotic changes in the vessel walls.

Hypertension does not directly decrease oxygen supply to the tissues, but it is a risk factor for the development of arteriosclerosis. Controlling hypertension is an essential component of preventing arteriosclerotic changes to the blood vessels. However, because hypertension does not directly affect oxygenation, it will not be reviewed in this book.

CORONARY ARTERY DISEASE

Changes to the coronary arteries brought on by atherosclerosis can result in diminished blood flow to the myocardium. If the heart muscle does not receive an adequate blood supply with the necessary oxygen and nutrients, ischemia can result. Patients with myocardial ischemia often have chest pain or angina. If the ischemia is prolonged, tissue death occurs and the patient has a myocardial infarction (MI or heart attack).

Atherosclerotic changes in the coronary arteries develop silently until the lumen of the artery is blocked more than 70%. Then, the decrease in blood flow to the myocardial tissue becomes more evident when the patient exercises or increases his activity level, thus increasing the myocardial oxygen demands. The narrowed or obstructed coronary artery cannot supply enough blood to meet the myocardial demands, and the result is ischemia. The patient experiences chest pain or tightness that usually subsides once the activity level decreases and the demand for oxygen subsides.

When the myocardium is ischemic, the patient feels chest pain or angina. The Latin phrase *angina pectoris* means "strangling of the chest." Patients may describe their pain differently. Some common descriptions are tightness, burning, boring, or aching. Angina is classified into two groups:

- "Stable" angina—chest pain that occurs with exercise and disappears with rest.
- "Unstable" angina—chest pain at rest or with minimal exertion.

Angina is a clinical diagnosis based on a history of chest pain brought on by exertion and relieved by rest. Chest pain relieved by nitroglycerine is also characteristic of angina. Exercise stress tests and radionuclide scans may be performed to establish the diagnosis. EKG findings may occur during an episode of angina and disappear after the attack. Coronary arteriography may be used to examine the extent of the coronary artery disease and determine whether other interventions are necessary.

Patients with angina are at risk for unstable angina, myocardial infarction, and sudden death. Treatment involves modifying the risk factors, treating underlying coronary artery disease, if appropriate, and preventing and relieving the symptoms. Risk factors such as hyperlipidemia, excess weight, smoking, stress, and dietary fat intake are all modifiable. Patients are taught how to change their lifestyle to reduce these risk factors. Medical treatment includes long- and short-acting nitrates and beta-blockers. Patients are taught to carry sublingual nitroglycerine with them at all times. Antiplatelet drugs like aspirin are used to decrease platelet aggregation either in the full-strength tablet (325 mg) or the "baby aspirin" dose (80 mg) once a day. Nonpharmacologic treatment is directed at weight and stress reduction. Some ways to reduce stress include lifestyle modification, massage, yoga, and meditation.

The New York Heart Association has classified heart disease depending on the amount of dysfunction:

Class 1: Patient with heart disease without limitations in physical activity. Ordinary activity does not cause any symptoms.

Class 2: Patient with heart disease with slight physical limitations. Ordinary activity results in dyspnea, fatigue, palpitations, or anginal pain. Patient is comfortable at rest.

Class 3: Patient with heart disease with marked limitation of physical activity. Less than ordinary activity causes symptoms. Patient is comfortable at rest.

Class 4: Patient with heart disease not able to carry on any activity without discomfort. Symptoms of anginal syndrome or cardiac insufficiency may be present even at rest.

Unstable angina is treated more aggressively because of the increased risk of myocardial infarction and sudden death. Aspirin and heparin may be used to prevent MI.

Coronary artery bypass surgery (CABG) may provide excellent relief if the patient has localized disease and is a good candidate for surgery. CABG surgery is discussed later in this chapter.

Myocardial ischemia can progress to a myocardial infarction if a coronary artery is narrowed or occluded for too long. This may happen if a plaque ruptures, blocking a coronary artery, if platelets clump or aggregate on irregular surface (like an atherosclerotic plaque) inside the artery, or if a thrombus develops and occludes the artery. If a coronary artery is 80% to 90% occluded, then ischemia develops in the myocardium distal to the blockage. If the ischemia continues and the blood flow is not returned, then tissue necrosis or death occurs. This is called a myocardial infarction.

A myocardial infarction develops over several hours and quick treatment may limit the extent of tissue death. Early treatment is essential to improving the survival of patients with MIs. Ventricular dysrhythmias are common early in the course of a MI and can lead to cardiac arrest. The most common cause of death prior to hospitalization is cardiac arrest. Patients with chest pain should be brought into the health care system as soon as possible so that life-threatening dysrhythmias can be detected and treated quickly, and myocardial oxygenation can be improved. Early supportive treatment can increase the likelihood of survival for patients experiencing a MI.

MIs begin with necrosis of the subendocardial layer of the heart and can progress to other layers of the myocardium. If the infarction spreads to all three layers of the heart, this is called a *transmural* ("through the wall") MI. Transmural MIs can affect ventricular wall motion and cardiac output. Left ventricular wall damage can result in heart failure and cardiogenic shock. Around the actual zone of necrosis is a zone of injury and further

> Nitroglycerine is light-sensitive. It should be stored in a tinted container in the refrigerator and replaced every 3 to 5 months.

out, a zone of ischemia (Figure 7-2). Prompt treatment may provide oxygen to the outer two zones of an infarction and reduce the extent of myocardial necrosis.

Depending on the location and extent of the tissue death, the conduction system of the heart may be damaged, the cardiac output diminished, or the heart may stop beating. The type of response to an MI depends on which arteries are occluded (Figure 7-3). The three most common coronary arteries that are obstructed are:

- **Left anterior descending (LAD) artery**—usually produces anterior and septal MIs because this is the area that it perfuses. Anterior wall MIs account for 25% of all infarctions and have the highest mortality rate. The left ventricular wall is frequently damaged in anterior MIs, resulting in ventricular failure and dysrhythmias.
- **Circumflex artery**—also supplies part of the left ventricular wall and portions of the conduction system.
- **Right coronary artery (RCA)**—perfuses the SA and AV nodes, and obstructions of this artery produce bradycardias and heart blocks. Blockage of the RCA usually causes an inferior MI.

Assessment of the patient with chest pain who may be having an MI is divided into two parts. One is the immediate assessment of the presenting pain. The second part, the family history and risk factors, is done when the patient is more comfortable.

Rapid assessment is necessary when a patient has chest pain. The nurse should quickly but completely assess the nature of the discomfort. This often is done in collaboration with the physician.

- Type of pain should be described (ie, burning, aching, stabbing, pressure, or tightness).

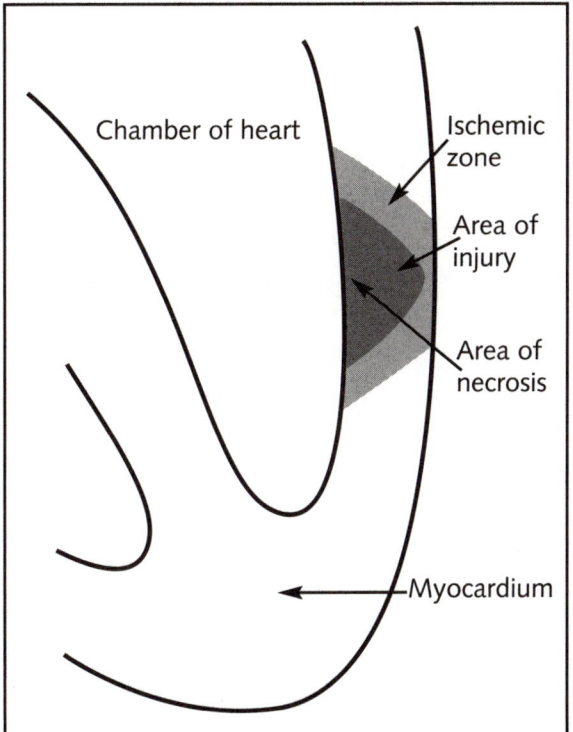

Figure 7-2. Zones of myocardial infarction.

Chamber of heart

Ischemic zone

Area of injury

Area of necrosis

Myocardium

- Location of the pain (eg, chest, left shoulder, left arm, or jaw should be noted). Radiation of the pain to the jaw, shoulder, and back is more common in MI than in angina.
- Intensity of the patient's pain should be graded on a scale of 1 to 10.
- Pain duration—pain from a myocardial infarction usually lasts more than 30 minutes and is relieved only by opioids. Chest pain from angina is usually relieved by nitroglycerine and rest.
- Relieving factors—how the patient has tried to relieve the pain and what has worked (eg, nitroglycerine under the tongue will relieve anginal pain but not MI pain). Rest may relieve anginal pain but not MI pain.
- Precipitating factors—what makes the pain come on or become more intense. Anginal pain may be brought on by exertion or stress. MI pain may occur without cause and commonly starts early in the morning.

Patients with chest pain may have additional symptoms such as nausea, vomiting, diaphoresis, dizziness, palpitations, shortness of breath, and headache. Note any additional symptoms that are not necessarily classic chest pain. It is important to remember that women may experience chest pain and describe it differently from men. Women more often report other symptoms that are more general, resulting in overlooked cardiac problems. Careful screening questions and an open mind are important in accurately assessing all patients with chest pain.

Physical assessment should proceed quickly and perhaps during questioning:

1. Vital signs—blood pressure, heart rate, respiratory rate, temperature, and oxygen saturation. In patients with an MI, decreased cardiac output may be manifested by hypotension, tachycardia, diaphoresis, diminished peripheral pulses bilaterally, and

Figure 7-3. Coronary arteries.

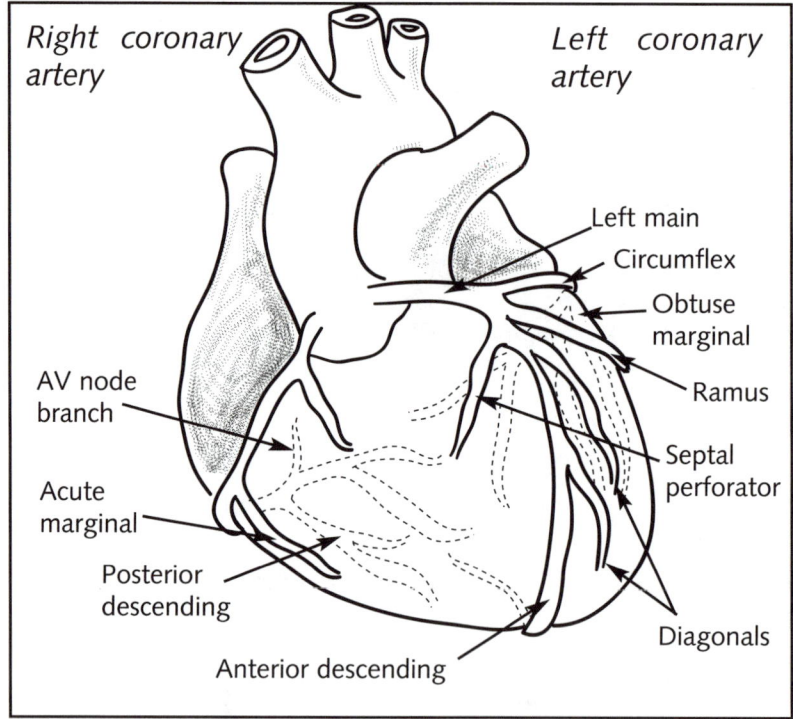

Right coronary artery

Left coronary artery

Left main

Circumflex

Obtuse marginal

Ramus

Septal perforator

AV node branch

Acute marginal

Posterior descending

Diagonals

Anterior descending

cool skin. Temperature may be elevated to as high as 102°F (38.9°C) for several days after an MI.

2. Cardiac monitor and 12-lead EKG—the patient should be connected to a cardiac monitor to assess for dysrhythmias. Sinus tachycardia with frequent premature beats occurs early in the course of an MI due to ischemia. A 12-lead EKG provides further information about the location of ischemia and necrosis. Changes in the S-T segment, T and Q waves may be seen on the EKG during an MI. (Indepth analysis of EKGs is beyond the scope of this book. See Chapter 6 Bibliography.

3. Vascular access—the patient should have an IV placed as soon as possible for intravenous medications and fluids.

The diagnosis of myocardial infarction is based on symptoms, history, EKG changes, and cardiac isoenzyme elevations. MIs are usually caused by blockage of a coronary artery by a plaque or thrombus, but they can also be caused by vasospasm of a coronary artery, prolonged hypotension, and excessive metabolic demands. MIs are often divided into Q wave and non-Q wave infarctions. The Q wave is seen on the EKG and its presence is associated with prolonged myocardial ischemia and necrosis. Non-Q wave MIs are associated with early reperfusion of the ischemic myocardium and better outcomes.

Diagnostic tests for MI include laboratory blood work, exercise stress test, thallium scan, and cardiac catheterization. Cardiac enzymes are useful laboratory blood tests that can confirm that an MI has occurred. Creatine kinase (CK) is a cardiac enzyme that rises within 3 hours of an MI, peaks in 24 hours, and returns to normal in 48 to 72 hours. CK is released when muscle tissue has been damaged. A specific component of CK, the CK-MB isoenzyme, is released into the bloodstream when the cardiac muscle is damaged. CK-MB levels are elevated for 24 hours after an MI. Lactic dehydrogenase (LDH) also rises after an MI and remains elevated for a week after the MI. A complete blood count is also done to rule out other disorders like anemia. White blood cells may be elevated (up to 1500/mL) on days 2 to 7 after an MI. Troponin is a newer serum indicator of myocardial damage. Troponin I and T may rise earlier than the CK and remain elevated longer than CK-MB, allowing for diagnosis of MI after the initial 24 hour peak of CK-MB.

Exercise stress tests may be done after the acute stage of an MI to assess the extent of ischemia and necrosis, and to determine the need for more invasive therapies like cardiac catheterization, angioplasty, or bypass surgery. Thallium scans are also useful in imaging the areas of ischemia and necrosis. Thallium is injected intravenously and is "picked up" by the perfused myocardium. Areas of decreased perfusion in the heart pick up less thallium and are imaged as "cold spots" on the scan.

Cardiac catheterization (as described in Chapter 6) is used to visualize the coronary arteries and locate occlusions. Not only does cardiac catheterization provide visualization of the coronary arteries, it can also be a route for invasive interventions like angioplasty, stent placement, and laser removal of obstructions. These interventions and coronary artery bypass surgery will be discussed starting on page 200.

Treatment of angina and MI begins in a similar manner while the presence of a MI is being evaluated. The goals of treatment are:

- Relieve pain.
- Increase myocardial oxygen supply.
- Decrease myocardial oxygen demand.
- Minimize damage to myocardium.

Pain relief is an essential part of early treatment. The experience of pain results in a catecholamine release that increases the heart rate, blood pressure, and myocardial oxygen demand. The first treatment for chest pain whether from angina or infarction is nitroglycerine (under the tongue) 0.3 to 0.4 mg sublingually. Intravenously, nitroglycerine is a potent vasodilator and can rapidly decrease the blood pressure. It may also be given topically in an ointment for longer-acting relief than sublingually. Nitroglycerine vasodilates the coronary arteries and increases collateral blood flow. If the pain is from ischemia (anginal pain), sublingual nitroglycerine will bring prompt relief. If the pain is not relieved and the systolic blood pressure remains above 100 mmHg, then the sublingual dose may be repeated every 5 minutes for a total of three doses. Side effects of nitroglycerine include rapid onset of hypotension and headache. Patients should be instructed to lie down before taking nitroglycerine. For many patients with angina, sublingual nitroglycerine and cessation of activity bring rapid relief of their chest pain.

If three doses of nitroglycerine do not relieve the pain or if the pain is very severe, then intravenous morphine is given to decrease the pain and diminish the myocardial oxygen demand. Side effects of morphine include respiratory depression, hypotension, and vomiting. Morphine is given intravenously because it provides prompt relief, can be titrated to achieve adequate pain control, and it does not damage muscle tissue as an intramuscular injection. Remember that damaged muscle tissue releases creatine kinase (CK), one of the diagnostic measures for determining the occurrence of an MI.

Nursing interventions for the patient experiencing chest pain can be focused around the nursing diagnosis: pain related to myocardial ischemia (Table 7-2).

Increasing available oxygen improves the chances for recovery of ischemic and injured myocardium. Oxygen via nasal cannula is often administered at 2 to 4 L per min. If the patient is also in respiratory distress as evidenced by a rapid respiratory rate, low PaO_2, or O_2 Sat, then he may require intubation and mechanical ventilation to maintain adequate oxygen levels. The semi-Fowler's position is often the most comfortable for a patient with chest pain.

Table 7-2

Pain Related to Myocardial Ischemia

1. Assess signs and symptoms of chest pain. Include location, severity, radiation, onset, precipitating factors, relieving factors, and associated symptoms.
2. Relieve pain with collaborative interventions (nitroglycerine, morphine) and non-pharmacologic methods such as massage, deep breathing, and a calming atmosphere.
3. Provide supplemental oxygen at 4 to 6 L per min (if not contraindicated) to improve myocardial oxygenation.
4. Place the patient in the semi-Fowler's or high-Fowler's position to promote comfort and breathing.
5. Decrease myocardial oxygen demands by promoting rest, controlling pain, and talking with the patient and his family in a calm and reassuring manner.

Decreasing oxygen demands is accomplished through pain relief, rest, and reassurance. Pain and anxiety, as previously discussed, increase catecholamine release. The nurse should provide a calm atmosphere and reassuring manner to help relieve some of the patient's anxiety. Interventions should be explained to the patient. Try to stay with the patient and incorporate a family member in discussions about the patient's care.

Patients with myocardial infarctions are admitted to intensive care or the coronary care unit. Their care includes close cardiac monitoring, rest, analgesia, oxygen therapy, and treatment of dysrhythmias and heart failure. Medications are often used when caring for patients with myocardial infarction to decrease the myocardial oxygen demands, increase the cardiac output, and improve oxygenation of the myocardial tissue. Commonly used medications include the following:

*   Nitrates like sublingual and intravenous nitroglycerine can vasodilate coronary and other arteries. Side effects include hypotension and headache.
*   Isosorbide dinitrate promotes vasodilation. Side effects include hypotension and dizziness.
*   Beta-blockers like atenolol decrease heart rate, blood pressure, and cardiac output. The decreased heart rate allows for a longer period of diastole, which is when the heart perfuses itself. Side effects include bradycardia and bronchoconstriction. *Note*: Beta-blockers may contribute to the development of heart failure.
*   Aspirin and other antiplatelet agents decrease inflammatory response and prevent platelet aggregation. Side effects include gastric irritation and tinnitus (at high doses). Newer agents include platelet IIb and IIIa receptor blockers (sometimes called "super aspirin").
*   Angiotensin converting enzyme (ACE) inhibitors like enalapril are used to decrease the work of the heart by decreasing systemic blood pressure, and therefore afterload. They also affect ventricular remodeling after MI. Side effects include hypotension, cough, and edema. They are used in patients with left ventricular dysfunction but may not be indicated in routine postinfarction care.

- Sympathomimetics like dobutamine and dopamine increase blood pressure in heart failure if the patient is hypotensive but not in shock. Side effects include dysrhythmias, increased heart rate, and blood pressure. Sympathomimetics must be titrated in an intensive care setting with hemodynamic monitoring.

More invasive strategies may be used to treat myocardial infarction depending on the symptoms, EKG findings, catheterization results, or other diagnostic test findings. The goal is to promote perfusion of the ischemic tissue. Interventions include the administration of thrombolytic agents, percutaneous transluminal angioplasty (PTCA), stent placement, laser treatment of lesions in the coronary arteries, and coronary artery bypass surgery.

Thrombolytic Agents

Thrombolytic agents are used to dissolve thrombi that are occluding coronary arteries. Since myocardial infarctions evolve over a period of hours, there is often a window of opportunity to open the artery and reperfuse ischemic myocardium. Thrombolytic agents are most effective if given within 6 hours of the coronary event. These agents are administered intravenously or via a coronary route during cardiac catheterization. Some examples are streptokinase, tissue plasminogen activator (tPA), and anisoylated plasminogen-streptokinase activator complex (APSAC).

Nursing care for the patient receiving thrombolytic therapy entails understanding the nature of these medications. Thrombolytics affect the clotting mechanism of the blood all over the body. Clots form when platelets and fibrin threads create a mesh that captures red blood cells. Thrombolytics facilitate the breakdown of clots by accelerating the conversion of plasminogen to plasmin, a clot dissolver (Figure 7-4). Streptokinase in particular is not fibrin specific and can cause systemic bleeding problems. Because of this risk, patients with known bleeding in the gastrointestinal or cerebrovascular system are not candidates for this treatment.

Nursing interventions for patients receiving thrombolytic therapy include:

1. Assessing indications of reperfusion after injection of thrombolytic agent (ie, relief of chest pain, reversal of EKG changes, and sudden onset of ventricular ectopy, sometimes referred to as reperfusion dysrhythmias).

2. Observing for signs of hypersensitivity to the thrombolytic agent (eg, itching, hives). Premedication with steroids and antihistamines is often done, particularly before treatment with streptokinase.

3. Assessing for signs of bleeding that include neurological changes, abdominal pain, changes in color of urine and stool, changes in hemoglobin, and hematocrit values from pretreatment values.

4. Frequent assessment of blood pressure and heart rate during and after injection of the thrombolytic agent and comparison to pretreatment values.

After reperfusion, the physician usually prescribes heparin and intravenous nitroglycerine for several days to maintain the patency of the reopened coronary artery. Long-term therapy includes daily aspirin to decrease the incidence of platelet aggregation.

Cardiac Catheterization

Cardiac catheterization is frequently performed after the acute phase of angina or myocardial infarction has resolved. Using injected dye, the coronary arteries and their blockages or lesions can be visualized. If patients are shown to have a treatable lesion in a coronary artery, percutaneous transluminal angioplasty (PTCA) can be performed. The best candidates for PTCA have one or two vessel disease with proximal, noncalcified

Figure 7-4. Thrombolytic therapy.

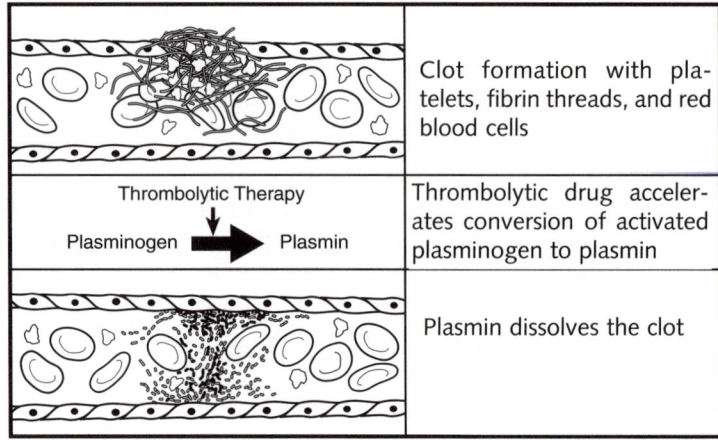

	Clot formation with platelets, fibrin threads, and red blood cells
Thrombolytic Therapy Plasminogen ➡ Plasmin	Thrombolytic drug accelerates conversion of activated plasminogen to plasmin
	Plasmin dissolves the clot

lesions. PTCA involves catheterization of the left side of the heart from the femoral artery and fluoroscopic insertion of a balloon-tipped catheter to the area of the lesion (Figure 7-5). The balloon is then inflated to compress the plaque against the vessel wall. Balloon inflation may be repeated to maintain the patency of the artery. A stent may be placed to maintain the opening by providing stiffer scaffolding in the newly opened artery (Figure 7-6). Laser angioplasty and arthrectomy may also be used to remove atherosclerotic plaque in the artery during cardiac catheterization.

Coronary Artery Bypass Grafting

Invasive surgery may be needed to perfuse the myocardium. Coronary artery bypass graft surgery (CABG) can bypass occluded vessels and provide blood flow to the myocardium. CABG may be needed when patients do not respond to medical management or when the symptoms or diagnostic tests show disease progression. Indications for coronary artery bypassing include:
- Unstable angina with severe two or three vessel disease.
- Left main coronary artery disease with angina.
- Acute myocardial infarction.
- Signs of impending MI after PTCA.
- Ischemia with heart failure.

Bypass surgery involves grafting a piece of blood vessel (the saphenous vein or internal mammary artery are common donor vessels) from the aorta to an area distal to the occlusion in the coronary artery (Figure 7-6). CABG surgery may be done on an immediate basis if the patient's condition warrants it or it may be scheduled after the acute phase of a myocardial infarction and the occlusions have been visualized during cardiac catheterization. Several vessels may be bypassed during the surgery.

CABG is accomplished by splitting the sternum (medial sternotomy) and opening the thoracic cage to reveal the heart. The surgery may be performed with the patient on cardiopulmonary bypass (extracorporeal circulation) or with the heart beating (so-called "beating-heart surgery"). If cardiopulmonary bypass is used, then the heart is stopped with a cold cardioplegia solution to decrease the metabolic (and oxygen) requirements of the heart. The body is also cooled to reduce its metabolic requirements. Electrodes are left on the atria and ventricles in case temporary pacing is needed after the surgery. Chest

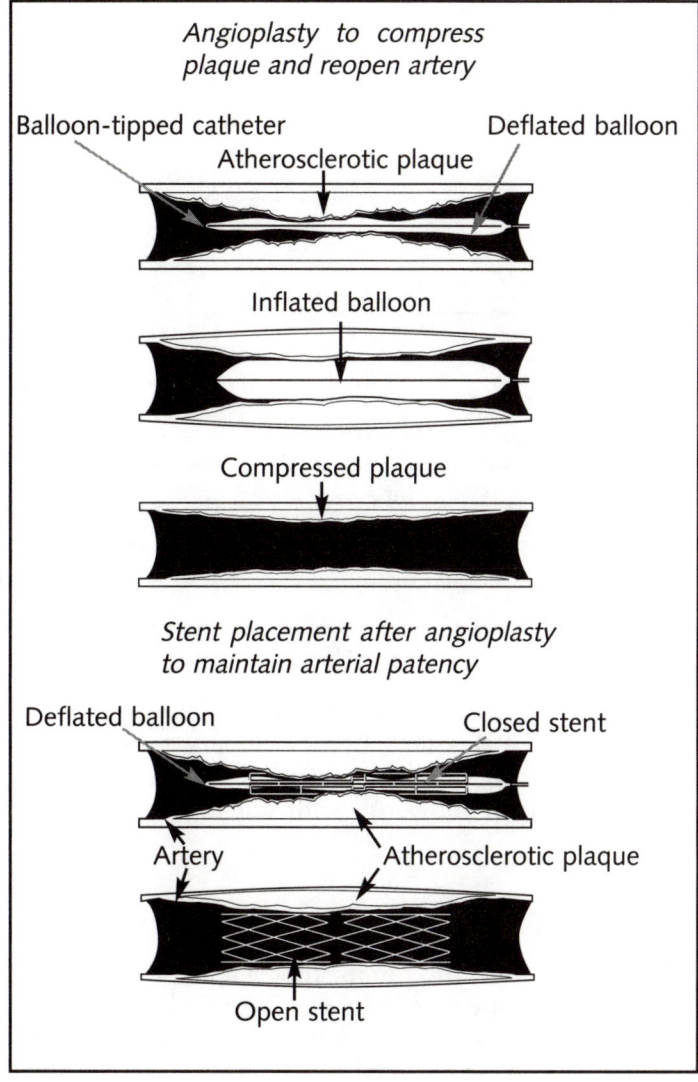

Angioplasty to compress plaque and reopen artery

Balloon-tipped catheter   Deflated balloon
        Atherosclerotic plaque

Inflated balloon

Compressed plaque

Stent placement after angioplasty to maintain arterial patency

Deflated balloon   Closed stent

        Artery   Atherosclerotic plaque

Open stent

Figure 7-5. Angioplasty and stent placement.

tubes are placed in the mediastinum and thorax to drain fluid and promote lung re-expansion. Postoperative complications include myocardial infarction, dysrhythmias, heart failure, cardiac tamponade (bleeding), pneumothorax, impaired renal function, thromboembolism, and cerebral vascular accidents.

Nursing care preoperatively involves allaying the patient's anxiety. Because surgery involves the heart, many patients fear dying during the surgery. Focusing on postoperative care may help the patient feel he is going to get through the surgery. Explain the unit, ventilator, chest tubes, intravenous lines, cardiac monitoring, and pain relief. Take time to explain the surgery to the patient and his family and show the family where to wait and how to contact their surgeon after the surgery. Families benefit from seeing their loved one as soon as possible after surgery.

Postoperatively, the patient undergoing bypass surgery will require careful care to maintain adequate cardiac and respiratory functioning, promote comfort, and prevent complications (Table 7-3).

Figure 7-6. Coronary artery bypass grafting.

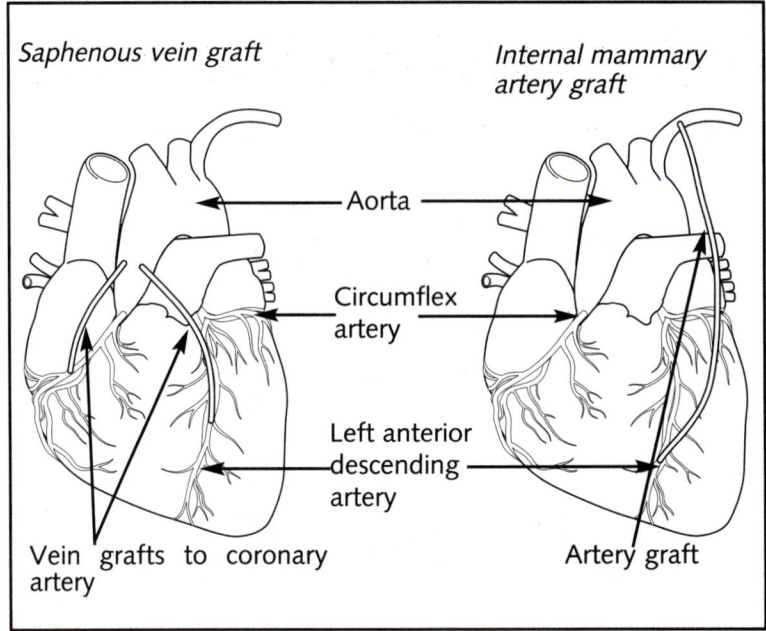

Saphenous vein graft

Internal mammary artery graft

Aorta

Circumflex artery

Left anterior descending artery

Vein grafts to coronary artery

Artery graft

The care of the patient undergoing coronary artery bypass grafting could and does fill entire books and is beyond the scope of this text. Bypass surgery does improve the oxygenation of the myocardium for patients with coronary artery disease. (Please see the Bibliography at the end of the chapter for books with nursing care plans for CABG patients.)

HEART FAILURE

Heart failure is the result of the heart's inability to pump sufficient amounts of blood to meet the metabolic needs of the body. There are many causes of heart failure, including myocardial ischemia and infarction, valvular dysfunction, hypertension, dysrhythmias, and constrictive pericarditis. If the body has compensated for the heart failure, sympathetic stimulation will increase the heart rate and blood pressure. Increased antidiuretic hormone (ADH) secretion will activate the renin-angiotensin-aldosterone system, resulting in salt and water retention. If the body can no longer compensate for the failing heart, the pulmonary artery pressures will increase and the ejection fraction will fall.

Heart failure can be divided in many ways, including right- and left-sided failure, backward and forward failure, and systolic and diastolic failure:

- Right-sided failure—reduced emptying of the right ventricle with systemic venous congestion and major organ engorgement.
- Left-sided failure—decreased emptying of the left ventricle with decreased tissue perfusion and back-up of blood in the pulmonary vasculature.
- Backward failure—inadequate emptying of the ventricle.
- Forward failure—caused by low cardiac output.
- Systolic failure—decreased ventricular emptying and ventricular dilation.
- Diastolic failure—impaired relaxation of the ventricle and decreased filling.

Table 7-3

Nursing Diagnoses Related to Bypass Surgery

1. Potential for Decreased Cardiac Output related to surgery, previous myocardial damage, fluid overload, hypothermia, impaired cardiac contractility and conductivity.
2. Impaired respiratory function:
   - Ineffective Breathing Pattern related to surgical incision, chest tubes, pain, decreased rate and depth of respiration.
   - Ineffective Airway Clearance related to increased mucus from endotracheal intubation and mucus stasis from weakened cough effort.
   - Impaired Gas Exchange related to atelectasis from general anesthesia, retention of secretions, pulmonary edema.
3. Altered Fluid and Electrolyte Balance related to fluid volume excess or deficit, electrolyte shifts during surgery, nasogastric tube drainage (hypokalemia, hypochloremia).
4. Pain related to surgical incisions (sternotomy, saphenous vein incision, chest tubes).
5. Knowledge Deficit related to follow-up care and postoperative activity levels.

Symptoms of heart failure are dependent on which side of the heart is failing and whether the failure is backward or forward. For the purposes of this chapter, heart failure will be classified as left- or right-sided failure, and treatment will focus on whether the failure is backward or forward.

Left-Sided Heart Failure

The left side of the heart is the pump for circulating oxygenated blood throughout the systemic vasculature. Effective pumping may be impeded if the walls of the left ventricle have areas of necrotic and inactive tissue from myocardial ischemia and infarction or degeneration. The first signs of left-sided heart failure are dyspnea, diffuse pulmonary crackles, and arterial hypoxemia (Figure 7-7). The crackles will be more pronounced in the dependent regions of the lungs. These signs develop as a result of blood backing up behind the left side of the heart and into the pulmonary vasculature. The pressure in the pulmonary vessels is so high that fluid leaks out of the capillaries into the alveoli, which is referred to as *pulmonary edema*. Systemic blood pressure may initially be elevated as a response to chest pain during MI but may decrease as the left ventricle fails. Compensatory mechanisms respond to the mechanoreceptors sensing low blood pressure, stimulating the sympathetic system to increase the heart rate. Gallop rhythms (S3) may develop as the heart fails. The patient may complain of fatigue at rest, weakness, cold intolerance, and difficulty breathing with mild exercise. He may be anxious and restless. His skin may be pale and clammy or overtly diaphoretic.

Left-ventricular failure may lead to gradual or abrupt onset of pulmonary edema. Pulmonary hypertension results in movement of fluid from the pulmonary capillaries into the alveoli. With less alveolar surface area for gas exchange, the patient becomes hypoxemic and may have signs of cyanosis. The pulse may be thready (weak and low pressure) and the blood pressure may be difficult to obtain.

Figure 7-7. Left-sided heart failure.

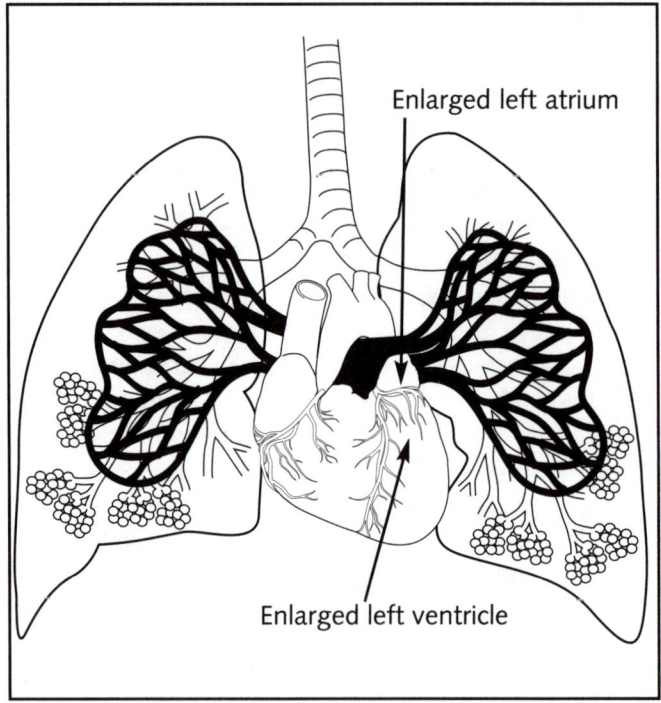

Enlarged left atrium

Enlarged left ventricle

Right-Sided Heart Failure

If left-sided heart failure and increased pulmonary pressures continue, then right-sided heart failure may develop. Left-sided heart failure is the most common cause of right-sided heart failure. The right ventricle wearies from pushing against the increased pressures in the pulmonary circulation. With pressures increasing behind a failing right side of the heart, the venous system becomes engorged, with the patient

> Afterload is the force resisting ventricular emptying and myocardial fiber shortening (ie, measured as the systemic vascular resistance). Preload is the force distending the myocardial fiber prior to contraction (ie, measured as the pulmonary artery end diastolic pressure).

experiencing related symptoms. He may complain of fullness in the neck (related to jugular venous distention), tenderness over the right upper quadrant (liver fullness), and ankle swelling (peripheral edema).

Treatment of heart failure involves identifying and treating the cause, reducing preload, supporting cardiac function, and improving oxygenation. Possible causes of heart failure are myocardial infarction, dysrhythmias, left ventricular hypertrophy, pericardial tamponade, fever, anemia, and pulmonary embolus. Collaborative interventions include:

- Diuretics to decrease preload and sodium and water retention.
- Positive inotropic agents (digitalis, dobutamine, amrinone) to increase myocardial contractility.
- Vasodilators (sodium nitroprusside, nitroglycerine, isosorbide, ACE inhibitors like captopril) to decrease vascular resistance and cardiac workload.

- Oxygen to improve arterial oxygenation or possibly mechanical ventilation.
- Balloon pump (counterpulsation) to improve cardiac output by assisting in left ventricular emptying.
- Salt-restricted diet (less than 2g per day) to reduce fluid retention.
- Rest to reduce the workload of the heart, including sedation with morphine or sedatives as needed.
- Complementary therapies to enhance relaxation, such as music therapy, massage and guided imagery.

Nursing diagnoses related to heart failure require careful assessment to determine the etiologies and defining characteristics, and a collaborative approach to establish the best interventions. The first step in the assessment is to be alert to the signs of heart failure, whether right- or left-sided. The following are the signs and symptoms of heart failure:

- Blood pressure—could be high or low depending on sympathetic stimulation, fluid volumes, and degree of failure.
- Respiratory pattern—dyspnea; rapid, shallow respiration; cough.
- Heart rate—tachycardia.
- Lung sounds—crackles, perhaps wheezes, decreased breath sounds.
- Heart sounds—S3 may be present.
- General symptoms—cool and clammy skin, fatigue, restlessness, dizziness.
- Circulation—cyanosis, decreased peripheral pulses, perhaps peripheral edema, jugular vein distention, abdominal tenderness over the upper right quadrant.

The nursing diagnosis of decreased cardiac output may be related to heart failure, decreased filling, or emptying of the ventricles. There are many etiologies for heart failure. The interventions require a collaborative approach and should be customized to the patient's diagnosis and functional abilities (Table 7-4).

Many patients with heart failure experience respiratory symptoms such as dyspnea and cough. Their impaired respiratory function could be categorized in any of three nursing diagnoses:

- Ineffective breathing pattern related to dyspnea.
- Ineffective airway clearance related to pulmonary edema.
- Impaired gas exchange related to pulmonary edema.

The interventions are similar because the etiologies are related to the heart failure. Interventions specific to heart failure and pulmonary edema include:

- Semi-Fowler's position to increase ventilatory capacity and comfort.
- Turning and repositioning every 2 hours to allow maximum ventilation and circulation in the lungs and help mobilize secretions.
- Incentive spirometry to inflate alveoli and improve gas exchange.
- Humidified oxygen to increase oxygen content of inspired air and keep secretions moist.
- Avoidance of large meals and gas-forming foods that compress the diaphragm and impede full inflation of the lungs.
- Medications such as morphine to decrease apprehension due to the dyspnea and to vasodilate the circulation, allowing pooling of blood in the periphery, thereby decreasing cardiac workload. Secondly, diuretics will decrease intravascular fluid volume and fluid accumulation in the lungs, and promote excretion of excess fluid.

Treatment of the patient with heart failure focuses on restoring cardiac function and decreasing excessive fluid in the body. The nursing diagnosis of altered fluid and electrolyte

Table 7-4

Decreased Cardiac Output (Related to Heart Failure)

1. Decrease the cardiac workload.
   - Place patient in the semi-Fowler's position, avoid Valsalva's maneuver, avoid breath-holding (increases venous return and the workload of the heart during exhalation). Administer nasal oxygen to increase inspired O_2 content.
   - Promote rest, both physical and emotional, and increase activity as ordered.
   - Provide small frequent meals to prevent excessive blood flow to the gastrointestinal tract. Avoid caffeine (a cardiac stimulant). Fluid and salt restrictions as ordered to reduce fluid volume excess. Monitor intake and output.
   - Do not allow smoking—nicotine is a cardiac stimulant and a vasoconstrictor.
2. Medicate to increase cardiac output and decrease fluid volume excess.
   - Positive inotropic agents (digitalis, dobutamine, amrinone) to increase myocardial contractility.
   - Vasodilators (sodium nitroprusside, nitroglycerine, isosorbide, ACE inhibitors) to decrease vascular resistance and cardiac workload.
   - Diuretics (furosemide) to decrease preload by decreasing sodium and fluid excess.
3. Balloon pump (counterpulsation) to increase left ventricular emptying.

balance related to fluid volume excess, is often used to focus the appropriate interventions. Fluid volume excess occurs because of a complex series of reactions to the heart failure. The glomerular filtration rate (GFR) in the kidneys decreases because of diminished blood flow, and sodium and water are retained. The renin-angio-tensin-aldosterone system is also activated due to decreased renal blood flow. These hormones contribute to sodium retention and peripheral vasoconstriction. The intravascular pressure increases because of the fluid volume excess. Third spacing of fluid into the tissues (edema) occurs because of the increased intravascular pressure. Low colloidal osmotic pressure (low albumin) due to nutritional deficiencies contributes to the movement of fluid out of the vascular serum prothrombin conversion accelerator (SPCA) and into the interstitial space. The serum sodium may become low (dilutional hyponatremia) because of fluid volume excess and treatment-related sodium restriction and diuretic-induced sodium loss.

> Signs of hyponatremia: Hyponatremia can be caused by diuretics and hormone fluctuations during heart failure. Signs and symptoms of hyponatremia include nausea, vomiting, lethargy, confusion, weakness, and seizures.

This complex series of interactions requires constant assessment and re-evaluation during the treatment of heart failure. The interventions for altered fluid and electrolyte balance are collaborative and focus on careful assessment and restoration of fluid and electrolyte balance (Table 7-5).

Table 7-5

Altered Fluid and Electrolyte Balance Related to Fluid Volume Excess

1. Assessment of fluid balance:
    - Daily weights—if greater than 2% increase, then a follow-up is required.
    - Vital signs—blood pressure, heart rate and rhythm (check for S3, tachycardia as signs of failure), respiratory rate (increase may indicate increasing failure).
    - Intake and output—imbalance may indicate fluid retention or kidney failure.
    - Pulmonary status—crackles (including a gravitational component), dyspnea, orthopnea (indicates failure or fluid volume excess).
    - Jugular venous distension (JVD) and central venous pressure to follow intravascular volume, preload, and right-sided pressures.
    - Third spacing—check edema and ascites.
    - Chest x-ray—shows pulmonary edema and cardiac dilation.
    - Laboratory results—hematocrit (low if blood diluted by fluid excess), potassium and sodium values (diuretics may result in depletion of these electrolytes).
2. Restore fluid balance:
    - Restrict fluid and sodium as ordered, carefully monitor intake and output measurement.
    - Medicate with diuretics as ordered to increase water excretion, watch serum potassium levels if using furosemide. Assess for signs of hyponatremia.
    - Medicate with vasodilators to increase cardiac output and improve renal blood flow.
    - Prevent third spacing—supplement dietary protein to increase serum albumin and increase colloidal osmotic pressure.
    - Thoracentesis to remove excessive pleural fluid.

There are many other nursing diagnoses that may apply to the patient with heart failure:
- Decreased Activity Tolerance.
- Altered Nutrition less than body requirements.
- Altered Comfort (nausea and vomiting) related to stimulation of visceral pathways or digitalis toxicity.
- Self-Care Deficit related to fatigue and dyspnea.
- Sleep Pattern Deficit related to orthopnea.
- Anxiety related to dyspnea and diagnosis of heart failure.

Complications of heart failure are related to the compromised cardiac functioning and fluid and electrolyte imbalance. Kidney function can be compromised because decreased cardiac output and fluid volumes can diminish renal blood flow. Fluid volume deficit can be treatment-induced by less than careful administration of diuretics. Cardiac dysrhythmias can occur as a result of impaired nodal function and decreased myocardial conductivity. Tachycardia can occur with stimulation of the sympathetic nervous system to compensate for decreased cardiac output. The heart can suffer structural changes such as ventricular hypertrophy.

Other complications from heart failure include thromboembolism and cardiogenic shock. Thromboembolism is a process that begins with vascular inflammation (phlebitis) or damage, hypercoagulability, and other risk factors like immobility, advanced age, obesity, and varicose veins. Clots form along the inflamed intima and later break away from the vessel wall and travel in the venous system to the heart and lungs. The clots can occlude pulmonary arteries (pulmonary embolism) and result in death of lung tissue.

Cardiogenic Shock

Cardiogenic shock occurs when the heart can no longer maintain perfusion of the vital organs. The reduction in cardiac output occurs as the result of factors other than hypovolemia. The tissues do not receive the necessary oxygen and nutrients to survive. Without the necessary oxygen, the cells begin anaerobic metabolism and produce lactic acid. The lactic acid build-up creates a metabolic acidosis. The respiratory rate increases to compensate for the hypoxia with a resulting alkalosis as carbon dioxide is blown off. Adult respiratory distress syndrome (ARDS) may develop in the lungs in response to the shock. Peripheral vasoconstriction shunts blood to the heart and lungs. Decreased renal perfusion from diminished cardiac output can result in renal failure.

Symptoms of cardiogenic shock are related to the physiologic compensation to decreased cardiac output. The patient's skin may be cool and clammy as a result of the vasoconstriction. Skin color may be pale or cyanotic with an increased capillary refill time. The patient may be restless, confused, or somnolent with a diminishing level of consciousness. The pulse may be rapid (tachycardia) and thready. The neck veins may be engorged and a third heart sound (S3) may be present. The blood pressure may remain normal at first due to compensatory mechanisms but drops in later stages of heart failure. Respiration is rapid and shallow due to hypoxia and metabolic acidosis. Crackles may be present on auscultation of the lung fields. Urinary output may drop as the kidneys fail. Untreated cardiogenic shock is fatal.

Treatment of cardiogenic shock revolves around maintaining vital functions: respiration and cardiac function. Interventions may be categorized using the nursing diagnosis, Decreased Cardiac Output:

1. Maintain an adequate airway (remove secretions) and give supplemental oxygen via mask or intubation as indicated by the patient's status and arterial blood gases.

2. Keep the patient warm and raise the legs to increase venous return to the heart.

3. Monitor vital signs and blood gases with hemodynamic catheters, continuous SVO_2 and cardiac output catheters, and arterial lines in an intensive care unit as soon as possible.

4. Medicate (intravenously) with vasopressors (norepinephrine, dopamine) to reverse hypotension.

5. Monitor urinary output hourly to assess renal function. Check blood urea nitrogen (BUN) and creatinine results.

6. Treatment of the underlying cause (myocardial infarction, pulmonary embolism, hemorrhage) is essential to reversing cardiogenic shock.

PERIPHERAL ARTERIAL DISEASE

Blockage of any artery can result in hypoxia of tissue distal to the occlusion. The blockage may be due to a clot or, more commonly, an atherosclerotic plaque. Peripheral arterial insufficiency, a decrease in blood flow to the extremities, is most commonly caused by atherosclerotic changes. The femoral artery is the most common site for arterial occlusion. Like coronary arteries with atherosclerotic changes, the tissues in the legs and feet receive less blood flow, and therefore less oxygen. Progressively, increased tissue demands for oxygen during activity cannot be met. The cells begin aerobic metabolism with subsequent lactic acid build-up in the tissues.

The signs and symptoms of peripheral arterial disease are related to the tissue hypoxia. One of the first symptoms is intermittent claudication. This refers to the pain or cramping that occurs in an extremity during activity that is relieved by rest. It occurs most commonly in the calf but can be felt in the foot, thigh, or hip. A common description of intermittent claudication is that a patient feels fine until he starts out for a walk and develops pain and cramping in his calves after 10 minutes. He stops and the pain subsides. He begins walking again and the same pain occurs. Ask the patient to describe the pain pattern—the onset, precipitating factors, quality, location, and alleviating factors. Note any rubbing of the affected extremity and facial expressions during activity. It is often useful to have the patient use a pain scale when describing his symptoms.

As the arterial occlusion progresses, the pain may occur earlier during exercise or at rest (so-called "rest pain"). Rest pain may be unrelenting, especially when the affected limb is elevated, such as at bedtime. The patient may get relief by hanging his leg over the bed (gravity increases the blood flow to the extremity). Nonhealing openings or ulcers may develop on the affected extremity as the result of long-term hypoxia. Severe disease may progress to gangrene of the extremity. Amputation may be the only solution to prevent life-threatening infection or gangrene of the extremity.

Assessment of the patient with suspected peripheral arterial disease provides physical evidence to the symptoms. Pulses in the extremity may be weak or absent. The extremity may pale when elevated for 1 to 2 minutes and develop rubor (bright red coloration) when placed in a dependent position again. If severe ischemia exists, then the foot may be pale and cool. The skin of the lower leg and foot may be hairless and scaly with poor nail growth.

In contrast to the gradual progression of atherosclerotic peripheral arterial disease, acute ischemia of an extremity occurs when an artery is suddenly blocked by a clot or ruptured plaque. The pain is sudden in onset and severe, with coldness and numbness of the extremity. Pulses are absent distal to the blockage. Immediate treatment with thrombolytics may dissolve the clot, PTA (percutaneous transluminal angioplasty) can reopen the artery, stents may be placed, or surgical treatment may be necessary.

A diagnosis of peripheral arterial disease is made by combining the patient's history of symptoms with the results of the diagnostic tests. Tests may include Doppler ultrasound of the artery, plethysmography, MRI, arteriography of the extremity, and segmental limb pressure measurements.

Conservative treatment of patients with peripheral arterial disease with intermittent claudication involves incorporating the patient in his own care. The nursing diagnosis, Altered Tissue Perfusion, is often used to focus the interventions and structure the documentation of the care. Like most nursing diagnoses, interventions require a collaborative response (patient, physician, nurse) and constant communication to optimize the effectiveness of the interventions (Table 7-6).

Table 7-6

Altered Tissue Perfusion Related to Peripheral Arterial Disease

1. **Foot care.** The patient should be taught the following steps:
    *   Inspect feet daily, including between the toes and the bottoms of the feet for cracks, calluses, ulcers, or fissures.
    *   Wash feet with lukewarm water and mild soap and gently pat dry.
    *   Moisturize with a lubricant like lanolin.
    *   Use a podiatrist to treat calluses, cut nails, and prescribe correctly fitting shoes if necessary.
    *   Use white cotton socks and change them daily. Loose wool socks may be used in the winter to keep feet warm.
    *   Avoid hot water bottles and electric pads.
    *   Always wear shoes (never go barefoot) and make sure they fit correctly.
2. **Walk for 60 minutes a day.** Stop if the pain develops and then begin again. (This can help develop better circulation and lessen the pain.)
3. **Eliminate all tobacco products.**
4. **Medications may improve circulation** such as pentoxifylline, calcium channel blockers, and thromboxane inhibitors.
5. **Control diabetes** carefully if this condition coexists with peripheral arterial disease, which it frequently does.
6. **Use analgesics** as necessary to control pain.
7. **Elevate the head of the bed 4 to 6 inches** (this allows gravity to increase blood flow to the extremity), or sleep in a recliner.

When conservative therapy fails to relieve the symptoms or the disease progresses, surgical intervention may be necessary to improve tissue perfusion. Worsening of the symptoms, pain at rest, and ischemic ulcers are all indications of significant arterial occlusion.

Invasive treatment involves surgically cleaning the plaque from the artery (endarterectomy) or bypassing the occluded artery with a synthetic or autogenous vein graft, such as the saphenous vein. Plaque removal or endarterectomy may be performed with lasers or surgical excision. Grafts are used to bypass the area of the occlusion beginning above the occlusion and then distal to the occlusion (Figure 7-8). The most common graft for peripheral arterial disease is the femoral-popliteal graft. Other types include the axillo-femoral, femoral-femoral, and axillo-bifemoral.

Care of the patient undergoing femoral-popliteal bypass grafting is focused on maintaining tissue perfusion of the extremity. Of course, maintaining comfort, allaying anxiety, and teaching about self-care after surgery are all important goals for nursing care for the patient undergoing surgery. Interventions for the patient with femoral-popliteal bypass surgery integrate the physiologic changes of peripheral arterial disease with improved perfusion and oxygenation of the extremity after surgery (Table 7-7).

Potential complications of bypass grafting include graft occlusion (by a clot or kink in the graft) and compartment syndrome (from swelling around the incision and in the reperfused muscles).

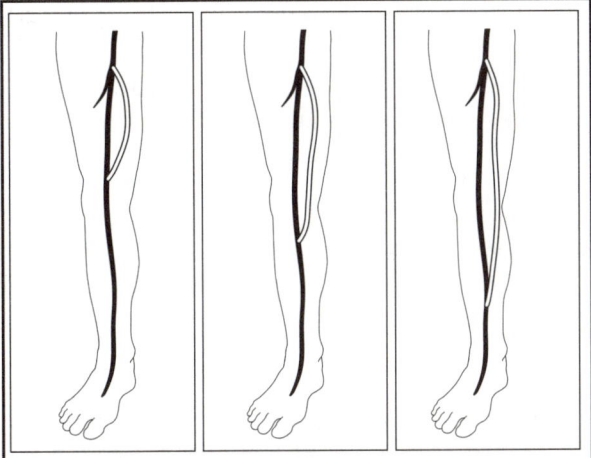

Figure 7-8. Femoral-popliteal bypass graft.

Table 7-7

Altered Peripheral Tissue Perfusion Related to Femoral-Popliteal Bypass

1. Assess for alteration in blood flow in the bypassed extremity:
    - Increased pain or intermittent claudication with less activity.
    - Diminished or absent pulses in the extremity.
    - Increasing pallor, coolness, or numbness.
    - Longer capillary refill time (greater than 3 seconds).
2. Prevent decreases in tissue perfusion:
    - Avoid crossing legs, pillows under the knees, sitting for long periods, 90-degree flexion at the hip.
    - Control pain and minimize stress (decrease sympathetic stimulation and vasoconstriction).
    - Eliminate all tobacco products.
    - Keep patient warm.
    - Progress activity as ordered, starting with foot exercises every 1 to 2 hours and progressing to short walks as ordered.
3. Implement measures to maintain graft perfusion:
    - Heparin intravenously for 24 to 48 hours—monitor PTT (partial thromboplastin levels).
    - Maintain a regular exercise program, such as short walks as ordered. Have patient time activities to establish predictable times to stop and rest. Medicate with analgesics as necessary to maintain comfort during activity.
    - Medicate with pentoxifylline if ordered.
    - Avoid constrictive stockings, like knee-highs and garters.
    - Teach patient signs of changing perfusion in the grafted extremity—increasing pain, numbness, tingling, coolness, paleness, or difficulty moving the extremity.
    - reduce cholesterol levels with a low fat diet and medication as ordered to prevent further atherosclerotic damage to the arteries.

The answers to the questions in the introduction are as follows:

- *What are the risk factors for coronary artery disease?*

The risk factors for coronary artery disease (CAD) include familial history of CAD, hypertension, diabetes, obesity, hypercholesterolemia, cigarette smoking, male gender, increased stress, and sedentary lifestyle.

- *Why does Al's pain subside after stent placement?*

Al's pain subsides after stent placement because the perfusion through the stenosed coronary artery has been re-established, allowing more oxygenated blood to reach the hypoxic cardiac muscle.

- *How does propanolol help patients with coronary artery disease?*

Beta-blockers like propanolol decrease the work of the heart by decreasing the heart rate, blood pressure, and myocardial contractility. With a diminished workload, the heart muscle also has decreased oxygen requirements.

- *What teaching will you do regarding the use of sublingual nitroglycerine?*

Al has been given a prescription for sublingual nitroglycerine (NTG) to use if his chest pain returns at home. He should carry it with him at all times. If rest does not relieve the chest pain, Al should take one NTG and wait 5 minutes. If pain is not relieved, he should take another NTG and wait 5 minutes. If the pain is still not relieved, he should take a third NTG and wait another 5 minutes. If the pain continues despite three NTGs in 15 minutes, he should dial 911 and/or his physician. Nitroglycerine can cause dizziness (orthostatic hypertension) and headache. Al should lie down if he feels dizzy. NTG should be kept in a dark bottle because it is light-sensitive. The prescription should be replaced every 3 to 5 months.

- *Which risk factors are modifiable, and how will you incorporate teaching about these to Al now that he has been diagnosed with coronary artery disease?*

Modifiable risk factors are those that Al can change to reduce his chances of having another MI. Al's teaching should include weight reduction, quitting cigarette smoking, reducing dietary fat intake, increasing his exercise level as prescribed by his cardiologist, and reducing stress.

- *What risk factors does Mrs. B have for coronary artery disease?*

Mrs. B's risk factors include hypertension and a history of diabetes and obesity.

- *What medications may be used immediately when Mrs. B arrives in the emergency department?*

Emergency medications for chest pain may include sublingual nitroglycerine, aspirin, and possibly morphine.

- *Why is oxygen administered to patients with chest pain?*

Increasing available oxygen in the blood may decrease myocardial ischemia and tissue death.

- *What is causing the premature ventricular contractions?*

The premature ventricular contractions may be the result of myocardial irritability from the ischemia in the heart muscle.

BIBLIOGRAPHY

Berkow R, Fletcher AJ. *The Merck Manual.* 16th ed. Rahway, NJ: Merck & Co, Inc; 1992.

Black JM, Matassarin-Jacobs. *Medical-Surgical Nursing: Clinical Management for Continuity of Care.* Philadelphia, Pa: W.B. Saunders; 1997.

Goldman L, Braunwald E. *Primary Cardiology.* Philadelphia, Pa: W.B. Saunders; 1998.

Ignatavius DD, Workman ML, Mishler MA. *Medical-Surgical Nursing—A Nursing Process Approach.* Philadelphia, Pa: W.B. Saunders; 1995.

Porth CM. *Pathophysiology: Concepts of Altered Health States.* Philadelphia, Pa: J.B. Lippincott; 1994.

Tierney LM, ed. *Current Medical Diagnosis and Treatment.* Norwalk, Conn: Appleton & Lange; 1995.

Ulrich SP, Canale SW, Wendell SA. *Medical-Surgical Nursing Care Planning Guides.* Philadelphia, Pa: W.B. Saunders; 1998.

MULTIPLE-CHOICE QUESTIONS

1. Atherosclerosis occurs because of all the following except:
   A. Accumulation of lipids in connective tissue
   B. Overgrowth of smooth muscle
   C. Formation of connective tissue in the intima of the vessel
   D. Hormonal response with peripheral vasoconstriction

2. Three risk factors for developing peripheral vascular disease are:
   A. Smoking, hypercholestorlemia, obesity
   B. Age, gout, smoking
   C. Hypertension, diabetes, smoking
   D. Prior surgery, age, gout

3. All of the following may be sign(s) of myocardial infarction except:
   A. Pain between the shoulder blades
   B. Nausea and vomiting with jaw pain
   C. Chest pain lasting more than 30 minutes
   D. Chest pain relieved by one nitroglycerin tablet

4. Treatment of suspected myocardial infarction includes:
   A. Oxygen, aspirin, morphine, nitroglycerin
   B. acetaminophen, bedrest, EEG
   C. Oxygen, cardiac catheterization
   D. Mechanical ventilation, CEA levels, acetaminophen

5. Thrombolytic agents are used to dissolve thrombi but have all the following side effects except:
   A. Reperfusion dysrhythmia
   B. Potential for bleeding
   C. Itching, hives, and hypersensitivity
   D. Renal failure

CHAPTER 7 ANSWERS

1. D
2. C
3. D
4. A
5. D

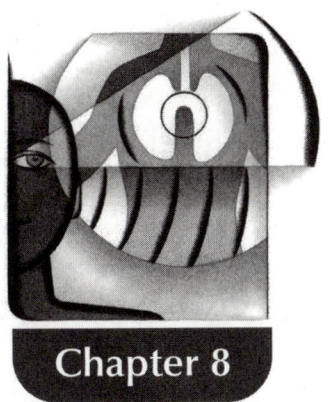

The Role of the Hematologic System in Oxygen Transport

When D. comes into the campus health office, she is moving slowly. She states that she has no energy and just wants to sleep all the time. D. is a 20-year-old college student and has been into the office before because of heavy menstrual periods. She is thin, 5 feet 6 inches, and 110 pounds. She has been skipping meals because of midterms, drinking diet soda, and eating popcorn in her room. Her blood work comes back with a hematocrit of 31 and a hemoglobin of 8.7.

- What lifestyle patterns would put D. at risk for anemia?
- What is the most common cause of anemia in young women?
- What interventions will improve D.'s energy levels?

Oxygen is transported throughout the body by the hematologic or hematopoietic system. This system is comprised of blood and lymph and the other components that circulate them. Blood is composed of plasma, red blood cells (erythrocytes), white blood cells (leukocytes), and platelets (thrombocytes). The hematologic system has three important functions:

- Gas exchange (oxygen and carbon dioxide).
- Nutrient delivery to the cells.
- Waste removal from the cells.

Additionally, the hematologic system is involved in acid-base balance, fluid and electrolyte balance, delivery of hormones, protection from foreign organisms, and temperature regulation.

The red blood cell (especially the hemoglobin molecule within the red blood cell) plays a crucial role in oxygen transport. The hemoglobin binds to oxygen in the pulmonary capillaries in the alveoli and transports the oxygen through the arterial system, releasing it at the cellular level. Readily available oxygen allows the cells to create energy aerobically.

Figure 8-1. Red blood cell development.

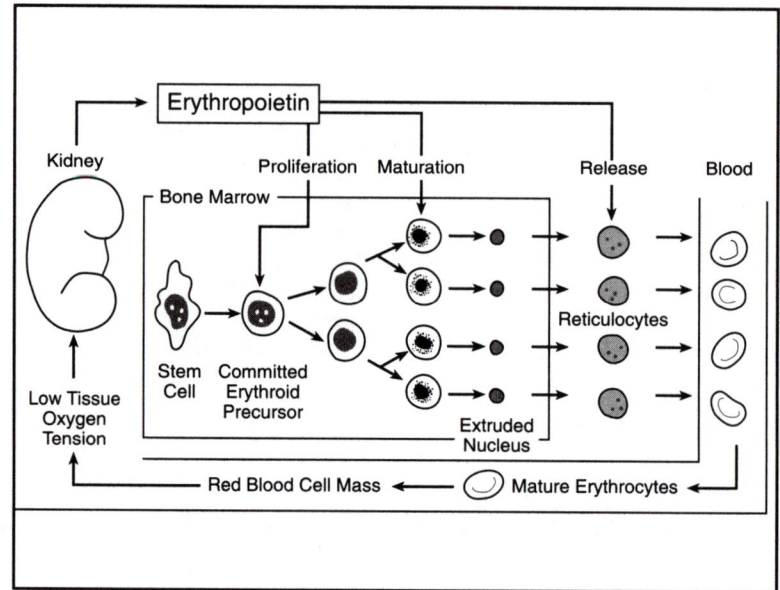

Without sufficient oxygen, the cells produce energy anaerobically, creating lactic acid as an end product. Sufficient oxygen for aerobic metabolism is referred to as critical oxygen (O_2 crit).

The red blood cell, or erythrocyte, is the most numerous of the formed elements in blood. Red blood cells (RBC) are of particular interest in a text on oxygenation because they carry hemoglobin, the molecule that binds to oxygen during transport. Approximately 98% of oxygen in blood is carried bound to hemoglobin as oxyhemoglobin. RBCs comprise about 40% to 50% of the total blood volume. This percentage is referred to as the *hematocrit*. RBCs are produced in the bone marrow and have a life span of about 120 days. Balanced production and destruction of red blood cells maintains a stable blood count. Every day, 1% of RBCs are produced by the bone marrow and another 1% are destroyed by phagocytic cells in the liver, spleen, and bone marrow. RBCs are released by the bone marrow as reticulocytes (immature RBC) and develop into erythrocytes in the circulating blood within 24 to 48 hours of their release from the bone marrow. The nor- mal percentage of reticulocytes in the circulating blood is 1% to 1.5% of the total RBCs. Abnormally high percentages of reticulocytes may occur during times of rapid RBC production.

The bone marrow is stimulated to produce red blood cells by the hormone erythropoietin (Figure 8-1). The kidneys produce this hormone when the capillary endothelial cells in the kidney sense hypoxia. Human erythropoietin is now produced using recombinant DNA technology (epoetin alpha). It is used to stimulate bone marrow production in severe anemia that occurs in conditions like chronic renal failure.

Hemoglobin is the master transporter of oxygen. It is comprised of two pairs of polypeptide chains, each attached to a heme unit. The heme unit is made of iron. If iron stores are low due to nutritional deficiencies, then the red blood cells contain low levels of hemoglobin (iron deficiency anemia). Hemoglobin also contains the red pigment, porphyrin. The iron pigment is the portion of hemoglobin that combines with oxygen and gives oxygenated blood the distinctive red color.

Hemoglobin carries the majority of the oxygen to the capillaries, where it moves out of the red blood cell, into the plasma, across the capillary wall, and into the interstitial fluid, becoming available to the cells. Only a small portion (1% to 2%) of the blood's oxygen is dissolved in plasma. The portion of oxygen that is dissolved in plasma can be measured as the PO_2. The oxygen that is combined with hemoglobin is measured as the percent of saturated hemoglobin (O_2 Sat).

The hemoglobin-oxygen bond (oxyhemoglobin) is a loose bond that is quickly reversed in the capillaries at the cellular level. Each gram of hemoglobin carries 1.34 mL of oxygen when it is saturated. In order for oxygen to become available to the cells, the oxyhemoglobin bond must be broken (dissociated). Hemoglobin's affinity for oxygen or its capacity to bind to oxygen depends on the pH of the blood and the presence of specific enzymes. It binds more strongly to oxygen when the blood is alkaline and releases it more easily when the pH is more acidic. This relationship or

Normal Hemoglobin Values for Adults		
	Males	**Females**
Hematocrit	40% to 54%	37% to 47%
Hemoglobin	13.5 to 17.5 g/100 mL	12 to 16 g/100 mL
Red blood cell count	4.2 to 5.4 million/µl	3.6 to 5 million/µl
Mean corpuscular volume (MCV): 87 to 103 fl/red cell for men and women		
Mean corpuscular hemoglobin concentration: 31 to 37 Hgb/dl for men and women		
Mean corpuscular hemoglobin (MCH): 26 to 34 picograms/cell		

affinity between hemoglobin and oxygen is described in the oxygen-hemoglobin dissociation curve. (Refer to Chapter 2 for more on this topic.) The enzymes 2-3-DPG and G6PD also affect hemoglobin's affinity for oxygen.

Red blood cells and hemoglobin also function to remove carbon dioxide and other waste from the cellular level. Carbon dioxide is a waste product of aerobic metabolism and is transported away from the cells in three ways: dissolved in the plasma as carbon dioxide, attached to hemoglobin (carbaminohemoglobin), and as bicarbonate (HCO_3^-). Seventy to 80% of the carbon dioxide in the blood is carried as bicarbonate or dissolved in plasma.

LABORATORY TESTS

The components of the hematologic system can be studied and measured in the laboratory. The hematocrit is the percentage of red blood cells in 100 mL of whole blood. A sample of blood is placed in a centrifuge and spun. The RBC, being the heaviest component of blood, falls to the bottom of the tube. The normal range for the hematocrit varies by age and sex. The hematocrit can be a deceiving measure of the actual RBC count because the amount of plasma, and the intravascular volume can vary. If the intravascular volume falls due to dehydration or increases due to fluid shifts into the intravascular space, then the percentage of RBCs will increase or decrease while the actual count is unchanged.

Hemoglobin levels can also be measured in the laboratory and are often considered a more reliable measure of the oxygen-carrying capacity of the blood. It is measured in grams per 100 mL of blood. Hemoglobin is measured to screen for anemia and evaluate polycythemia (too many RBCs). The RBC count measures the total number of RBCs in a cubic millimeter of blood. RBC indices are tests to distinguish the color and size of the RBCs. The mean corpuscular hemoglobin concentration (MCHC) is the average concentration of hemoglobin in the RBCs. It is often used to describe the color of the cells, but it is expressed as the ratio of the weight of hemoglobin to the volume of the RBC. For example, hypochromic anemia refers to RBCs of decreased color and is often a finding in iron deficiency anemia.

Another RBC index is the mean corpuscular volume (MCV). It refers to the relative size of the RBCs, such as normocytic (normal), microcytic (small), or macrocytic (large). It is used to classify different anemias.

Finally, the mean corpuscular hemoglobin (MCH) is an RBC index used to measure the weight of hemoglobin in the RBC. It is a calculated value with an increase associated with macrocytic (large RBC) anemias and a decrease associated with microcytic (small RBC) anemias.

DISORDERS OF THE HEMATOLOGIC SYSTEM

Disorders of the hematologic system can affect the oxygen-carrying capacity of the blood. While disorders can affect any component of the blood, this section will focus on problems with the RBC and hemoglobin: anemias and hemoglobinopathies.

Anemia reflects a reduction in the total hemoglobin concentration in the body. A decreased amount of hemoglobin diminishes the oxygen-carrying capacity of the blood. Anemia results from three main problems:

- Decreased production of erythrocytes (eg, iron deficiency, pernicious anemia, lead poisoning, and renal failure).
- Acute or chronic blood loss (eg, trauma, chronic gastrointestinal bleeding).
- Increased destruction of erythrocytes (eg, hemolytic anemias, physical trauma to blood like extracorporeal "bypass" circulation).

The signs of anemia do not usually present until there is a substantial drop in the amount of hemoglobin or circulating RBCs. The signs and symptoms reflect the decrease in oxygen-carrying capacity of the blood and tissue hypoxia. They include:

- Fatigue, weakness, and muscle cramps.
- Dyspnea and tachypnea.
- Pallor of skin, conjunctiva, and mucus membranes.
- Dizziness and syncope.
- Tachycardia and palpitations.
- Beefy red tongue, sore mouth, and anorexia.
- Jaundice in hemolytic anemias.
- Petechiae (small, red spots from bleeding) in aplastic anemia.

The most common cause of anemia is iron deficiency. Iron deficiency produces a microcytic, hypochromic RBC because insufficient iron is available to synthesize hemoglobin. Although body iron is retained from destroyed RBCs and reused, over time the iron stores can be depleted due to chronic loss. In postmenopausal women and men, the most common cause of chronic loss and iron-deficiency anemia is gastrointestinal bleeding from ulcers, tumors, or hemorrhoids. In menstruating women, monthly periods, especially heavy or prolonged periods, can lead to anemia. Pregnant women also have increased iron needs. People at risk for hookworm may also have chronic blood loss as the parasite removes blood from the intestinal tract.

Signs and symptoms of iron deficiency anemia are related to impaired oxygen transport: fatigue, dyspnea, palpitations, tachycardia, and angina. Treatment is aimed at controlling blood loss, increasing dietary intake of iron, and administering supplemental iron either orally or intramuscularly as needed. Although an adequate diet includes 12 to 15 mg of indirect iron, only 1 mg is absorbed daily and another 1 mg is lost. Supplemental iron may be necessary to rebuild the iron stores. Interventions are aimed at teaching the patient to increase intake of iron-rich foods and pacing activities until the fatigue subsides (about 3 to 6 months):

- Encourage an iron-rich diet with foods such as liver, lean red meat, egg yolks, raisins, spinach, apricots, beet greens, and whole wheat bread.
- Take supplemental iron (iron sulfate—$FeSO_4$ 325 mg one to three times daily) with food. Use a stool softener like docusate sodium or senna for constipation if this becomes a problem. Warn patient that stools will be black-colored while taking iron.
- Administer intramuscular iron if ordered, using the Z-track method to minimize skin staining and irritation. (See a nursing text for further explanation of this method.)

Two other nutritional deficiencies can result in altered RBC production. Folic acid and vitamin B12 are also needed for the synthesis of RBCs. Folic acid deficiency results from inadequate dietary intake, malabsorption syndromes like celiac sprue, or during times of increased bodily needs, such as during pregnancy and growth. Folic acid is necessary for RBC maturation. It is found in green leafy foods, liver, and yeast. Some drugs like phenytoin, phenobarbital (antiseizure drugs), methotrexate (antimetabolite used in chemotherapy), and triamterene (a diuretic) impair absorption of folic acid. Alcoholics frequently have folic acid deficiencies. Because folic acid deficiency is linked to birth defects like spina bifida, it is important that menstruating and pregnant women have an adequate intake or take a multivitamin supplement.

Vitamin B12 (cobalamin) deficiency can cause anemia not because of inadequate intake but because the body does not adequately absorb this nutrient. Intrinsic factor produced by the gastric mucosa is needed to absorb B12 from food. In cases of atrophy of the gastric mucosa, insufficient intrinsic factor is produced and B12 is not absorbed. Without B12, DNA synthesis of the RBC is impaired and anemia will result. Anemia due to B12 deficiency is sometimes referred to as *pernicious anemia*. The RBCs, when examined under the microscope, are abnormally large (macrocytic), oval shaped, and have thin membranes. Long-term effects of pernicious anemia include neurological manifestations, such as paresthesia of the hands and feet, and spastic ataxia. Treatment involves lifelong injections of B12 (100 mcg) to reverse the anemia and try to improve any neurological manifestations.

Anemias from bone marrow failure are referred to as *aplastic anemias*. Usually the production of all hematopoietic cells (red blood cells, white blood cells, and platelets) is affected and is called *pancytopenia*. The anemia results from the failure of the marrow to replace the old RBCs. The cells that are produced are of normal size and color but few in number. The patient presents symptoms of increasing fatigue and dyspnea. Aplastic anemia may develop slowly or acutely and at any age. Possible causes include exposure to toxic chemicals (like benzene) and high-dose radiation. Half the time the cause is never discovered. Treatment includes removal of the offending substance (if known), immunosuppressive therapy, blood transfusions, corticosteroids, and bone marrow transplantation in severe cases.

Anemia of chronic disease is a normocytic, normochromic anemia that is thought to result from uremic toxins destroying the kidney's ability to produce erythropoietin. Causes include diseases like cancer and chronic infections. The treatments are transfusions and erythropoietin injections (if the bone marrow is functioning.)

Transfusion therapy for chronic anemias does have complications. Blood transfusions can result in transfusion reactions and predispose the patient to iron overload. Transfusion reactions occur because surface antigens on the blood cells interact with antibodies in the patient's serum. Reactions can be quite serious and blood should always be administered very cautiously.

> Blood transfusions are used to treat anemias of various causes if tissue hypoxia is severe. Packed red blood cells are usually transfused, but whole blood may be used if there is acute bleeding. Blood comes from volunteer donors and is screened for ABO compatibility, Rh group, and blood-borne diseases, such as hepatitis and HIV. A crossmatch is done prior to transfusion to observe for agglutination, which would indicate incompatibility.

The two most common reactions are hemolytic and febrile reactions. The most serious and feared reaction is a hemolytic reaction from ABO incompatibility. The signs and symptoms are urticaria, flushing of the face, back pain, headache, chills, fever, nausea and vomiting, tachycardia, dyspnea, and hypotension. The transfusion is immediately stopped, and the remaining blood is saved for testing. Intravenous access is maintained for medications. Kidney function must be carefully followed to assess for renal damage from the hemoglobin released from the destroyed RBCs.

In a febrile reaction, the patient's blood reacts to the donor's white blood cells, causing fever and chills. Leukocyte-depleted blood is frequently used to avoid this reaction. (Leukocytes are depleted by irradiating the blood.) Antipyretics are used to treat the fever.

Multiple blood transfusions can lead to iron overload. The body metabolizes iron at a fixed rate and recycles it from destroyed RBCs. The iron balance in the body is usually maintained. Each transfusion adds another 200 mg of iron to the system, and iron overload can result. Iron can cause cardiac myopathies, liver fibrosis, skin discoloration, as well as endocrine and pancreatic dysfunction. The treatment for iron overload is chelation therapy.

> The most common cause of transfusion reactions is clerical error or misidentification. Always identify the patient and the transfusion source with another nurse.

Hemolytic anemia is caused by premature destruction of RBCs, shortened life span of RBCs, or failure of the marrow to replace RBCs.

Causes of hemolytic anemia include immune responses (antigen-antibody reactions, infections, lead poisoning, and chronic diseases like cancer and lupus). The treatment involves identifying the cause, maintaining renal function, steroids, and possibly splenectomy for refractory cases.

HEMOGLOBINOPATHIES

Defects in the structure of hemoglobin can lead to accelerated RBC destruction and blood vessel occlusion. Two hemoglobinopathies will be discussed: sickle-cell anemia and thalassemia.

Sickle-cell anemia is a congenital disorder affecting 0.1% to 0.2% of all African-Americans. It is a recessive characteristic that is transmitted either as a trait or as the disease. Almost 9% of all African-Americans carry the gene for the sickle-cell trait. In sickle-cell anemia, an amino acid is abnormally substituted for a chain in the hemoglobin molecule. The problem with the substitution arises when the hemoglobin deoxygenates and takes on a sickle shape. This deformed RBC can block vessels in the microcirculation, causing tissue ischemia. A crisis occurs when a blood vessel is blocked, causing damage to tissues and organs. Sickle-cell crises are often very painful for the patient. Common sites are joints, the abdomen, and chest. There is no known cure for sickle-cell anemia. Treatment focuses on increasing tissue oxygenation with supplemental oxygen. Patients are taught to avoid situations that could precipitate a crisis, such as infections, cold exposure, excess physical exertion, dehydration, and acidosis. Bone marrow transplantation, antisickling agents, and red cell exchange therapy are also being used to improve outcomes in patients who are unresponsive to other treatments.

Thalassemias are a group of inherited anemias. Occurring mostly in Mediterranean populations, they are sometimes called Cooley's anemia. In thalassemia, one of the two polypeptide chains in the hemoglobin molecule is defective. The anemia results from defective and reduced hemoglobin synthesis. Signs and symptoms are based on the severity of the anemia and include hepatomegaly, splenomegaly, growth retardation in children, bone thinning, and bone marrow expansion with facial changes. The severity of the disease depends on the number of defects in the hemoglobin molecule. The treatment for thalassemias is transfusion therapy and genetic counseling.

The answers to the questions from the introduction are as follows:
- *What lifestyle patterns would put D. at risk for anemia?*

D. is at risk for anemia because of her diet (low in calories, nutritional value, and probably iron) and her history of heavy periods.

- *What is the most common cause of anemia in young women?*

The most common cause of anemia in young women is an iron-poor diet.

- *What interventions will improve D.'s energy levels?*

D.'s energy levels will improve over time with rest, increased iron-rich foods in her diet, and iron supplementation.

BIBLIOGRAPHY

Fischbach F. *A Manual of Laboratory & Diagnostic Tests*. Philadelphia, Pa: J.B. Lippincott; 1992.

Porth CM. *Pathophysiology: Concepts of Altered Health States*. Philadelphia, Pa: J.B. Lippincott; 1994.

Swearingen PL, Keen JH. *Manual of Critical Care Nursing: Nursing Interventions and Collaborative Management*. St. Louis, Mo: Mosby Inc; 2001.

MULTIPLE-CHOICE QUESTIONS

1. A normal hematocrit for women is:
    A. 40% to 48%
    B. 37% to 47%
    C. 35% to 40%
    D. 30% to 40%

2. The immature form of red blood cells released by the bone marrow is:
    A. Reticulocytes
    B. Erythrocytes
    C. Monocytes
    D. Granulocytes

3. Anemia occurs because of all of the following except:
    A. Renal failure
    B. Chronic blood loss
    C. Increased destruction of erythrocytes
    D. Congestive heart failure

CHAPTER 8 ANSWERS

1. B
2. A
3. D

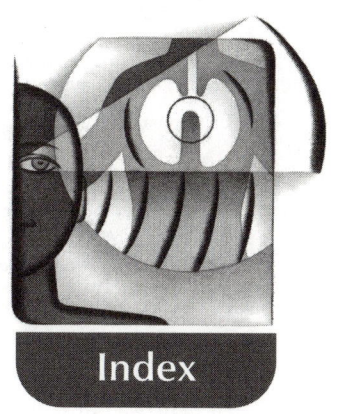

Index

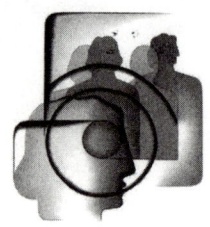

Keep up with the Latest in Nursing!

Other Exciting Books in the Nursing Concepts *Series Include:*

Title	Author	Book #	Price
❏ Nursing Concepts: Ethics and Conflict	Perrin	25171	$24.00
❏ Nursing Concepts: Pain	Kazanowski	25228	$24.00
❏ Nursing Concepts: Mobility	Durette	25201	$24.00
❏ Nursing Concepts: Symptom Management in the Acute Care Setting	Laccetti	25198	$24.00

Subtotal $_____
NJ, CA, and CO Sales Tax* $_____
Handling Charge $ 4.50
Total $_____

ORDER TODAY!

Name: _____

Address: _____

City: _____ State: _____ Zip Code: _____

Phone: _____ Fax: _____

Charge my: ❏ [American Express] ❏ [MasterCard] ❏ [VISA] Account#:_____

Exp. date: _____ Signature: _____

Prices are subject to change. Shipping charges may apply. Shipping and handling charges are non-refundable.
*Purchases in NJ, CA, and CO are subject to tax. Please add applicable state and local taxes.

CODE: 2A719

Mail Order Form To

SLACK Incorporated
Professional Book Division
6900 Grove Road
Thorofare, NJ 08086-9864

OR

Call 800-257-8290 or 856-848-1000
Fax 856-853-5991
Email Orders@slackinc.com

Visit Our World Wide Web: www.slackbooks.com